Innovation in HealthTech

Sophisticated data analysis is revolutionizing healthcare decision-making, personalized treatments, and operational efficiency. *Innovations in HealthTech* covers this impact and highlights the significance of robust security measures in safeguarding sensitive medical data and ensuring patient confidentiality. The book provides insights into the development, implementation, and future potential of telemedicine infrastructure. It is primarily written for senior undergraduates, graduate students, and academic researchers in the fields of electrical engineering, electronics and communications engineering, computer engineering, and biomedical engineering.

- Explores the role of wearable technology in promoting patient engagement and wellness and addressing the critical issue of data security.
- Offers practical technical insights that provide a deeper understanding of the real-world applications and challenges in the healthcare technology landscape.
- Examines the role of telehealth and remote monitoring in healthcare accessibility, and use of artificial intelligence in augmenting clinical decision-making processes.
- Discusses frameworks and guidelines that enable different health technologies and systems to work together seamlessly, ensuring efficient data exchange and improved patient care.
- Presents the essential measures and strategies in place to protect sensitive healthcare data, ensuring the confidentiality and integrity of information.

Advancing Science and Engineering through Artificial Intelligence, Machine Learning, and Mathematical Modeling
Series editor: Manoj Saini

Innovation in HealthTech: *A Roadmap for Empowering Healthcare*
Edited by Rakesh Kumar and Meenu Gupta

Sustainable Smart Composites: *Technology and Applications*
Edited by Hiral Parikh, Piyush P. Gohil

For more information about this series, please visit: https://www.routledge.com/Advancing-Science-and-Engineering-through-Artificial-Intelligence-Machine/book-series/ASEAIMLMM

Innovation in HealthTech

A Roadmap for Empowering Healthcare

Edited by
Rakesh Kumar and Meenu Gupta

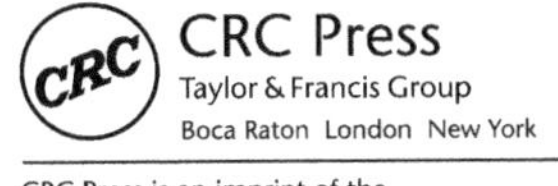

CRC Press is an imprint of the
Taylor & Francis Group, an **informa** business

Front cover image: raker/Shutterstock

First edition published 2025
by CRC Press
2385 NW Executive Center Drive, Suite 320, Boca Raton, FL 33431

and by CRC Press
4 Park Square, Milton Park, Abingdon, Oxon, OX14 4RN

CRC Press is an imprint of Taylor & Francis Group, LLC

ISBN: 978-1-032-85027-6 (hbk)
ISBN: 978-1-032-85028-3 (pbk)
ISBN: 978-1-003-51616-3 (ebk)

DOI: 10.1201/9781003516163

Typeset in Times
by Newgen Publishing UK

Contents

Preface

In today's fast-evolving healthcare landscape, technology integration has opened up new possibilities for enhanced patient care, accessibility, and innovation. *Innovation in HealthTech: A Roadmap for Empowering Healthcare* offers a comprehensive guide to understanding and implementing the emerging technologies shaping healthcare's future.

CHAPTER 1: INTRODUCTION: PIONEERING THE FUTURE OF CLINICAL CARE

We begin by exploring integrative technologies and the emerging trends that lay the foundation for transformative advancements in clinical care. This chapter sets the stage, emphasizing how innovative technologies are beginning to reshape patient outcomes, medical practices, and healthcare delivery worldwide.

CHAPTER 2: THE LANDSCAPE OF HEALTHTECH: A COMPREHENSIVE OVERVIEW

To contextualize these innovations, this chapter provides an overview of the current HealthTech ecosystem, covering key players, the scope of existing solutions, and the technological frameworks redefining healthcare. This landscape analysis is a roadmap to understanding the dynamic forces at play.

CHAPTER 3: TECHNOLOGY AND DIAGNOSTICS: ADVANCEMENTS IN CLINICAL MEDICINE

Precision medicine is at the forefront of modern healthcare, and this chapter explores how advancements in diagnostic technologies allow for more personalized and accurate treatments. It examines how these tools empower healthcare providers to tailor therapies, enhancing outcomes and minimizing side effects.

CHAPTER 4: DIGITAL HEALTH RECORDS: ENHANCING DATA-DRIVEN CLINICAL DECISIONS

The digitization of health records has transformed clinical decision-making by making vast amounts of patient data accessible to providers. This chapter discusses the impact of digital records in improving diagnostics, treatment planning, and patient care.

CHAPTER 5: TELEMEDICINE AND REMOTE MONITORING: EXPANDING ACCESS TO CARE

With the rise of telemedicine and remote health monitoring, healthcare has become more accessible than ever. This chapter explores the transformative power of these technologies, particularly in reaching underserved and rural populations and supporting continuous patient monitoring.

CHAPTER 6: ARTIFICIAL INTELLIGENCE AND MACHINE LEARNING IN CLINICAL CARE: REVOLUTIONIZING DECISION SUPPORT

Artificial intelligence (AI) and machine learning are critical in assisting clinicians with data-driven decision support. This chapter delves into the impact of AI in diagnostics, prognosis, and treatment recommendations, offering insights into its role in reshaping the future of healthcare.

CHAPTER 7: WEARABLE HEALTHTECH: EMPOWERING PATIENTS AND PREVENTIVE CARE

Wearable devices are redefining patient engagement, enabling individuals to take a proactive role in their health. This chapter discusses the impact of wearables in monitoring vital health metrics, encouraging preventive care, and allowing for early intervention.

CHAPTER 8: BLOCKCHAIN AND DATA SECURITY: SAFEGUARDING PATIENT INFORMATION

With increased digitalization comes the need for enhanced data security. This chapter explores how blockchain technology provides solutions for safeguarding patient information, ensuring data integrity, and supporting secure patient–provider interactions.

CHAPTER 9: ETHICAL CONSIDERATIONS IN HEALTHTECH: BALANCING INNOVATION AND PRIVACY

Developing and deploying health technologies present ethical challenges, especially concerning patient privacy. This chapter examines the ethical considerations that must guide HealthTech innovation, including maintaining patient trust and ensuring equitable access.

CHAPTER 10: THE FUTURE OF CLINICAL TRIALS: ACCELERATING DRUG DEVELOPMENT

Innovations in HealthTech are also transforming clinical trials, with AI and digital monitoring accelerating drug development. This chapter explores how technology enables faster, safer, and more effective clinical trials, reducing time-to-market for critical treatments.

CHAPTER 11: CHALLENGES AND ROADBLOCKS: NAVIGATING THE HEALTHTECH ECOSYSTEM

Despite its promise, the HealthTech ecosystem faces several challenges. This chapter addresses these roadblocks, including regulatory, financial, and operational hurdles, and discusses strategies to overcome them, paving the way for successful technology adoption.

CHAPTER 12: REAL-WORLD EXAMPLES OF HEALTHTECH EMPOWERMENT

In this chapter, we explore real-world HealthTech applications, illustrating how innovations have successfully empowered providers and patients. These case studies offer practical insights into how HealthTech is making an impact.

CHAPTER 13: REVOLUTIONIZING HEALTHCARE: THE IMPACT OF WEARABLE HEALTH TECHNOLOGY ON PROACTIVE AND PREVENTIVE CARE

This chapter provides an in-depth look at how wearable health technology drives proactive care, enabling early detection, lifestyle adjustments, preventive measures and fostering a healthier population through technology-driven self-care.

CHAPTER 14: ARTIFICIAL INTELLIGENCE IN HEALTHCARE: FROM DIAGNOSIS TO TREATMENT

The application of AI in healthcare goes beyond diagnostics, extending into treatment planning and patient management. This chapter discusses AI's role in developing personalized treatment plans and delivering care tailored to each patient's needs.

CHAPTER 15: THE ROAD AHEAD: FORECASTING THE FUTURE IMPACT OF HEALTHTECH INNOVATIONS

With an eye toward the future, this chapter forecasts the anticipated impact of emerging HealthTech innovations on clinical practice, healthcare delivery, and patient outcomes, providing insights into what lies ahead for HealthTech.

CHAPTER 16: EMBRACING HEALTHTECH FOR A HEALTHIER TOMORROW

In the concluding chapter, we discuss the transformative potential of health technology and encourage stakeholders to embrace these advancements for a healthier, more equitable future. This chapter serves as a call to action for all readers to contribute to realizing this vision.

Innovation in HealthTech: A Roadmap for Empowering Healthcare is a guide and an inspiration to drive innovation, foster patient empowerment, and build a sustainable healthcare system equipped for future challenges. We hope this book serves as a comprehensive resource for those eager to participate in this HealthTech revolution.

About the Editors

Rakesh Kumar is an Associate Director at the UIE-CSE Department, Chandigarh University, India. He is pursuing his Post Doc Fellowship from MIR Labs, USA. He has completed his PhD in Computer Science and Engineering from Punjab Technical University, Jalandhar, India, 2017. He has more than 20 years of teaching experience. His research interests are IoT, machine learning, and natural language processing. He has edited more than 7 books with the reputed publishers such as Elsevier, Springer, and Taylor and Francis and authored 5 books. He works as a reviewer for several journals, including *Big Data*, *CMC*, *Scientific Reports*, *TSP*, *Multimedia Tools and Applications*, and *IEEE Access*. He is a senior member of IEEE. He has authored or co-authored more than 170 publications in various national/international conferences and journals. He is also an organizer and editor of many international conferences under the aegis of IEEE and AIP.

Meenu Gupta is an Associate Professor at the UIE-CSE Department, Chandigarh University, India. She is pursuing her Post Doc Fellowship from MIR Labs, USA. She has completed her PhD in Computer Science and Engineering from Ansal University, Gurgaon, India, in 2020. She has more than 16 years of teaching experience. Her research areas cover machine learning, intelligent systems, and data mining, with a specific interest in artificial intelligence, image processing and analysis, smart cities, data analysis, and human/brain–machine interaction (BMI). She has edited more than 17 books and authored 4 engineering books. She reviews several journals, including *Big Data*, *Artificial Intelligence Review*, *CMC*, *Scientific Reports*, and *Digital Health*. She is a life member of ISTE and IAENG. She is also a senior member of IEEE. She has authored or co-authored more than 37 book chapters and 200 papers in refereed international journals and conferences. She has also organized many conferences technically sponsored by the IEEE Delhi Section, AIP, etc.

Contributors

Shakeel Ahmed
School of Computer Science (SCS), Taylor's University, Subang Jaya, Selangor,, Malaysia

Ashok R.
ECE Department, Kamaraj College of Engineering & Technology, Virudhunagar, Tamilnadu, India

Vidhu Baggan
Chitkara University Institute of Engineering and Technology, Chitkara University, Baddi, Himachal Pradesh, India

Gauri Bansal
Department of Computer Science and Engineering, Chandigarh Group of Colleges, Landran, Mohali, Punjab, India

E. Bijolin Edwin
Division of Computer Science and Engineering, Karunya Institute of Technology and Sciences, Coimbatore, Tamilnadu, India.

Robert Cep
Department of Machining, Assembly and Engineering Metrology, Faculty of Mechanical Engineering, VSB-Technical University of Ostrava, Ostrava, Czech Republic

Divyashree Duggegowda
School of Science and Computer Studies, CMR University, Bengaluru, Karnataka, India

V. Ebenezer
Division of Data Science and Cyber Security, Karunya Institute of Technology and Sciences, Coimbatore, Tamilnadu, India

Ushaa Eswaran
Department of ECE, Mahalakshmi Tech Campus, Chennai, Tamilnadu, India

Vishal Eswaran
CVS Health Centre, Dallas, Texas, The United States

Vivek Eswaran
Tech Lead at Medallia, Austin, Texas, The United States

Fathimathul Rajeena P.P.
Department of Computer Science, College of Computer Sciences and Information Technology, King Faisal University, Al-Ahsa

Parth Gharat
Department of Pharmacognosy, Regional Ayurveda Research Institute CCRAS Ministry of Ayush, Pune, Maharashtra, India

Anjuli Goel
Chitkara University Institute of Engineering and Technology, Chitkara University, Chandigarh, Punjab, India

Ashwini Dattatraya Gopwad
Department of CSIT &Animation, M.S.P. Mandal Deogiri college, Chhatrapati Sambhaji Nagar, Aurangabad, Maharashtra, India

Meenu Gupta
Department of Computer Science and Engineering, Chandigarh University, Chandigarh, Punjab, India

Shubham Gupta
Model Institute of Engineering and Technology, Jammu, J&K, India

Hemanth K.S.
Department of Computer Science, Christ University, Bangalore, Karnataka, India

M. Robinson Joel
Department of Information Technology, KCG College of Technology, Chennai, Tamilnadu, India.

Gurleen Kaur
Department of Computer Science and Engineering, Chandigarh Group of Colleges, Landran, Mohali, Punjab, India

Rajnish Kohli
Chandigarh University, Punjab, India

Anurag Kumar
Department of Biochemistry, Regional Ayurveda Research Institute, CCRAS Ministry of Ayush Pune, Maharashtra, India

Manoj Kumar
Department of Orthopedics, PGIMER, Chandigarh, Punjab, India

Rakesh Kumar
Department of Computer Science and Engineering, Chandigarh University, Chandigarh, Punjab, India

Ritesh Kumar
CSIR – Central Scientific Instruments Organization, Chandigarh, Punjab, India

Vishal Kumar
Department of Orthopaedics, PGIMER, Chandigarh, Punjab, India

Shalini Kumari
Chitkara University Institute of Engineering and Technology, Chitkara University, Chandigarh, Punjab, India

K. Martin Sagayam
Division of Electronics and Communication Engineering, Karunya Institute of Technology and Sciences, Coimbatore, Tamilnadu, India

M. Mary Shanthi Rani
The Gandhigram Rural Institute (DTBU), Gandhigram, Chinnalapatti, Tamilnadu, India

Rahul Maurya
Department of Pharmacy, Central Ayurveda Research Institute CCRAS Ministry of Ayush, Jhansi, Uttar Pradesh, India

Kapil Mehta
Department of Computer Science and Engineering, Chandigarh Group of Colleges, Landran, Mohali, Punjab, India

Shaik Khaja Mohiddin
Department of CSE, Koneru Lakshmaiah Education Foundation, Vaddeswaram, Andra Pradesh, India

Anuradha More
Department of Pharmaceutics, Modern College of Pharmacy Nigdi, Pune, Maharashtra, India

Keerthna Murali
Dell EMC | CKAD | AWS CSAA, Austin, Texas, The United States

P. Nagaraja
GITAM Deemed to be University, Bengaluru, Karnataka, India

Nagashruthi, M.K.
School of Computer Science and Application, REVA University, Bangalore, Karnataka, India

A. Nithya
The Gandhigram Rural Institute (DTBU), Gandhigram Chinnalapatti, Tamilnadu, India

Chander Prabha
Chitkara University Institute of Engineering and Technology, Chitkara University, Chandigarh, Punjab, India

S. Prasanth
Division of Computer Science and Engineering, Karunya Institute of Technology and Sciences, Coimbatore, Tamilnadu, India.

Sridhar Raj S.
ECE Department, Mepco Schlenk Engineering College, Sivakasi, Tamilnadu, India

Saumya Rajvanshi
Department of Computer Science and Engineering, Chandigarh Group of Colleges, Landran, Mohali, Punjab, India

Umadevi Ramamoorthy
School of Science and Computer Studies, CMR University, Bengaluru, Karnataka, India

Belfin Robinson
Department of Neurology, School of Medicine, BRIC, University of North Carolina, Chapel Hill, North Carolina, The United States

M. Roshni Thanka
Division of Data Science and Cyber Security, Karunya Institute of Technology and Sciences, Coimbatore, Tamilnadu, India.

P. Shanmugavadivu
The Gandhigram Rural Institute (DTBU), Gandhigram, Chinnalapatti, Tamilnadu, India

Palvi Sharma
Department of Computer Science and Engineering, Model Institute of Engineering & Technology, Jammu, J&K, India

Shaik Sharmila
Department of IT, VNITSW, PedaPalakalur, Guntur Andhra Pradesh, India

Gaurav Kumar Singh
Department of Forensic Science, Sharda School of Allied Health Sciences (SSAHS), Sharda University, Greater Noida, Uttar Pradesh, India

Ujjwal Srivastava
Department of Microbiology, Sharda School of Allied Health Sciences (SSAHS), Sharda University, Greater Noida, U.P., India

S. Stewart Kirubakaran
Division of Computer Science and Engineering, Karunya Institute of Technology and Sciences, Coimbatore, India.

1 Introduction

Pioneering the Future of Clinical Care – Integrative Technologies and Emerging Trends

Kapil Mehta, Gauri Bansal, Gurleen Kaur, and Saumya Rajvanshi

1.1 INTRODUCTION

Artificial intelligence (AI)-based analytics have considerably progressed in a range of technical study domains, such as natural language processing (NLP), imaging classification, and signal processing. AI is revolutionizing clinical research as well [1], and new technology is being added to the traditional research paradigm. Traditionally, evidence-based treatment plans have dominated medical decision-making by taking advantage of the average treatment effect in a group [2]. Nonetheless, it is commonly acknowledged that a patient community is often diverse, meaning that a single size does not suit everyone. Stated differently, even though a particular therapeutic approach has been shown to benefit the majority of people, it may not be useful for certain patients' category. To address the problem of differentiating therapy effects in a varied population, the concept of customized treatment is put forth. The majority of patients in emergency and critical care settings are diverse, and their clinical conditions often fluctuate [3, 4]; this emphasizes the significance of customized care and early risk assessment. In the context of emergency and critical care, AI can be used in three ways. Risk stratification prediction models for critical care situations were established in a number of studies. Various clinical hazards are described across a range of study populations, including the risk of coagulopathy in sepsis, risk of blood transfusion in liver transplant patients, and mortality prediction in surgical intensive care unit (ICU) patients. Together, these experiments trained a prediction model by utilizing the supervised learning technique. Clear definitions of the clinical measures of attention and tags are required. Misclassification in the database causes model uncertainty or forecast inaccuracy in subsequent samples. The second area of research involves employing unsupervised machine learning (ML) methods to separate heterogeneous populations into more homogeneous groupings. The algorithms are not dependent on the samples having been labeled beforehand, which sets them apart from supervised learning techniques. Rather, they utilize the characteristics to categorize samples into

DOI: 10.1201/9781003516163-1

distinct subgroups or subtypes. There may be prognostic and predictive enrichment in the patient subgroups. While predictive enrichment shows that distinct subgroups may respond differently to a given intervention, predictive enrichment shows that the risks of clinical outcome events varied throughout subgroups. Applying an algorithm for reinforcement learning to recommend a medication plan in a step-by-step fashion is the third category of clinical scenarios. The fundamental tenet of this application is that the treatment plan should be modified gradually in response to the patient's changing circumstances. To optimize the reward in the end, the relationships between the therapy action, the patient's condition, and the incentive are codified in a dynamic procedure. The dynamic treatment regime (DTR) model, on the other hand, leverages the concept of reinforcement learning to estimate a series of decision rules, one for each step of intervention, which specify how to tailor treatments to patients according to their changing needs and covariate histories. DTR models are more palatable in the field of medical epidemiology because they reduce model complexity. This model has been used in critical care settings to customize ventilation plans for acute respiratory failure and fluid resuscitation in sepsis.

1.2 ARTIFICIAL INTELLIGENCE ROLE IN HEALTHCARE

AI has several benefits for the healthcare sector employees and the patients that use it on a regular basis. Due to improved decision-making and more efficient automated services, healthcare professionals can use technology to diagnose illnesses and develop personalized treatment plans more quickly and accurately than they could on their own. This can also result in cost savings on operating expenses. As more cost-effective health treatments result in lower prices, patients may anticipate possibly better health outcomes. The role of AI in healthcare that is shown in Figure 1.1, includes early(timely) disease detection, clinical decision-making, hospital operation management, patient care monitoring, expanded access to medical services, and use of wearables for health checking.

1.2.1 Timely Disease Detection and Diagnosis

It takes years of medical training and hands-on experience for a doctor to skillfully and correctly diagnose a disease. A diagnostic process involves the assessment of symptoms and the analysis of test results. Diagnosis is an extremely time-consuming

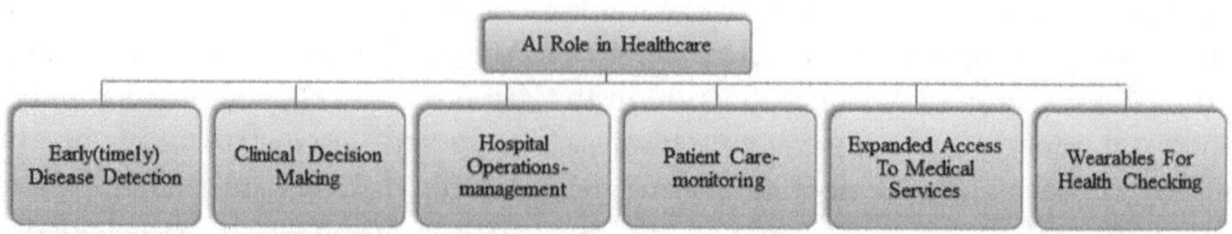

FIGURE 1.1 AI Role in Healthcare.

and important part of medical care. Even in developed nations, there is a great demand for expert physicians in many fields of human science. A key role is played by AI-driven ML and deep learning algorithms in this regard. Clinical diagnostics supported by AI are accurate, inexpensive, and convenient.

It is possible to detect even the smallest changes in a patient at an initial stage using AI systems. Whether it is the detection of cancer or the analysis of electrocardiograms (ECGs), electroencephalograms (EEGs), or even X-rays, ML and AI techniques are paving the way for healthcare advancements. Similar to a physician who must recognize patterns to diagnose a condition, ML algorithms are pre-trained with datasets to recognize patterns. AI clinical diagnosis makes use of deep neural networks (DNNs) and a variety of predictive analysis methods. Accurate diagnosis can be aided by ML algorithms that have been developed by knowledgeable specialists. ML powered by AI is now being used to conduct diagnosis such as computed tomography (CT) scans to identify stroke and lung cancer, measure blood flow to predict cardiovascular risks, diagnose disease using ECG and cardiac magnetic resonance imaging (MRI) image use patterns, take photos of the skin to categorize skin lesions, analyze retinal images to identify diabetic retinopathy, and use MRI imaging to locate tumor-containing or healthy tissue areas.

Computer vision and ML are fields of AI that involve training the AI system's algorithm to see and process images just like a human would. The system is trained using digital images, videos, and other visual inputs. The supervised or unsupervised AI system then takes actions or makes a recommendation. When it comes to healthcare, computer vision is applied in tumor and cancer detection, medical imaging, and the fight against health monitoring. X-rays, CT scans, MRIs, ultrasound images, and others provide rich ground for the creation of AI-based solutions that help therapists identify various anomalies. Let us take a brief look at the most potential usage scenarios. When diagnosing brain tumors, MRI provides the clearest images of soft tissues, such as the brain. The primary difficulty in this case is that these tumors can vary widely in size and shape. The likelihood of a successful course of treatment increases with the early detection of the condition. Furthermore, there's a chance that ML methods could significantly accelerate tumor localization [5]. Different algorithms trained to segment tumors in MRIs have reported accuracy ranging from 73–79% to 92%. Even if they are far from ideal, AI techniques can nonetheless help physicians in their decision-making. To stop the infection from spreading, early identification of coronavirus symptoms using chest X-rays is essential. It makes sense that ML models have been the subject of intensive research worldwide as a potential diagnostic tool. Nearly 97% accuracy was achieved by the most powerful AI programs [5]. The following AI disciplines and techniques are used to implement clinical diagnosis using AI:

1. Time series and predictive techniques. When gathering observational data over a period of time, time series analysis is helpful. It is useful in forecasting possible risk factors and a patient's prognosis. This area of AI is producing precise forecasts, ranging from tools for anticipating cardiac arrest to those for forecasting brain tumors, as well as the prognosis of respiratory ailments and

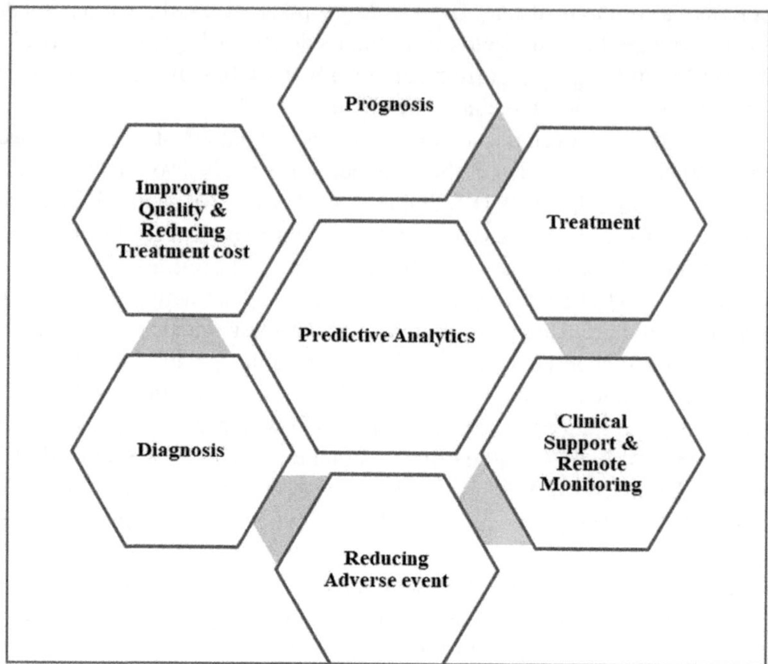

FIGURE 1.2 Notable Instances of Predictive Analytics.

COVID-19 patients. Predictive analytics can help at every step of a patient's journey, including diagnosis, prognosis, and treatment. Predictive analytics can also enhance remote patient monitoring and reduce negative incidents. On a larger scale, predictive analytics has promise for cost reduction and improved quality of treatment.

Using predictive analytics can assist in addressing inquiries such as what kind of care is most appropriate for any patient and patient reviews about outcome from the specific procedure. Instances of predictive analytics that can be applied in the healthcare industry at different stages of the patient experience are shown in Figure 1.2. First is diagnosis; in a patient cohort, diagnoses of malignant mesothelioma have been predicted using predictive analytics. Early diagnosis allows patients to begin treatment right once, increasing their chances of survival, which makes prediction a vital tool [6]. Second is prognosis. Researchers identified which patients were most likely to be readmitted after a hospital stay by using predictive analytics on physiological data from patients with congestive heart failure. With that knowledge, doctors might start treating patients early to avoid the anticipated readmissions [2]. Third, treatment physicians have employed predictive analytic models based on ML to ascertain the best course of action for patients with chronic pain [7]. Improving quality and reducing treatment cost, remote monitoring are some other instances of predictive analytics.

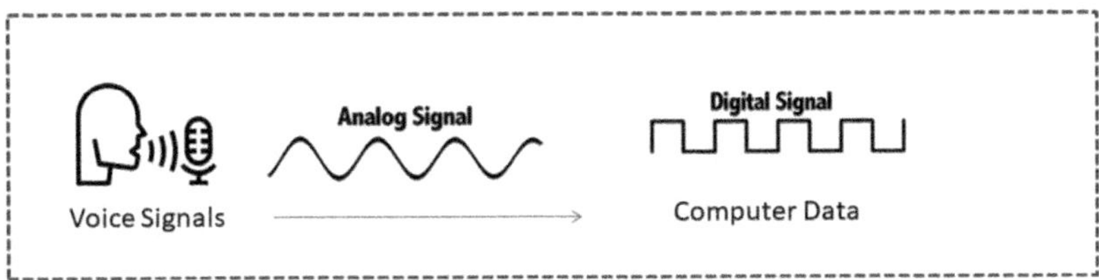

FIGURE 1.3 Speech Reorganization.

2. Speech recognition is an electronic equipment to comprehend spoken words. A microphone records the subject's voice first, and circuitry then transforms the signal from analog sound waves to digital audio. Figure 1.3 shows the process of converting voice signals to digital signals.

   Afterward, software processes the audio data and separates the sounds into distinct words. Technology is assisting in the delivery of more effective outcomes in the healthcare industry, both in clinical settings and administration [8]. Healthcare uses speech recognition software to boost efficiency. Clinicians and frontline staff are already able to concentrate on patients because there is less paperwork. Speech recognition techniques are utilized in clinical diagnostics to diagnose neurological diseases. Amazon has filed for a patent recently for voice-based user characteristic and physical feature detection. Researchers hope to employ speech analysis in diagnostics for anything from forecasting a person's risk of suicide to diagnosing sore throats. Speech recognition solutions covering a wide range of clinical and administrative demands are being supplied by software development companies to hospitals and healthcare providers on an increasing basis. Voice-based technology is improving the experiences of patients, clinicians, and support personnel with everything from intricate programs to one-stop-shop apps [2]. For many patient groups, voice-activated software offers a major improvement in diagnosis and treatment. A case in point is those living with dementia or cognitive impairment, who might get advantages from innovative apps that employ speech recognition technology. These apps enable users to access well-being data, communicate securely, and link with well-known tools like Alexa. Note-taking for clinicians is a voice recognition software that has been a game changer for medical professionals who are overworked and short on time. Doctors can now enter notes into their organization's records without ever picking up a pen by employing speech recognition technology as a virtual scribe. Time is money, as they say, and medical dictation software helps physicians make the most of their time by providing precise transcriptions of their own words. Solutions for hearing-impaired software are used because elderly individuals are more likely to need medical attention; there is a disproportionately high rate of patients with hearing issues. Advancements in voice recognition technology; these patients to now take advantage of innovative solutions like applications that provide subtitles for live discussions, preventing them from losing important information during sessions. One's chances of receiving high-quality care are significantly increased when they can speak with medical personnel. Healthcare providers are similarly investing substantially in "Patient Engagement," as is the corporate sector when it comes to improving the consumer experience. In this regard, the emergence of voice-activated assistants is critical, as it is becoming less necessary to divert or hold patient calls. Busy patients can more quickly and easily request appointments, confirm prescriptions, or update information via voice-based technologies [9].

3. NLP is the AI-based chatbots can interpret natural language and do a preliminary assessment of a patient's symptoms. NLP is also helpful in extracting data from digital health record data made using Optical Character Recognition (OCR), Named Entity Recognition (NER), Sentiment Analysis, Text Classification, and Topic Modeling. OCR is the process by which a computer "reads" handwritten or printed text and transforms it into a digital format known as optical character recognition, or OCR. One example of this process is scanning a paper document and turning it into a PDF. OCR is also used to extract text and tables from unstructured data sources, including text files or photos, and present the information in an understandable manner. After formatting, this data can be entered into an NLP pipeline for additional examination. OCR is frequently used in the healthcare sector to digitize medical test results, clinical notes, patient intake forms, discharge summaries, and medical history records, among other documents. The greatest benefit of OCR technology is that it gives consumers access to data around the clock. Patients can avoid treatment delays because the data is digitally stored and the data extraction process is simple. Figure 1.4 includes the benefits of OCR in healthcare, like text results, clinical notes, patient intake form, discharge summaries, and medical history records.

   NER is a technique for extracting information that splits named entities (i.e., actual subjects like an individual, place, business, or product) into pre-established groups. NER is also referred to as entity identification, entity chunking, or entity extraction [10]. Additionally, custom entities can be used to train NER to recognize and extract custom tags such as medication names, disease names, and symptom names. Several pre-trained NER engines are available in the Spacy and not libraries for labeling content using generic labels. Modern transformer models with a robust NER library, like

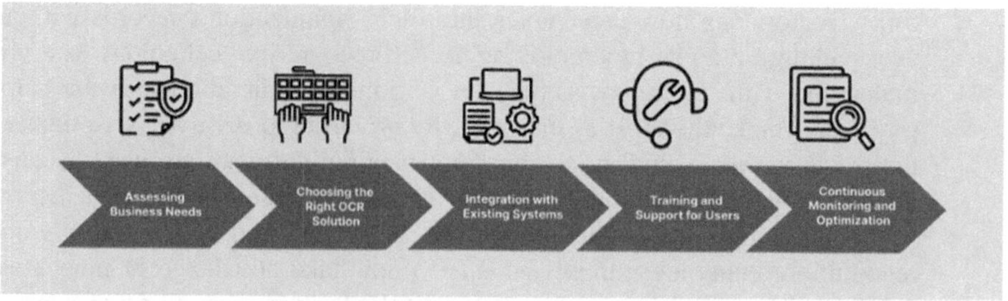

FIGURE 1.4 Benefits of OCR in Healthcare.

Bidirectional Encoder Representations from Transformers (BERT), are also capable of extracting generic entities. There are variants of models like BERT that are trained using unique data. Pre-trained on biomedical datasets from PubMed, Bio-BERT is a BERT model. To categorize the retrieved tokens into entities, a classifier model is constructed on top of the Bio-BERT model [11].

Sentiment analysis includes three vital steps: identifying, extracting, and analyzing. To determine if patient sentiment is positive, negative, or neutral, sentiment analysis requires a three-step process that involves patient identification, data extraction, and analysis. The next stage is to act accordingly depending on the conclusions that have been formed. Healthcare providers can better establish a long-lasting patient–provider relationship and enhance their brand image by getting to know their patients, learning about their opinions, and evaluating their needs through the study of those opinions and the actionable insights that follow. To determine the underlying sentiment of a text, sentiment analysis combines NLP, text analysis, computational linguistics, and biometrics. Because of this, sentiment analysis is also frequently called opinion mining or sentiment detection.

A patient sentiment analysis framework powered by AI/ML is shown in Figure 1.5. The healthcare professional is to analyze the patient's behavior, a patient's emotions in relation to a service they have received, request a sentiment analysis report for patients, and react promptly to any service-related course corrections that are required to provide the patient with more proactive service recommendations.

Text classification is the NLP technique, sometimes referred to as text categorization, that is used to evaluate text input and apply labels or tags to various semantic units or phrases according to predetermined categories. A healthcare professional might, for instance, utilize text categorization to pinpoint patients who are at risk based on certain phrases or keywords used in their medical documents. Some key points about its applications and

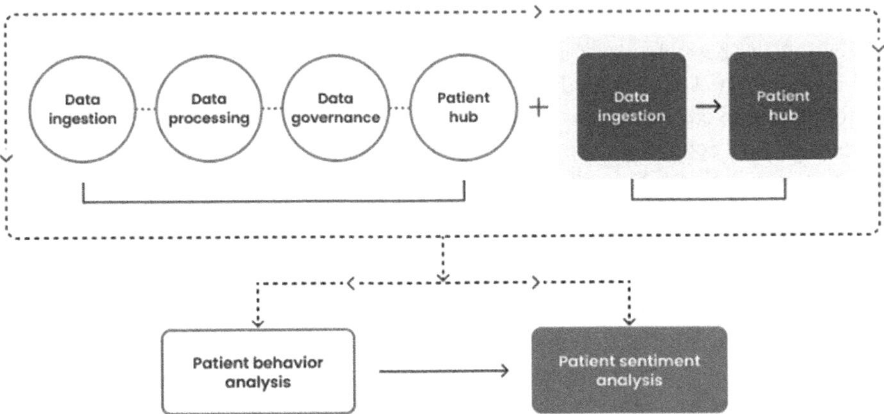

FIGURE 1.5 AI/ML Driven Patient Sentiment Analysis.

methods are Clinical Decision Support is used in text classification to facilitate decision-making by assisting in the identification of pertinent clinical data from patient records. For instance, categorizing a patient's symptoms to recommend potential diagnosis [12]. Medical coding is another significant application in the automatic assignment of International Classification of Diseases (ICD) numbers to medical records. This supports statistical analysis, insurance claims, and billing [13]. Deep learning is used to identify intricate patterns in the data; sophisticated models like Convolutional Neural Networks (CNNs) and Attention-based Models (like Attention) are utilized to increase the accuracy of text classification.

Topic Modeling: To find semantic structures, or "topics," collections of documents are categorized using a type of statistical modeling and NLP called topic modeling. This technique groups documents together based on common words or phrases. Latent Dirichlet allocation is the most popular type of topic modeling, grouping words and phrases based on their semantic links, which are found by algorithms. OCR and NER are the most widely used NLP techniques in the healthcare sector out of the five.

1.2.2 Clinical Decision-Making

Interactive computer programs known as clinical decision support systems or software (CDSS) are made to help doctors and other health professionals make decisions. A dynamic (medical) knowledge base and an inference mechanism – typically a collection of guidelines generated from experts and evidence-based medicine – are the fundamental parts of a CDSS, and they are carried out by means of medical logic modules [14].

In the modern healthcare setting, CDSSs are indispensable instruments that improve patient outcomes and physician decision-making. Currently, the incorporation of AI is further modernizing CDSS. The ways that AI technologies are changing CDSS, how they are being applied in healthcare decision-making, the difficulties that they present, and the possible path toward achieving the full potential of AI-CDSS. For this, picture yourself with a digital assistant at your side, prepared to aid you in making the best choices for your patients and armed with the most recent medical information. That is exactly what CDSS – computer programs that help medical professionals make decisions – represent: a significant breakthrough in healthcare that combines technological innovation with medical knowledge to enhance clinical decision-making procedures. These systems are intended to improve patient outcomes, treatment efficacy, and diagnostic accuracy by giving medical personnel at the point of care meaningful insights, evidence-based recommendations, and patient-specific information. To close the gap between a wealth of medical data and prompt, well-informed clinical judgments, CDSS relies on patient data, algorithms, and medical knowledge as shown in Figure 1.6.

Fundamentally, CDSS is a cognitive aid that helps doctors make sense of the complex world of contemporary medicine. To give healthcare practitioners individualized recommendations, prompts, and warnings throughout the administration of treatment,

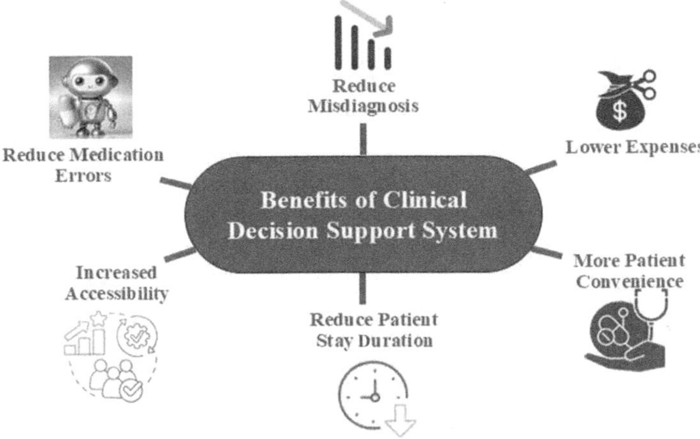

FIGURE 1.6 Benefits of CDSS.

it evaluates patient data, medical literature, and best practices. The potential of CDSS to minimize diagnostic errors, optimize treatment regimens, lower healthcare costs, and ultimately enhance patient safety and care quality makes it significant. The Agency for Healthcare Research and Quality (AHRQ) states that CDSS interventions have been demonstrated to improve the quality of healthcare by avoiding adverse drug events, decreasing medication errors, and facilitating adherence to clinical standards. Furthermore, the adaptability and broad applicability of CDSS, illustrating its usefulness in a variety of healthcare settings, including ICUs and primary care clinics have been highlighted [15].

Some examples of CDSS involvements by aim area of care are given in Table 1.1. It is authoritative for clinicians to integrate a vast array of clinical data while managing competing demands to reduce costs, patient hazards, and uncertainty in diagnosis. Choosing what data to collect, what tests to conduct, how to analyze and integrate this data to make diagnoses, and what recommendations for treatments [16]. Upon assessing a patient, medical professionals typically need to respond to the following inquiries for the physical examination and history point to any particular diagnoses, checking for any “red flags” that point to a pressing social or medical concern that should be resolved before a diagnosis is confirmed, checking the necessity to conduct testing or seek advice. Clinicians typically make these judgments reflexively in simple or common settings; testing and therapy are started based on standard practice; diagnoses are made by identifying illness patterns. For example, in the event of a flu pandemic, a healthy adult who presents with fever, acute myalgia, orbital pain, and a harsh cough for a period of 2 days is probably going to be diagnosed with influenza again and simply receive the necessary symptomatic treatment. Although this type of pattern recognition is effective and simple to use, it may be prone to inaccuracy due to the lack of systematic or significant consideration given to alternative diagnostic and therapeutic options. A patient with that flu pattern and low oxygen

TABLE 1.1
Examples of CDSS Involvements by Aim Area of Care

Target	Example
Precautionary care	Guidelines for disease management, screening, and immunization for secondary prevention
Diagnosis	Recommendations for potential diagnoses that fit the symptoms and indications of a patient
Making treatment plans or carrying them out	Drug dosage recommendations, treatment protocols for particular diseases, and notifications of drug–drug interactions
Monitoring	Reminders and corollary instructions for medication adverse event monitoring
Efficiency of hospitals and providers	Plans for minimizing the duration of stay and order sets
Lower expenses and more patient convenience	Drug formulary guidelines and alerts for duplicate testing

saturation, for instance, could actually have COVID-19 or bacterial pneumonia and need antibiotics. Physicians need to be conscious of the possibility of biases being introduced throughout the diagnostic procedure [17].

1.2.3 Hospital Operations and Management

Numerous jobs in healthcare operations can be made better or more efficient by carefully integrating AI. One of the quickest ways AI can impact healthcare is frequently mentioned as being the improvement of administrative processes and back-office productivity. It requires more than half of a nurse's time on average, for example, and puts a strain on staff resources. However, operations management personnel already have the technological infrastructure required to use AI sooner rather than later. AI has many more uses in healthcare, both now and in the future. However, clinical settings present greater challenges in terms of user confidence and technological engagement [18]. This piece will focus on useful ways AI can enhance hospital operations management.

1.2.3.1 Efficiently Schedule Equipment and Providers

One of the most important aspects of operations management is scheduling doctors' visits, expensive equipment, and other services [19]. Healthcare scheduling done well can give a company a financial edge over competitors, while poorly done scheduling might have the opposite effect [20]. AI-enhanced scheduling has been used for a while by healthcare organizations, particularly in medical specialties where scheduling is crucial. One such specialization where scheduling is difficult but crucial is home healthcare; a home health operation's ability to maximize patient time and reduce travel time is critical to its success [21].

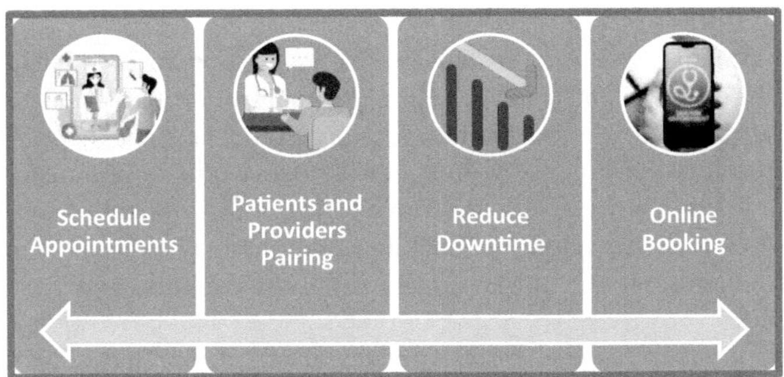

FIGURE 1.7 Healthcare Scheduling.

TABLE 1.2
Schedule Equipment and Providers

Scheduling KPIs	How AI Can Help
Patient wait time	AI programs that facilitate efficient scheduling and, where necessary, take travel time into consideration minimize needless waiting periods for emergencies and scheduled visits.
Utilization rate	AI-assisted scheduling reduces downtime for life-saving devices like ventilators and MRI machines while optimizing the safe use of each healthcare worker.
Time to schedule	Self-service scheduling enables patients to make their own appointments, while automated scheduling technologies assist staff in booking appointments more efficiently utilizing "suggested" time frames.
Adherence to treatment plan	When an appointment is not rescheduled after a predetermined number of days, AI-enhanced scheduling software can notify staff members and push the scheduler to contact the patient, thereby decreasing the likelihood that they would discontinue their treatment plan.

AI has a number of useful uses in healthcare scheduling (Figure 1.7), including:

1. Schedule Appointments: Make appointments using a system that takes into consideration the duration of each service type, staff availability, necessary travel time, and other internal Key Performance Indicators (KPIs).
2. Patients and Providers Pairing Effectively: It matches patients with providers according to the patient's preferences or the provider's qualifications, geography, or past interactions with the patient.
3. Reduce downtime of facilities (such as surgery suites), skilled labor, and equipment to increase utilization and save costs.
4. Online Booking: More than 90% of healthcare clients indicate they would utilize online self-service booking if their supplier offered it; enable it. Table 1.2 is about patient scheduling.

1.2.3.2 Simplify Internal Communication

Frequent communication is essential to healthcare operations management with suppliers, employees, clients, and internal departments. Fortunately, nonclinical communication is one area where AI can have a big influence right soon. With chatbots and intelligent virtual assistants that can answer frequently asked customer queries, AI is already helping businesses improve their marketing and public relations efforts and expand their 24/7 reach [22]. AI-enabled solutions can help healthcare operations workers communicate more effectively and simply in a number of ways, like

1. Create drafts of routine correspondence for food suppliers, cleaning services, maintenance firms, medtech suppliers, and other partners, such as welcome letters and account status updates.
2. Simplify accounting and billing duties by verifying calculations are correct and pulling important data from budget reports and invoices to expedite staff work.
3. Create graphs and reports on the KPIs that are being tracked, such as patient satisfaction, staff utilization, efficiency, and expenses over time.
4. Requests for proposals (RFPs) can be made simpler by providing pertinent staff members with a summary of the essential information.

1.2.3.3 Minimize Administrative Tasks That Require Human Labor

Running a health organization requires performing administrative duties, such as managing and safeguarding patient records, supervising staff, negotiating with vendors, managing facilities, and ensuring healthcare activities comply with legal and professional requirements. Administrative work is crucial, but if every step of the process is carried out by hand, staff time and resources could be better used on initiatives that improve health and generate income. Healthcare operations teams can benefit from using AI to automate certain simple administrative duties. Automate laborious data entry tasks, such as manually transcribing visit notes to update patient records or produce discharge summaries. Simplifying the process of managing health insurance claim is as follows:

Scripted AI assistants can help cut down on the amount of time spent on the phone with patients, providers, and pharmacies.

Minimize time spent on medical coding. Make the most of the text and picture recognition AI capabilities available to reduce the amount of time spent on medical coding and other billing duties.

1.3 HEALTHCARE-SPECIFIC NATURAL LANGUAGE PROCESSING APPLICATIONS

1.3.1 Clinical Assertion Application

Healthcare professionals can examine clinical notes to determine whether a patient is having a problem and whether it is present, absent, or conditional by using clinical assertion modeling. Clinical assertion models are so frequently employed to aid in patient diagnosis and treatment. For instance, a patient may report to her doctor that she has been experiencing headaches for the previous 2 weeks and that she gets nervous when she walks quickly. Following an examination, the physician may observe that the patient does not seem to be in any discomfort and that she does not exhibit any alopecia symptoms. The physician might examine the clinical notes from that visit using NER and text categorization, marking "pain," "headache," "anxious," and "alopecia" as PROBLEM items. The headache would be present, the anxiety would be conditional, and the alopecia and pain would be absent. Based on the doctor's declarations, the conditions may then be further classified as present, conditional, or absent. This example shows how NLP may be used in healthcare to help doctors identify the most urgent patient problems and treat them right away, resulting in improved patient care.

1.3.2 Clinical De-Identification Application

This application provides healthcare services, health plans, and other covered entities must "protect sensitive patient health information from being disclosed with the patient's consent or knowledge," according to the Health Insurance Portability and Accountability Act (HIPAA). Data that has been de-identified, or from which specific individual identifiers, such as name, address, phone number, and so forth, have been removed, is the exception to this rule. Since de-identified data does not contain any information that would jeopardize patient privacy, it is no longer regarded as Protected Health Information (PHI). In fact, healthcare practitioners can employ NLP to identify potentially PHI-containing text and replace PHI with semantic tags to de-identify or obfuscate it. Healthcare companies can prevent HIPAA non-compliance by doing this.

1.3.3 Clinical Entity Resolver

Healthcare professionals can assign an ICD-10 Clinical Modification (ICD-10-CM) code to various diseases and diagnoses by extracting information about them from patient records using NLP. ICD-10-CM codes are a useful tool that enables doctors to make more informed judgments by allowing them to cross-reference diagnoses and symptoms with one another. Therefore, doctors may keep an eye on quality outcomes, mortality statistics, healthcare statistics, and more for a certain disease by giving the correct ICD-10-CM number. As a result, they are better equipped to comprehend medical difficulties, create treatments, and assess the effectiveness of care.

1.3.4 Clinical Named Entity Recognition General

Healthcare providers can use this form of NER, which is similar to the Clinical Assertion Model, to analyze clinical notes, extract keywords, and assign those keywords to particular entities, such as problem, test, or treatment. For instance, "insulin drip" and "reduction" would be flagged as treatments, "Educa" and "HTG" as PROBLEMs, and "the anion gap" and "triglycerides" as TESTs if a patient received an insulin drip for Educa and HTG with a reduction in the anion gap to 13 and triglycerides to 1400 mg/dL within a day. The Clinical NER General Model is expanded upon by the Clinical Named Entity Recognition Posology, as depicted in the illustration below. Clinical studies can identify patients through drug and dose filtration using either version of this program.

1.4 CONCLUSION AND FUTURE SCOPE

AI advancements have the potential to revolutionize healthcare by providing a more personalized, accurate, predictive, and portable future. These technologies can help healthcare professionals return to patients and focus on what matters most. They can use a globally democratized set of data assets, including the highest levels of human knowledge, to work at the limits of science and provide a high standard of care. AI has the potential to enhance health equity globally. It is increasingly ingrained in areas like radiology, pathology, cancer, and surgery. AI can influence medical professionals' decisions and ensure safety during the COVID-19 pandemic. The next decade will focus on analyzing the value and insights society can derive from digital assets, improving clinical outcomes with AI, and developing new data assets and tools. We are at a turning point in medicine and technological application, but there are enormous obstacles that must be addressed.

REFERENCES

[1] F. Grignaffini et al., "The use of artificial intelligence in the liver histopathology field: A systematic review," *Diagnostics*, vol. 14, no. 4, pp. 388, Feb. 2024. doi:10.3390/diagnostics14040388.

[2] X. Zhang et al., "Automated detection of cardiovascular disease by electrocardiogram signal analysis: A deep learning system," *Cardiovascular Diagnosis and Therapy*, vol. 10, no. 2, pp. 227–235, Apr. 2020. doi:10.21037/cdt.2019.12.10.

[3] D. A. Hashimoto, E. Witkowski, L. Gao, O. Meireles, and G. Rosman, "Artificial intelligence in anesthesiology," *Anesthesiology*, vol. 132, no. 2, pp. 379–394, Feb. 2020. doi:10.1097/aln.0000000000002960.

[4] A. Lal, Y. Pinevich, O. Gajic, V. Herasevich, and B. Pickering, "Artificial intelligence and computer simulation models in critical illness," *World Journal of Critical Care Medicine*, vol. 9, no. 2, pp. 13–19, Jun. 2020. doi: 10.5492/wjccm.v9.i2.13.

[5] K. Mehta, Aayushi, C. Singh, H. Chugh, and M. Kumar, "Revolutionizing healthcare by accessing the opportunities for virtual and augmented reality," *2023 7th International Conference on Intelligent Computing and Control Systems (ICICCS)*, IEEE, pp. 836–841, 2023.

[6] G. Lippi, F. Sanchis-Gomar, and G. Cervellin, "Global epidemiology of atrial fibrillation: An increasing epidemic and public health challenge," *International Journal of Stroke*, vol. 16, no. 2, pp. 217–221, Jan. 2020. doi:10.1177/1747493019897870.

[7] C. Yang, N. D. Aranoff, P. Green, and N. Tavassolian, "A binary classification of cardiovascular abnormality using time-frequency features of cardio-mechanical signals," *2018 40th Annual International Conference of the IEEE Engineering in Medicine and Biology Society (EMBC)*, vol. 11, pp. 5438–5441, Jul. 2021. doi:10.1109/embc.2018.8513644.

[8] A. J. Jacob et al., "AI-based, automated chamber volumetry from gated, non-contrast CT," *Journal of Cardiovascular Computed Tomography*, vol. 17, no. 5, pp. 336–340, Sep. 2023. doi:10.1016/j.jcct.2023.08.001

[9] T. A. Retson, E. M. Masutani, D. Golden, and A. Hsiao, "Clinical performance and role of expert supervision of deep learning for cardiac ventricular volumetry: A validation study," *Radiology: Artificial Intelligence*, vol. 2, no. 4, p. e190064, Jul. 2021. doi:10.1148/ryai.2020190064.

[10] L. Alzubaidi et al., "Review of deep learning: Concepts, CNN architectures, challenges, applications, future directions," *Journal of Big Data*, vol. 8, no. 1, p. 53, Mar. 2021. doi:10.1186/s40537-021-00444-8.

[11] M. Yazdimamaghani, P. J. Moos, M. A. Dobrovolskaia, and H. Ghandehari, "Genotoxicity of amorphous silica nanoparticles: Status and prospects," *Nanomedicine: Nanotechnology, Biology and Medicine*, vol. 16, pp. 106–125, Feb. 2020. doi:10.1016/j.nano.2018.11.013.

[12] M. B. Khorrami et al., "Antioxidant and toxicity studies of biosynthesized cerium oxide nanoparticles in rats," *International Journal of Nanomedicine*, vol. 14, pp. 2915–2926, Apr. 2019. doi:10.2147/ijn.s194192.

[13] X. Zhao et al., "Autophagic flux blockage in alveolar epithelial cells is essential in silica nanoparticle-induced pulmonary fibrosis," *Cell Death and Disease*, vol. 10, no. 2, pp. 214–220, Mar. 2021. doi:10.1038/s41419-019-1340-8.

[14] P. Huang et al., "RTMS improves dysphagia by inhibiting NLRP3 inflammasome activation and caspase-1 dependent pyroptosis in PD mice," *npj Parkinson's Disease*, vol. 10, no. 1, p. 156, Jan. 2024. doi:10.1038/s41531-024-00775-2.

[15] P. Khoury et al., "A framework for augmented intelligence in allergy and immunology practice and research – a work group report of the AAAAI Health Informatics, Technology, and Education Committee," *Journal of Allergy and Clinical Immunology: In Practice*, vol. 10, no. 5, pp. 1178–1188, May 2022. doi:10.1016/j.jaip.2022.01.047.

[16] S. M. Rappaport, "Response to 'the role of the exposome in promoting resilience or susceptibility after SARS-COV-2 infection,' " *Journal of Exposure Science and Environmental Epidemiology*, vol. 30, no. 6, pp. 905–905, Sep. 2020. doi:10.1038/s41370-020-00274-5.

[17] O. Olsson et al., "Efficient, automated and robust pollen analysis using deep learning," *Methods in Ecology and Evolution*, vol. 12, no. 5, pp. 850–862, Mar. 2021. doi:10.1111/2041-210x.13575.

[18] L. Li, B. Chen, G. Li, S. Chen, and J. Zhang, "Anti-inflammatory nanotherapies based on bioactive cyclodextrin materials," *Advanced NanoBiomed Research*, vol. 3, no. 12, Nov. 2023. doi:10.1002/anbr.202300106.

[19] X. Sun, A. Tan, and B. J. Boyd, "Magnetically-activated lipid nanocarriers in biomedical applications: A review of current status and perspective," *WIREs Nanomedicine and Nanobiotechnology*, vol. 15, no. 3, p. e1863, Nov. 2022. doi:10.1002/wnan.1863.

[20] A. Huguet-Casquero, E. Gainza, and J. L. Pedraz, "Towards green nanoscience: From extraction to nanoformulation," *Biotechnology Advances*, vol. 46, p. 107657, Jan. 2021. doi:10.1016/j.biotechadv.2020.107657.

[21] R. Kavya, J. Christopher, S. Panda, and Y. B. Lazarus, "Machine learning and XAI approaches for allergy diagnosis," *Biomedical Signal Processing and Control*, vol. 69, p. 102681, Aug. 2021. doi:10.1016/j.bspc.2021.102681.

[22] S. N. Bukhari, J. Webber, and A. Mehbodniya, "Decision tree based ensemble machine learning model for the prediction of Zika virus T-cell epitopes as potential vaccine candidates," *Scientific Reports*, vol. 12, no. 1, p. 7810, May 2022. doi:10.1038/s41598-022-11731-6.

2 The Landscape of HealthTech

A Comprehensive Overview

P. Nagaraja, P. Shanmugavadivu, M. Mary Shanthi Rani, and A. Nithya

2.1 INTRODUCTION

Health technology, otherwise known as "HealthTech," is an emerging large industry that aims to improve quality of life and well-being of everyone by incorporating cutting-edge technology into the practices of healthcare professionals, payers, and providers. It includes a range of technology-driven innovations to improve the administration and provision of healthcare services, including instruments, software, packages for disease diagnosis, and data analytics. HealthTech has gained significant momentum due to its ability to transform healthcare practices and thereby has brought about a thorough paradigm shift in boosting access, reliability, and resilience in healthcare, optimizing patients' outcomes, and streamlining procedures. HealthTech has exhibited enormous scope to resolve crucial issues in the healthcare sector, such as early detection and classification of diseases and robotic surgery, in the light of technology. The intervention of technology in healthcare has brought out new vistas, namely telemedicine, remote patient monitoring (RPM), and electronic health records (EHR), which have enabled the incorporation of digital solutions into conventional healthcare systems and practices. These developments hold great promise in terms of cost saving, enhanced patient satisfaction, and improved efficacy and efficiency of healthcare services. The envisaged developments in HealthTech are expected to influence the field of medicine in medical instrument design, patient care, diagnostic precision, and overall healthcare outcomes [1, 2].

2.2 OVERVIEW OF HEALTHTECH

The field of health technology is broad and ever-changing due to the unforeseen developments in electronics and digital innovations, real-time/remote monitoring, personalized healthcare services, personalized drug design, and communication The applications of artificial intelligence (AI) models for healthcare have redefined the dimensions of disease diagnosis, prediction, and classification. The contemporary HealthTech trends in real-time processes are depicted in Figure 2.1.

DOI: 10.1201/9781003516163-2

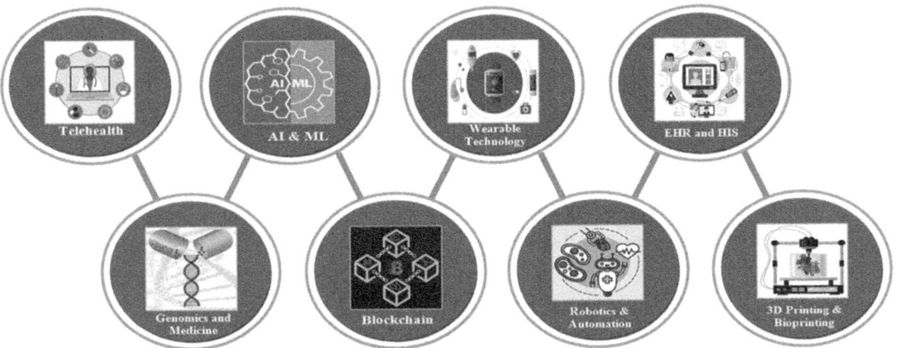

FIGURE 2.1 Trending Technologies in HealthTech.

2.2.1 Telehealth

The use of communications technology to deliver medical care to remotely located patients is known as telehealth. The convergence of breakthroughs in medical technologies, computer science, informatics, and communications has made telehealth an invaluable resource in technology-enabled healthcare. The key components of telemedicine's growth include mobile health applications, remote monitoring tools, and video-conferencing platforms. A common practice in telehealth is the remote monitoring of blood pressure, heart rate, and other vital health-monitoring parameters using a patient-worn gadget that electronically transmits real-time data to medical experts. The surge in use of smart phones and other smart personal gadgets is becoming increasingly common worldwide, without any exception, even in isolated and underprivileged sections of the community. These devices seamlessly generate enormous data, which serves as a vital source for health monitoring and analytics. Since the outbreak of the COVID-19 pandemic, virtual consultations between physicians and patients have been increasingly common. The likelihood of virtual medical care as a choice in healthcare depends on the perception and belief of the stakeholders, namely, doctors, patients, and other healthcare service providers [3].

Healthcare ideologies have been redefined due to the increased demand for teleconsultations, which allow doctors to offer consultancy services over the phone or by sending medical images like CT, MRI, or ultrasound scans. The well-structured EHRs provide detailed insights into the records of medical information, which would enable specialists to diagnose and prescribe treatments with reliable accuracy. This practice has popularized RPM, which calls for sending real-time sensor data of a patient observed at home to medical personnel. For instance, a patient with chronic health conditions due to diabetes can be uninterruptedly monitored on real-time glucose readings and provide preventive medical care as well as life-saving assistance during emergencies. Telehomecare deals with offering the physical and emotional comfort of being at home along with monitoring a patient's health and providing timely medical care during unforeseen issues, risks, and threats, for instance, patients with dementia or chronic diseases. When emergencies arise, Telehomecare sensors can identify problems like gas leakage, fire, or falls and promptly notify emergency service providers. In addition to these developments, point-of-care (PoC) medicine makes use of diagnostic tools that are used for patients at home, in clinics, or in isolated locations to receive medical care and healthcare delivery [4].

2.2.1.1 HealthTech Services in Vogue

1. *Paper-Based HIV Test:*A ten-dollar test uses a mobile phone for RNA extraction, reaction, and result analysis to quantify the HIV viral load in the blood in 15 minutes. The results can be digitally stored in the cloud and be ideally made available for PoC infectious illness diagnosis.
2. *Wearable System for Knee Osteoarthritis:* This adaptable system uses sensors placed in insoles and sleeves to track and manage the biomechanics of muscle movement. The analysis of data generated by sensors when the patient feels pain due to osteoarthritis helps in the customization of individualized therapeutic strategies for rehabilitation,
3. *Smartphone-Based Anemia Test*: AnemiaPhone uses a smartphone attachment to measure iron, vitaminB, and inflammatory levels from a drop of blood sample. In remote areas, mobile-based blood analysis has proved to be handy and a boon to diagnose anemia, which is commonly observed among rural women.
4. *Mobile Device for Heart Congestion:* This gadget combines a smart ring and wristband that tracks the variations in heartbeat and identifies the early symptoms of cardiac congestion effortlessly. The real-time analytics of the collected medical data helps the cardiologists to continuously monitor the trend of the ailment, based on which medication modifications can be done from time to time. This device helps in avoiding hospitalization in emergencies and in monitoring slow progression of heart failure.

2.2.2 Artificial Intelligence and Machine Learning

AI is a branch of science that aims to mimic human cognitive skills of human in machines. The AI models under the umbrella of machine learning (ML) and deep learning (DL) are designed to outsmart human intelligence in data-driven prediction, classification, translations, text summarization, music composition, art creation, and many more. ML is an AI methodology that builds a computer algorithm–a collection of guidelines and instructions to evaluate and forecast data that is fed into the system.

In recent years, ML technology driven solutions and services are widely used in various day-to-day activities, such as customized news feeds and traffic prediction maps. Artificial neural networks (ANNs) designed after the mechanics of biological neurons have shown reliable precision in object identification/recognition and forecasting. DL is a branch of ML that intends to extract hidden non-linear patterns/associations from the vast volume of complicated, unstructured data by utilizing multiple layers of computing. Self-driving cars that can recognize traffic signs and voice-activated virtual assistants are products of deep neural networks [5, 6].

2.2.2 Impact and Influence of Artificial Intelligence Technologies in Healthcare

It is evident that AI is unprecedentedly transforming healthcare research in many ways, boosting interdisciplinary innovations and smart strategies to optimize workflow, supply chain management, and data analytics. A few important domains where AI has impacted in a significant way are listed herein under:

1. *Predictive Analytics:* AI models are used to predict the occurrence of disease outbreaks, patients' outcomes, and disease trends by mining the past trends/patterns of patients' data. These predictions are observed to improve the efficacy of therapy and treatment and reduce relapse rates.
2. *Medical Imaging:* Most of the medical image modalities such as X-rays, mammograms, CT scans, and MRIs are handled by AI systems for automated disease diagnosis. The latest AI models, such as Generative Adversarial Network (GAN), offer a newer solution for image pre-processing, such as noise removal and image augmentation. The extension of AI models, such as Explainable AI (XAI), helps to understand the rationale behind the performance behavior of AI models.
3. *Personalized Medicine:* AI offers another breakthrough in medicine for personalized drug design based on the genetic, clinical, and lifestyle data of patients. The success of this effort shall bring about newer directions in treatments and outcomes, primarily to minimize the side effects due to overdosage/irrelevant prescription of medication.
4. *Clinical Decision Support:* AI facilitates the clinicians to derive data-driven decisions, which could help to contain diagnostic errors and prevent the cascading ill effects on the patients.
5. *EHRs:* The EHRs are the primary source of data on the patients, which are systematically created and augmented with vital data from time to time during every visit of the patients. These records provide a wider scope for automated data acquisition, feature extraction, dimensionality reduction, and processing for expected outcomes such as disease prediction/classification. AI tools are vibrantly used to handle missing data, duplicate data, irrelevant data, data normalization, data encoding, etc. Natural language processing (NLP) also plays an inevitable role in handling medical unstructured data to augment the precision of data understanding and decision-making.
6. *Remote Patient Monitoring:* AI can analyze information collected from remote sensors and wearables to constantly monitor patients' health conditions. It can instantly capture and/or forecast abnormal conditions andhealth deteriorations from the online real-time data and notify medical professionals for appropriate medication and remediation.
7. *Virtual Health Assistants:* AI-powered chatbots and virtual assistants play a very important role in managing and treating patients'chronic conditions by providing medical information, arranging appointments, and reminding patients to take their medications. These services increase patient engagement.

8. *Precision Medicine and Genomics:* AI analyzes genomic information to identify genetic markers linked to illnesses and predict patient reactions to therapies. This is in favor of precision medicine strategies that focus on certain genetic characteristics.
9. *Health Data Integration:* AI combines and explores the health data generated from diverse sources, viz., clinician notes, clinical test reports, inferential reports, and data generated by wearable devices, and thereby offers a holistic understanding of the patients' case history. This heterogeneous data serves as a rich repository for new research directions aiming at innovative healthcare solutions and services.
10. *Simulation and Modeling*: AI-driven simulations and models in real-world settings serve as a precursor for the researchers to validate the hypotheses, computational workflow related to investigations on disease causes and effects, trials on therapy, and forecast the outcomes in virtual environment.

In other words, AI is fueling rapid advancements in technology-enabled healthcare services research, ensuringutmost precisionin disease diagnoses, treatments, and improved patient care. The AI models exhibit an unbounded capacity to analyze and learn from voluminous datasets, the ability to handle new data, and deliver actionable insights, thereby propelling innovations in transformative healthcare.

2.2.3 Wearable Technology Promoting HealthTech

Wearable devices are a path-breaking innovation, especially in the healthcare sector, which are designated to read health-related parameters and communicate the readings to medical experts. These gadgets can be in many forms, such as clothing, accessories, specialized jewelry, and special-purpose medical equipment. The terminology "wearable computing" advocates high-order computing and communication capabilities of wearables in the form of specialized and sophisticated devices. Some of the most advanced wearable technology examples are virtual reality (VR) headsets with holographic computers, Google Glass, Microsoft's HoloLens, and AI hearing aids. A simple example of wearable technology is a throw-away skin patch that has wireless sensors to transmit a patient's data to the designated receiver [7].

2.2.3.1 Developments in Wearable Technology

To tackle and mitigate health-related issues and challenges, wearable health technology serves as a boon, assuring the following functional features:

1. *Improved Sensitivity and Accuracy:* The sophisticated sensors with increased sensitivity and precision can monitor a wider range of health parameters, including uncommon ailments. The biochemical sensors are designed to monitor intricate signals such as changes in hormone levels, blood pressure, heartbeat, or pre-disease symptoms.
2. *Integration of Emerging Technologies:* Utilization of advanced AI models for customized health suggestions, forecasting health trends, and improved data

analysis. Utilization of Internet of Things (IoT) connection to build all-in-one health ecosystems that offer a comprehensive picture of a person's health.

3. *Personalization and Adaptability:* Refinement of health suggestions using adaptive algorithms in response to patient data and thereby evolving medical solutions. Creation of user interfaces and notifications that is customizable to meet individual health needs and preferences.
4. *Extended Data Monitoring:* Optimization of wearables to facilitate ongoing, extended data monitoring with the least amount of user intervention. Provision of automated systems to examine past health datato unveil hidden trends and patterns over a time frame.
5. *Enhanced Wearability and Comfort:* Usage of innovative fabrics that are breathable, light, and cozy for prolonged use. Availability of subtle and adaptable wearable devices to cater to the preferences of hobbies and lifestyles.
6. *Security and Privacy of Data:* Protection of sensitive health data against vulnerability and security threads using robust and novel encryption and security measures. Consumers are provided with strong privacy controls to regulate and safeguard data sharing and privacy preferences.
7. *Integration with Healthcare Systems:* Provision of an exhaustive overview of a patient's health data, making sure wearables can easily link with EHRs and other healthcare systems. Provision of real-time alerting systems so that, in the event of an anomaly, healthcare providers may access data right away.
8. *Accessibility and Affordability:* Promises quality-assured service at a reduced cost is the key aspect of increased accessibility and affordability to wearable technologies. Creation of items that adhere to regionally specific legislation and a range of healthcare needs.

Wearable devices provide accurate, tailored, and integrated healthcare solutions and services, thereby offering leverage to harness technological advancements and align them with future health concerns. Table 2.1 represents the various notable wearable technologies and their applications in HealthTech.

2.2.4 Electronic Health Records and Health Information Systems

EHRs are pivotal to the development of health information systems. They encompass a multidisciplinary approach to improve the functionalities of patient care and usability, thereby creating user-centric interfaces that are simple to use and adaptable to diverse operational environments. Effective communication across various systems depends on ensuring interoperability through the use of standards like Health Level 7 Fast Healthcare Interoperability Resource (HL7 FHIR); also, improving data integration with other complementing health technologies like wearables and lab systems is critical. The validation tools and routine audits help to ensure data quality in terms of coherency and consistency that conform to its reliability and data protection. Ensuring patient data security and privacy is of utmost mandate, demanding the use of strong encryption techniques and strict access controls to limit access to sensitive information only to authorized personnel. The practice of creating and

TABLE 2.1
The Wearable Technologies and Applications in HealthTech

S.No.	Name	Year	Country	Applications
1	Fitness Tracker	2009	USA	Tracks sleep patterns; promotes healthy habits, and keeps an eye on physical activity
2	Smart Watche (iWatch)	2015	USA	Monitors vital health parameters (heart rate, ECG), fitness tracking, and seamless connectivity
3	Continuous Glucose Monitor (CGMs)	2006	USA	Enables real-time blood glucose monitoring, for diabetes management
4	Wearable ECG Monitor	2015	USA	Tracks heart rhythms, detects arrhythmias, and provides critical cardiovascular data
5	Wearable Sleep Monitor	2015	USA	Analyzes sleep quality and patterns, helping improve sleep health
6	Smart Clothing	2015	Canada	Monitors vital signs and muscle activity during exercise, enhancing performance insights
7	Hearing Aid	2010	Denmark	Enhances hearing capabilities, providing better auditory health management
8	Oura Ring	2018	Finland	Tracks sleeping pattern and other activities, providing insights into recovery and overall health
9	WHOOP Strap	2016	USA	Monitors strain, recovery, and sleep factors to optimize athletic performance
10	Smart Patch	2020	USA	Monitors various health metrics based on real-time data

maintaining patient portals, offering instructional materials, and assisting patients in comprehending their EHRs can enhance patients' participation and involvement. Predictive analytics models and decision support systems can benefit from the integration of data analytics techniques to help detect and treat health problems early [8]. Compliance with evolving regulations and standards, such as the Health Insurance Portability and Accountability Act (HIPAA), must be maintained through systematic documentation and regular updates. Finally, gathering user feedback and conducting pilot tests of new features are critical to refine and improve the EHR systems.

2.2.4.1 Considerations of Electronic Health Records in HealthTech

Future health technology improvement of EHRs will require multiple strategic developments aimed at improving EHR functionality, interoperability, security, and user experience. Here is a thorough strategy for improving the efficacy and innovation of EHRs:

1. *Enhanced Interoperability:*EHR systems in the future ought to put a high priority on smooth interoperability across various platforms and healthcare environments. Data interchange between various EHR systems, wearable technology, and other health technologies will run more smoothly with the adoption and advancement of standards like HL7 FHIR. This will enable a patient care strategy that is more cohesive and well-integrated.
2. *Advanced Data Analytics:*EHRs serve as a one-stop solution to train ML algorithms in the scenario of an ever-increasing patient population, improved health management systems, tailored treatment plans, and early diagnosis of health disorders. To improve clinical decision-making and offer meaningful insights, EHR systems ought to incorporate real-time data analysis.
3. *Improved User Experience:* Future EHRs should entail streamlining navigation minimizing the effort of data entry by utilizing NLP and voice recognition. The customizable dashboards can meet the requirements of individual users for data acquisition and management. Ergonomic design specifically suited to various professions and specializations in healthcare will also contribute to an improved user experience.
4. *Patient-Centric Features*: The EHR systems should place a greater emphasis on patient participation and self-management, which will enhance the features, including integrated telehealth choices, direct access to health data, appointment scheduling, and secured communication. In future, patient-generated data from wearable technology and home monitoring gadgets shall beincorporated into the EHRs.
5. *Robust Security Measures:* Future EHR systems must have cutting-edge security features in place against cyber attacks as data breaches are becoming more common. This comprises AI-driven threat detection systems, multi-factor authentication, and end-to-end encryption. To protect sensitive patient data, adherence to current regulations and regular security updates are also essential.
6. *Integration with Emerging Technologies:* EHR systems should be built to work smoothly with new technologies like AI, Blockchain, and the IoT. AI can improve diagnosis accuracy, automate repetitive procedures, and offer healthcare decision support. IoT devices can feed real-time health data into EHRs, and Blockchain technology can facilitate safe and transparent data sharing.
7. *Enhanced Customization and Adaptability:* Future EHR systems ought to be more flexible to accommodate the different requirements of different healthcare professionals and environments. The usage of modules that can be customized and adaptable procedures will enable the design of healthcare systems with unique needs, increased relevance, and efficiency.
8. *Streamlined Data Entry and Management:* It will be essential to use automation and cutting-edge technology like speech recognition and NLP to lessen the workload associated with data entry. Reducing clinician stress, increasing data accuracy, and eliminating manual data entry should be the prime goals of future EHR systems.

9. *Continuous Learning and Feedback:* Mechanisms for continuous learning and adaptation based on users' input and new best practices should be incorporated into EHR systems. Processes for continuous improvement, such as routine updates and user training, will make sure that the system adapts to the patients' and healthcare professionals' evolving demands.
10. *Global Health Integration:* International collaboration and healthcare service and deliverables can be enhanced by extending EHR capabilities to enable global health efforts and cross-border data exchange. This calls for the support of worldwide patient care coordination, enabling global health research and modifying systems to adhere to international standards and laws.

EHRs in health technology have a revolutionary future that can improve patient care, operational effectiveness, and overall healthcare outcomes if these areas are prioritized.

2.2.5 Genomics and Personalized Medicine

The research on the exploration of individuals' genetic profiles from genomics for personalized drug design and customized medicine is a revolution of technology in healthcare. Advances in genomic sequencing innovations the intrinsic patterns like next-generation sequencing (NGS), which, when combined with EHRs, can reveal the profile of genetic susceptibilities of a wide range of illnesses. These innovative approaches make it easier to design targeted medicines and pharmacogenomics, which tailors the drug selections based on an individual's genetic composition, attributing to improved treatment outcomes and reduced side effects [9]. Through the risk assessment for critical ailments like cancer and cardiovascular disorders, predictive and preventive healthcare measures vigorously use genomic data to enable early intervention and recommendations on customized lifestyle. The accuracy of the genetic testing methods is expected to improve the correctness of the identification of genetic problems, enabling early detection of illness, using appropriate genetic markers. Clinical decision support systems and sophisticated patient portals are examples of personalized medicine platforms that assist medical professionals and provide access to patients for customized health information. The major concerns on privileged access to patient's data and the right use of genetic data call for appropriate provisions for data security and privacy. The major challenge of discovery/identification of patterns in massive genomic data is addressed by AI predictive and analytics models. Genetic databases and customized clinical trials serve as vital data sources for promoting innovative and collaborative research. Healthcare technology can progress toward a more accurate and customized approach by utilizing genetics and personalized medicine, which will enhance patient treatment outcomes and their quality of life post treatment.

2.2.5.1 Scope and Promises of Genomics and Personalized Medicine

Future innovations in genomics-based customized medicine are expected to trigger significant advancements in a number of critical areas of therapy and treatment with improved precision, accessibility, and integration. The key concerns in these fields are listed below.

1. *Enhanced Genomic Sequencing:*
   - Cost Reduction: The availability of a broader spectrum of genomic data and the development of cost-effective, comprehensive genomic analysis will open up new vistas in genomic sequencing and economies of scale.
   - Speed and Accuracy: The availability of error-free genomic data and the accuracy of genomic sequencing discovery are the two major influential factors in this domain of research.
2. *Integration into EHRs:*
   - Seamless Integration: The provision of a unified view of a patient's profile, elicited and integrated from the medical records, genetic data into EHRs, shall help in the standardization of medical data in different formats and shall enhance the interoperability of EHR systems.
   - Data Interpretation: The development of effective EHRs' built-in tools and algorithms shall help in a great way to effectively interpret the genomic data and offer a detailed insight into medical data.
3. *Advanced Data Analytics and AI:*
   - Predictive Analytics: This approach gives the scope for personalized gene-based treatment plans, disease risk prediction, and prediction of disease progression based on time-series analysis/trend analysis. The advancements in data analytics and ML offer enormous scope to analyze the patterns of genomic data for medical diagnosis and treatment.
   - AI Algorithms: The leverage of enormous hidden patterns in voluminous data is effortlessly brought out with the AI models based on the statistical and probability measures, depicting the correlations and trends portrayed by the genetic data that may result in novel discoveries and individualized treatment plans.
4. *Personalized Treatment and Drug Development:*
   - Targeted Therapies: The research on expediting the development of personalized, targeted medicines based on each person's genetic profile provides an edge over generalized treatments and therapy. These approaches payoff in precision oncology as well as other areas where treatment outcomes are greatly impacted by genetic variants.
   - Pharmacogenomics: The effective utilization of pharmacogenomics plays a pivotal role in prescribing personalized medicines according to the genetic profile of the patients, targeting the bifold benefit of enhancing the medication efficacy as well as minimizing unfavorable drug responses.
5. *Patient-Centric Tools and Education:*
   - Genomic Portals:The increased use of such patient portals offers pinpointed informatics on the genomic data, which is proven to have a groundbreaking impact on healthcare services.
   - Education: The knowledge of the exploration and utilization of genomics for data-driven decisions has fueled paramount transformation in disease diagnosis, cure, and therapeutic choices.

6. *Ethical and Privacy Considerations:*
    - Data Security: The increased use of medical records and data and sharing them across the networks ideally call for the establishment of strong security policies, procedures, and measures to combat unanticipated breaches and unethical access, which has emerged as a challenge in the digital era. The increasing popularity of telemedicine underscores the need to evolve novel safety and security strategies for improved data access and storage.
    - Informed Consent: The increase in the knowledge and awareness of patients on the implications of genetics-based diagnosis has motivated the patients to opt forgenomic data-driven diagnostic approaches. These transformative approaches have radically increased the responsibility and concern of consent over protecting and preserving the privacy of those data.
7. *Collaboration and Data Sharing:*
    - Global Databases: Based on the proven medical advantages, the efforts on the creation of global genomic databases have drastically intensified the research studied on objective exploration and inferential comprehension of genetic patterns of patients.
    - Research Partnerships: The increasing advancement of personalized medicine and genomics has seamlessly promoted collaboration and partnerships among researchers, technocrats, healthcare providers, and businesses.
8. *Integration with Emerging Technologies:*
    - Blockchain: This technology has the potential to provide innovative strategies for genomic data management, assuring data security, privacy, and integrity, along with transparency.
    - Wearable Devices: The smart wearable devices are designed to collect genomic data, which are unboundedly utilized for individualized healthcare recommendations and services, in addition to real-time healthcare monitoring.
9. *Regulatory and Policy Development:*
    - Standards and Guidelines: The increased use of ICT-enabled healthcare services, technology-enabled health monitoring, and data-driven decisions in disease diagnosis and treatment has led to the creation, standardization, and implementation of guidelines, standard operating procedures (SOPs), which has augmented the reliability and accountability of such procedures and practices.
    - Policy Frameworks: The healthcare sectors have evolved policy frameworks that ensure fair access and responsible usage of medical records and data, aligned with the ethical, legal, and social concerns on the usage of genomics for many applications, including patient-specific medicine.
10. *Personalized Preventive Measures:*
    - Early Detection: The AI-based models are capable of identifying the onset of any disease well before the emergence of symptoms using genomic or healthcare data. The early detection/prediction of disease is proven to facilitate timely treatment and increased outcomes.

- Lifestyle Integration:The integration of environmental, lifestyle, and genetic data ids in offering comprehensive individualized consultation on healthcare toward disease preventive strategies.

It is evident that the domain of genomics and personalized medicine is proven to have a wider scope in providing more accurate, efficient, and customized healthcare services, which is a revolutionary advancement in the field of medical treatment and therapy.

2.2.6 Blockchain Technology in Healthcare

The unprecedented developments in Blockchain technology and its application in data security have drastically impacted the healthcare industry. Its decentralized access control system limits access to patient data, and its immutable ledger guarantees the accuracy, coherency, and consistency of all transactions. Blockchain technology offers a universal, decentralized record-keeping system that guarantees safe data sharing across heterogeneous platforms, facilitating interoperability across the various healthcare systems. The automation of medical records management using Blockchain technology has lowered the risk of breaches and restricted unethical access, thereby assuring enhancing data security and privacy. The use of advanced cryptography algorithms for data security and decentralized storage has proved to be a boon to EHR management. Further, Blockchain prevents data manipulation and conforms trust in research data integrity and transparent reporting of results of clinical trials and reassures regulatory compliance through open record-keeping, strengthens traceability, and prevents counterfeit medications, attributing to better pharmaceutical supply chain management [10].

Blockchain minimizes errors and administrative costs by automating transactions using smart contracts, which also streamlines billing and payments. It can expedite the process of validating the credentials of medical practitioners and help patients establish safe digital identities. Blockchain-enabled decentralized health networks allow patients to gain more control and security over their health data while encouraging collaborative innovations of payers, providers, researchers, and patients. In general, Blockchain technology has proven its potential for data security by strengthening the reliability, trust, and efficiency of healthcare systems and services.

2.2.6.1 Future of Blockchain Health Technology

Future healthcare technology may draw plenty of benefits from advancements in Blockchain in terms of integration, scalability, security, and usability, attributing to better quality of services.

1. *Enhanced Scalability and Performance:*
   - Optimized Consensus Algorithms: The incorporation of consensus algorithms helps to speed up transactions and boost throughput. Enhancing scalability without compromising on security concerns is made possible with innovations like proof-of-stake (PoS) sharding.

- Layer 2 Solutions: The Layer 2 scaling options help in managing high transaction volumes more effectively and in minimizing congestion on the main Blockchain, such as side chains or payment channels.

2. *Integration with Existing Systems:*
   - Interoperability Standards: The integration of Blockchain technology in healthcare is expected to ensure seamless data flow and interoperability of Blockchain technology into EHRs and health information exchanges (HIEs) management by establishing and accepting the standards.
   - Application Programming Interfaces (APIs) and Middleware: Incorporation of Blockchain networks into conventional healthcare systems find a place while creating reliable APIs and middleware.
3. *Enhanced Security and Privacy:*
   - Advanced Encryption: The use of cutting-edge cryptographic techniques like multi-party computing and zero-knowledge proofs offer safety measures by enhancing the privacy and security of patient data stored in the shared platform.
   - Access Controls: Enhancing access control and permissions to healthcare systems guarantee that only systems and people with the proper authorization can handle the sensitive data with due data integrity and confidentiality.
4. *User-Friendly Interfaces and Tools:*
   - Intuitive Platforms: Development of user interfaces and platforms facilitate communication between Blockchain systems and healthcare providers, patients, and administrators. The efficient and wider adoption of Blockchain technology can be achieved by streamlining these interfaces.
5. *Educational Resources:* The knowledge and awareness of the scope and potential of Blockchain technology among healthcare providers, patients, and other stakeholders are deemed essential for adoption with better clarity.
6. *Interdisciplinary Collaboration:*
   - Partnerships: The cooperation among researchers, policymakers, healthcare professionals, and tech developers is to be encouraged to accelerate innovation and resolve operational obstacles.
   - Consortiums: Participation in Blockchain-focused consortiums of the healthcare industry to exchange best practices and understand and create new standards can help in adopting Blockchain technology.
7. *Enhanced Data Management and Usability:*
   - Data Integration: Enhancing the potentiality of the protocol by integrating the Blockchain with different data sources so that Blockchain systems may manage a variety of health data, such as clinical trial data and patient information.
   - Data Usability: Integrating Blockchain in the development of tools for data querying, analysis, and visualization without negotiating on the security aspects opens up new directions and perspectives in healthcare services.
8. *Patient-Centric Solutions:*
   - Patient Control: The Blockchain-based management systems for health informatics and analytics have equally empowered patients with greater

control over their health data, thereby involving them in the decisions on data access permissions and privacy.

9. *Personalized Health Management*: The integration of lifestyle data, genetic information, and other vital health parameters is well-supported by Blockchain technology to draw individualized recommendations and interventions in accordance with Global Standards and Data Sharing. The integration of the latest advanced technologies and procedures is aimed to eventually enhance patient care, data management, and healthcare results in a holistic manner
   - International Collaboration: The creation and adoption of Global Blockchain Standards for the healthcare industry promote cross-border collaboration endeavors and facilitate the freedom of interoperability.
   - Global Health Networks: Blockchain technology empowers global healthcare networks with secured and transparent data sharing, leading to international alliances on global healthcare initiatives and research.

2.2.7 Robotics and Automation in HealthTech

Through the integration of cutting-edge technologies, robotics and automation are transforming the HealthTech sector in improving the effectiveness, precision, and caliber of healthcare services. The aspirations for improved patient care, disease diagnosis, and medical procedures have resulted in many innovative and resilient practices, including robotics-based healthcare services. HealthTech has enabled robots to play a pivotal role in a variety of healthcare contexts, such as surgery, consultation, counseling, patient rehabilitation, diagnostics, and pharmacy operations [11]. Robotic systems in surgical settings allow for minimally invasive operations with improved control and precision, which lowers surgical risks and speeds up recovery. By offering dependable and efficient therapy, rehabilitation robots help patients to restore their strength and movement. AI is used in diagnostic automation to evaluate medical data and images, increasing the precision and speed of diagnosis. Pharmacy automation systems reduce human error and enhance patient safety by efficiently managing medication distribution and inventory. In particular, for the elderly and for those patients with chronic diseases, patient care robots monitor health conditions and assist in day-to-day tasks while providing personalized care and assistance. Automating repetitive procedures helps in boosting accuracy and throughput; laboratory automation speeds both research and clinical testing. The use of remote monitoring technologies improves the management of chronic diseases and patient care by enabling timely interventions and continuous observation of patient's health conditions [12].

2.2.7.1 Improving Robotics and Automation in Health Technology

A multidisciplinary strategy encompassing technological, governmental, and human elements is needed to improve robots and automation in healthcare services. The following are some crucial areas for future development:

1. Enhanced AI and ML: Advanced AI-based models are seamlessly developed by researchers aiming to improve quality and optimize the operability of

patient-specific treatment plans, as well as to enhance the predictive and diagnostic accuracy of diseases. Robotic systems that are more adaptive can learn from real-time data and be more robust through reinforcement learning.

2. Miniaturization and Portability: The research on reducing the size, weight, and portability of robotic devices has augmented the scope of their application in a range of contexts of providing improved patient care and healthcare access, assuring inclusivity and equity.
3. User-Friendly Interfaces: The user interfaces have simplified the operational procedures and thus have enabled both patients and healthcare professionals to effortlessly use the automated healthcare system. Simplification of the degree interactions with complex robotic systems can drastically reduce the training time and boost overall productivity.
4. Cost Reduction: Prioritizing innovations in low-cost robotics technologies has resulted in improved access to the advanced healthcare system by everyone, breaking economic barriers.
5. Safety and Reliability: Increased dependency and safety aspects of robotic systems have opened up new avenues in healthcare, such as guaranteed patient safety, real-time monitoring, and fail-safe procedures.
6. Customization and Personalization: The power of AI models and the latest research outcomes in healthcare-related domains, namely genomics, has led to the emergence of personalized healthcare, drug design, and delivery based on the profile and requirements of a patient. By customizing interventions pertaining to particular medical situations and patient preferences, personalized robotic systems might enhance the outcomes.
7. Ethical and Regulatory Frameworks: It is essential to provide regulations and explicit ethical standards to control the applications of automation and robotics in healthcare. Automation of medical decision-making directly raises the demand for improving the standards of data security, privacy, and its moral ramifications.
8. Human–Robot Collaboration: The research study on improving human–robot cooperation aims to enhance the human services and functional ability of robots rather than replacement. Application-specific tools are being developed to assist healthcare providers with experimentation and decision-making.
9. Training and Education: The medical personnel are skilled to utilize and oversee advanced technology-driven robotics by earmarking funds for training and educational initiatives.
10. Telemedicine Integration: Telemedicine platforms can be integrated with robots and automation to facilitate remote consultations and processes. This modality can make it easier to get healthcare services, particularly in geographically deprived rural locations.

By addressing these aspects, the future of robotics and automation in health technology can be shaped further to offer more effective, efficient, and equitable healthcare solutions. Table 2.2 presents the robotics and automation technologies and their applications in HealthTech.

TABLE 2.2
Robotics and Automation Technologies in HealthTech

S.No.	Name	Country	Year	Applications
1	Surgical Robotics	USA	2000	Minimally invasive surgeries (e.g., prostatectomy, hysterectomy).
2	Robotic Exoskeletons	USA	2010	Rehabilitation for stroke patients, aiding movement for spinal cord injury recovery.
3	Telemedicine Robots	USA	2015	Remote patient consultations, particularly in rural areas.
4	Automated Medication Dispensing	USA	2005	Pharmacy automation, improving accuracy in medication delivery.
5	Robotic Process Automation (RPA)	USA	2017	Streamlining administrative tasks like billing and scheduling.
6	Patient Monitoring Systems	The Netherlands	2010	Continuous vital sign monitoring, remote patient management.
7	Robotic Assistants in Care Facilities	Japan	2016	Providing companionship and assistance in elderly care settings.
8	3D Printing in Surgery	USA	2015	Custom implants and prosthetics, surgical planning models.
9	Artificial Intelligence Integration	Global	2020	AI-driven diagnostics and personalized treatment plans.
10	Autonomous Delivery Robots	USA	2016	Delivering medical supplies to remote locations using drones.

2.2.8 Three-Dimensional Printing and Bioprinting

The cutting-edge technologies of bioprinting and three-dimensional (3D) printing have a big impact on health technology. By layering materials according to computer plans, 3D items are created using additive manufacturing, often known as 3D printing. This technique is utilized in the healthcare industry to create prosthetics, anatomical models, and personalized medical gadgets. For example, 3D printing makes it possible to create orthotic devices and prosthetic limbs that are customized for each patient, improving their comfort and functionality. Additionally, it enhances surgical accuracy and results by enabling physicians to prepare and rehearse preoperatively using anatomical models unique to each patient. Furthermore, biocompatible materials are used in the production of patient-specific implants and medical equipment via 3D printing to guarantee their compatibility with the human body [13].

Bioprinting is a specialized type of 3D printing that creates tissue and organ structures using bioinks, which are made of living cells, growth hormones, and biomaterials. Through the creation of functional biological tissues, this approach seeks to revolutionize tissue engineering and regenerative medicine. Tissue structures for research and possible therapeutic applications, such as skin, cartilage, and muscle tissues for medication testing and illness modeling, are created using bioprinting. Bioprinting has the potential to generate functional organs, such as kidneys and livers, for transplantation by fusing printed tissues together, but the technology is still in its experimental stages. Bioprinting also helps personalized medicine by making it possible to create patient-specific tissue models for more precise medication testing and treatment planning. This could minimize the need for animal testing and enhance the effectiveness of therapeutic interventions. With the advancements in materials science and biological understanding, 3D printing and bioprinting are expected to progress much further, offering improved patient outcomes, simpler medical procedures, and new avenues for study and therapy [14].

2.2.8.1 Role of Three-Dimensional Printing and Bioprinting in Health

To enhance 3D printing and bioprinting in healthcare, several key areas should be addressed, which would overcome the contemporary limitations and unlock the full potential of these technologies:

1. *Enhancing Material Diversity and Quality*
   Research should concentrate on creating a wider range of biocompatible materials that more closely resemble the mechanical and biological characteristics of human tissues and organs for use in bioprinting and 3D printing. Furthermore, improving these materials' strength and endurance is essential to guarantee the long-term functionality and safety of implants and prosthetics.
2. *Advancing Printing Techniques*
   Investing in technologies that improve the precision and resolution of 3D and bioprinting processes is essential for producing more complex and detailed structures at a microscopic level. Additionally, advancements should focus on accelerating printing techniques to shorten production times without

compromising quality, which is crucial for both clinical applications and large-scale manufacturing.

3. *Expanding Clinical Applications*
The goal of developing bioprinting technology is to create viable tissues and organs that can be used as models for disease research and drug testing or as organs for transplantation. Furthermore, efforts ought to be directed toward improving the capacity to design prosthetics and implants that are specifically customized to meet each patient's unique anatomical and functional requirements.
4. *Scaling Up Production*
Making bioprinting and 3D printing more affordable should be the main focus of efforts to promote their widespread adoption and reduce total healthcare expenses. Furthermore, to manage large volumes of 3D-printed and bioprinted products while preserving quality, investments in scalable production technology and infrastructure are essential.

TABLE 2.3
Applications of Bioprinting

S. No.	Name	Country	Year	Applications
1	NovoGenBioprinter	USA	2007	Liver and kidney tissue models for drug testing and disease modelling.
2	INKREDIBLE series	Sweden	2016	Bioinks, bioprinter series, and tissue constructs for research.
3	RX1 Bioprinter	Canada	2013	Microfluidic tissue constructs for drug discovery and disease modelling.
4	Discover 3D Printer	Switzerland	2013	3D-printed scaffolds and tissues for regenerative medicine applications.
5	Bioprinter	USA	2016	Bioprinted heart tissues aimed at creating full heart models for transplantation.
6	PrellisBioprinter	USA	2016	Human tissues and organoids for drug testing and research applications.
7	Bioprinting solutions	USA	2015	Bioprinting systems and scaffolds for various tissue engineering applications
8	Bioprinter	USA	2010	3D-printed bone and cartilage structures for orthopedic applications
9	J750 (with biocompatible materials)	USA	1989	Biocompatible materials for 3D printing, including anatomical models for medical use.
10	Biofabricated Systems	USA	2014	Biofabricated materials, including leather-like products made from living cells.

5. *Promoting Collaboration and Knowledge Sharing*
   Encouraging collaboration among engineers, biologists, medical professionals, and researchers is crucial for advancing innovation and addressing complex challenges in 3D printing and bioprinting. Additionally, offering education and training programs on the latest technologies is expected to promote interdisciplinary and multidisciplinary collaboration and bring together healthcare professionals and researchers to lead to innovations.

Table 2.3 presents the leading 3D bioprinting companies and their applications in HealthTech. By focusing on these areas, the future of 3D printing and bioprinting in healthcare can be significantly advanced, offering innovative solutions that improve patient outcomes and expand the possibilities of medical treatments and research.

2.3 CHALLENGES AND FUTURE DIRECTIONS FOR HEALTHTECH

HealthTech holds the promise of revolutionizing the industry, but attaining its fullest potential requires overcoming the challenges. The key obstacles include technology adoption, regulatory complexities, data privacy concerns, and ensuring equitable access. As digital health devices become more common these days, data security has become increasingly crucial. Protecting patient information and complying with legal standards necessitate robust data protection measures to address the challenges of security breaches due to unauthorized access. Additionally, the regulatory landscape is complex, making it difficult for innovators to navigate. Adapting regulations to keep pace with technological advancements and streamlining approval processes can accelerate the deployment of new technologies while ensuring safety and efficacy. Integrating new health technologies into existing workflows often faces resistance due to reluctance to change, the need for extensive training, and compatibility issues with current systems. Addressing these challenges requires strategic planning, support for healthcare professionals, and user-friendly design. Finally, ensuring that technological advancements benefit all segments of society is essential, as disparities in access can be exacerbated, particularly in underserved or rural areas. Efforts to promote equitable access should focus on affordability, infrastructure development, and targeted outreach.

2.3.1 Future Directions

Future developments in healthcare technologies tend to focus on improving the strategies of technology-enabled healthcare systems and services. To achieve this, better interoperability and smoother data interchange between various platforms would be needed to provide a more unified and effective healthcare experience. Furthermore, greater emphasis will be placed on patient-centered care, with technology developed to empower patients via tailored treatment plans, self-management tools, and enhanced contact with medical professionals. To address the current obstacles, sustained development is needed to institute state-of-the-art security protocols and encourage technology adoption via instruction and training, thereby guaranteeingimproved quality of services to everyone, irrespective of social and economic limitations. By addressing the challenges and focusing on emerging technologies, the HealthTech sector may maximize its potential to enhance patients' outcomes, healthcare delivery, system equity, and effectiveness.

2.4 CONCLUSION

The HealthTech environment's rapid technological innovation and integration have the potential to completely transform healthcare delivery and outcomes. Because telehealth makes real-time consultations and monitoring possible, it has completely changed the way that people may obtain healthcare, particularly those who live in distant or underdeveloped locations. Nonetheless, there are also issues with guaranteeing fair access and telehealth's smooth integration into established healthcare systems. Advances in AI, ML, and DL are proven to revolutionize personalized treatment planning and outcomes, disease prediction, and its trend, with greater accuracy. Healthcare efficiency and results could be greatly enhanced by these technologies, but many issues such as algorithmic bias and data privacy. Users can take proactive control of their health with the help of wearable technology, which offers real-time data and continuous health monitoring. Future advancements will focus on enhancing system interoperability and better usage of EHR data for patient care and research. EHR and HIS ease data administration and improve healthcare coordination. The field of personalized medicine is rapidly evolving due to advancements in genomics, which are enabling customized treatments based on an individual's genetic profile. However, these advancements pose ethical and genetic data privacy problems. Blockchain technology offers possibilities for transparent and safe data management, which could enhance data integrity and traceability. However, integrating Blockchain technology into current systems and putting it into practice are still difficult tasks. Hospital operations and surgical precision are being advanced by robotics and automation, and future developments are expected to increase these technologies' affordability and capabilities while maintaining their efficacy and safety. Last but not least, despite the technological and legal challenges, 3D printing and bioprinting are modernizing the production of implants, prostheses, and even tissue, offering more individualized and efficient medical solutions. Furthermore, to overcome obstacles and optimize the advantages of new technologies, interdisciplinary cooperation between technologists, healthcare professionals, and legislators will be necessary for successful deployment.

REFERENCES

[1] Vilcahuamán,L.andRivas,R.,2017.*HealthcareTechnologyManagementSystems:Towards a New Organizational Model for Health Services*. New York: Academic Press.

[2] Mosnaim, G., Safioti, G., Brown, R., DePietro, M., Szefler, S.J., Lang, D.M., Portnoy, J.M., Bukstein, D.A., Bacharier, L.B. and Merchant, R.K., 2021. Digital health technology in asthma: A comprehensive scoping review. *Journal of Allergy and Clinical Immunology: In Practice*, 9(6), pp.2377–2398.

[3] Manocchia, A., 2020. Telehealth: Enhancing care through technology. *Rhode Island Medical Journal*, 103(1), pp.18–20.
[4] Brennan, D.M., Holtz, B.E., Chumbler, N.R., Kobb, R. and Rabinowitz, T., 2008. Visioning technology for the future of telehealth. *Telemedicine and e-Health*, 14(9), pp.982–985.
[5] Chen, M. and Decary, M., 2020, January. Artificial intelligence in healthcare: An essential guide for health leaders. In *Healthcare Management Forum* (Vol. 33, No. 1, pp. 10–18). Los Angeles, CA: SAGE Publications.
[6] Johnson, S.L., 2019. AI, machine learning, and ethics in health care. *Journal of Legal Medicine*, 39(4), pp.427–441.
[7] Dinh-Le, C., Chuang, R., Chokshi, S. and Mann, D., 2019. Wearable health technology and electronic health record integration: Scoping review and future directions. *JMIR mHealth and uHealth*, 7(9), p.e12861.
[8] Jardim, S.V., 2013. The electronic health record and its contribution to healthcare information systems interoperability. *Procedia Technology*, 9, pp.940–948.
[9] Tarkkala, H., Helén, I. and Snell, K., 2019. From health to wealth: The future of personalized medicine in the making. *Futures*,109, pp.142–152.
[10] Attaran, M., 2022. Blockchain technology in healthcare: Challenges and opportunities. *International Journal of Healthcare Management*, 15(1), pp.70–83.
[11] Okamura, A.M., Matarić, M.J. and Christensen, H.I., 2010. Medical and health-care robotics. *IEEE Robotics & Automation Magazine*, 17(3), pp.26–37.
[12] Guntur, S.R., Gorrepati, R.R. and Dirisala, V.R., 2019. Robotics in healthcare: an internet of medical robotic things (IoMRT) perspective. In *Machine Learning in Bio-Signal Analysis and Diagnostic Imaging* (pp. 293–318). Academic Press.
[13] Combellack, E., Jessop, Z.M. and Whitaker, I.S., 2018. The commercial 3D bioprinting industry. In *3D Bioprinting for Reconstructive Surgery* (pp. 413–421). Woodhead Publishing.
[14] Jovic, T.H., Combellack, E.J., Jessop, Z.M. and Whitaker, I.S., 2020. 3D bioprinting and the future of surgery. *Frontiers in Surgery*, 7, p.609836.

3 Technology and Diagnostics

Advancements in Clinical Medicine

Chander Prabha, Shalini Kumari, and Vidhu Baggan

3.1 INTRODUCTION

In the past 50 years, medicine has undergone major changes because of advancements in technology and diagnostics. As the world moves forward in the healthcare sector, the trend is now toward enhancing patient outcomes, bringing about cost savings, and boosting the efficiency of care delivery; as a result, new diagnostic tools and technology have gained prominence. These technological breakthroughs have an overarching effect on how diseases are diagnosed and tracked; they additionally enable doctors to tailor treatments more individually and accurately [1, 2]. In this all-case study, the authors have analyzed the possibilities of using state-of-the-art technologies, such as artificial intelligence (AI), machine learning (ML), advanced imaging, genomics, and wearable devices, in clinical diagnostics. Here, technology is a positive and important area for consideration. Diagnostic procedures in traditional healthcare settings usually involve manual processing and the subjective opinions of experts. This can result in complications, which are hard to predict, and diagnostic errors. Nevertheless, the introduction of AI and ML technologies has caused a significant change in the methodology of diagnostic systems. These systems are the most data-driven and automated, allowing for built-in checks for accuracy [3, 4]. When it comes to the likes of AI, these are computer systems that have been trained using really large sample sets which are using software to recognize patterns and specific information that Experience Management (XM) technicians cannot pick up, the absence of human specialists, and the possible use of specialist machines for diagnostic purposes are the subject of discussions [5]. ML models are similarly used in steering the course of diseases and testing the success of therapies, thus creating the basis for developing future proactive healthcare models and personalized medications.

One of the main achievements in the field of genomic technologies has been the connection through which full genetic screening and the identification of mutations associated with diseases [6], thus promoting advancements in medical practice. The application of bioinformatics tools, along with the use of high-throughput sequencing

DOI: 10.1201/9781003516163-3

technologies, has resulted in the detection of disease-causing genes and the personalization of drugs for each of the patients, thereby creating a treatment profile for each person one hundred percent matching their unique genes, followed by the administration of those drugs, etc. This is the most significant development in the diagnosis part of precision medicine [7, 8]. Furthermore, the development of the innovations of wearables and remote monitoring tools allows patients to be actively involved in their healthcare. These tools provide patients with information in real time, viz, their vital signs and other health factors. This capability helps in the earlier discovery of emerging health concerns and the provision of early medical intervention.

On the other hand, adopting and deploying modern diagnostic tools come with its own challenges. Challenges, including data protection, ensuring smooth usage of technology in various healthcare systems, controlling costs, and setting out verification and standardization, are the main challenges that must be addressed. Moreover, it is crucial to underline that accessibility to technological tools should be granted to the entire population, and they should be able to benefit from it, thus preventing the exacerbation of small health differences.

The chapter's main purpose is to present a thorough summary of the latest diagnosis technology and its impact on clinical medicine. The main issue is to stress the extraordinary capability of tools, the use of new procedures in raising diagnostic efficiency, and the time it takes to get the correct diagnosis and patient outcomes. Moreover, the text will also emphasize the barriers and problems that must be resolved to make the best of the advantages of these innovations in the clinical area. This examination is expected to increase the ongoing debate about the future of medical diagnostics and the influence of technology on healthcare delivery.

The chapter is structured as follows: Section 3.2 presents the historical perspective of clinical medicine, specifying the tools and technologies. Section 3.3 briefly describes imaging technologies. Section 3.4 presents the integration of digital pathology with AI. Section 3.5 briefly discusses genomics and personalized medicine. Further, Section 3.6 gives a detailed insight into the advancements in clinical medicine. Section 3.7 presents challenges faced and future work. Finally, Section 3.8 concludes the chapter.

3.2 HISTORICAL PERSPECTIVE

The progress made in the technological sectors of medicine and clinical diagnosis is reflected in the quality of the available diagnostic tools. The main method of early diagnosis was usually the physical examinations and basic tools. Using the stethoscope in the 19th century was a significant step forward that allowed doctors to listen to the inside sounds of the body audibly. The arrival of X-rays in the late 19th century was a revolution in diagnostic imaging, allowing the doctor to see inside the human body down to a level that had never happened before. The 20th century emerged as a time of extreme advancement and modernization. Incorporating tools, viz., ultrasound, computed tomography (CT), and magnetic resonance imaging (MRI) machines, led to technological improvement. Furthermore, these instruments provide detailed images of internal systems, thereby greatly helping determine various diseases. Moreover, blood tests and biochemical analyses have advanced so that diseases can now be diagnosed at the molecular level.

3.2.1 Molecular Diagnostics

Molecular diagnostics completely revolutionize the identification and description of diseases at molecular and genetic levels. Techniques, viz., polymerase chain reaction (PCR), next-generation sequencing (NGS), and microarrays, are governing factors enabling the detection of genetic mutations, infections, and biomarkers that are extremely precise and sensitive.

3.2.2 Polymerase Chain Reaction

Developed in 1983 by Kary Mullis, PCR has become a widely used and significant technique for various biological research laboratory applications. PCR allows the replication of DNA without a living organism. The PCR process allows the amplification of a small quantity of the DNA molecule numerous times, thus following an exponential pattern, as shown in Figure 3.1. In Step 1, the availability of larger quantities of DNA at one's disposal facilitates the analysis process, making it more convenient and less challenging. Step 2 deals with annealing at 55°C, which gives nucleotides. In Step 3, synthesizing is done at 72°C. The whole process is repeated 20–40 times. PCR is widely utilized in medical and biological research laboratories. Examples are identifying hereditary diseases, genetic fingerprinting, infectious diseases diagnosis, gene cloning, paternity testing, computing DNA, etc. The real-time variant of PCR, quantitative PCR (qPCR) enables quantitative measurement of DNA or RNA, providing insights into the severity and progression of diseases [4–6].

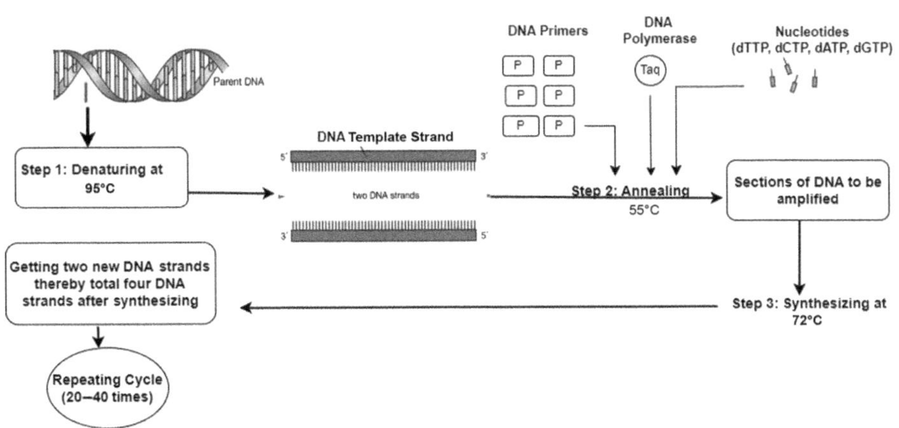

FIGURE 3.1 The PCR.

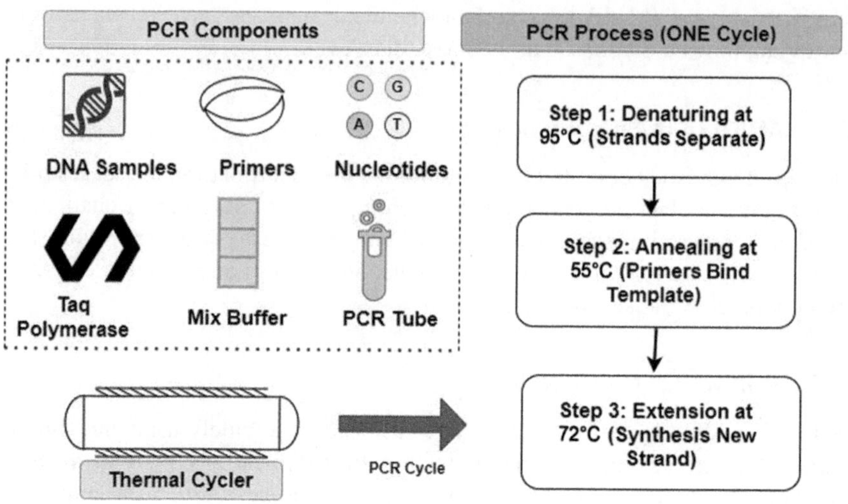

FIGURE 3.2 PCR Components and Process in One Cycle.

3.2.2.1 Prerequisites of Polymerase Chain Reaction

A PCR consists of the target double-stranded DNA, two primers that bind to adjacent sequences on opposite strands of the target, a DNA polymerase, all four deoxyribonucleoside triphosphates, buffer, enzyme co-factors, and water, as shown in Figure 3.2. During the process, it relies on the utilization of a heat-stable DNA polymerase due to the intermittent elevation of temperature. Figure 3.2 presents various components of PCR and the process involved in one cycle.

3.2.2.2 Applications of Polymerase Chain Reaction

PCR is a versatile technique that can be employed to diagnose numerous human diseases and conduct a wide range of analyses and experiments. PCR is a crucial diagnostic tool used to confirm the presence of infectious diseases, viz., HIV, tuberculosis, cytomegalovirus (CMV), hepatitis, mycoplasma, protozoal and fungal diseases, and certain types of cancers, including lymphoma and leukemia. It also detects malaria, Staphylococcal bacteremia, tuberculosis, and *Toxoplasma gondii* infections. PCR is crucial for genetic profiling and determining paternity. PCR exhibits a high level of sensitivity (95–100%) and specificity (100%) [9, 10].

3.2.2.3 Challenges in Polymerase Chain Reaction

PCR necessitates costly apparatus that may only be financially feasible for some laboratories, including a thermal cycler, an agarose gel electrophoresis tray, a DNA purification kit, and various chemicals and reagents. Furthermore, there is a potential for acquiring erroneous positive and negative results, reducing the precision and dependability of the tests.

3.2.2.4 Developments in Polymerase Chain Reaction

The fast and widespread occurrence of pandemic diseases has resulted in global attention to the need for quick, timely, and accurate molecular diagnostics. It is remarkable that ultra-fast PCR technology has been achieved in a relatively short time. Microfluidic on-chip PCR devices are the most efficient for point-of-care diagnostic applications. This is possible through the use of this technique, which ensures that it is possible to quickly and accurately diagnose at the point of care. Glass nanopillar arrays, doped with microfluidic channels and Au nanoislands to make the plasmofluidic PCR chip, are gas permeable, thus allowing the gas to pass through. The open chambers are equipped with arrays of microchambers designed for the reactions, a pre-charged vacuum cell, and a barrier restricting vapor escape. The integrated circuit design facilitates the entry of samples and PCR procedures actuation while effectively preventing the formation of microbubbles.

The sample loading process, taking less than 3 minutes, is the starter for a two-step PCR that promptly speeds up the lambda-DNA and plasmids. The amplification results are obtained in 264 seconds for lambda-DNA and 306 seconds for the plasmids after 40 cycles. Furthermore, identifying amplicons in their original position in real time highlights amplification efficiencies beyond 91%. This PCR strategy serves diagnoses as quickly as needed at the treatment location to help handle the fast spread of the pandemic.

3.2.3 Next-Generation Sequencing

NGS has made genome sequencing accessible to a broader population, allowing for profound examination of genetic material in much less time and at lower costs than traditional methods. The roles of NGS entail personalized medicine, where treatment recommendations are determined based on an individual patient's genetic makeup [11]. This, in turn, has led to a more cost-effective and efficient DNA sequencing method compared with the Sanger sequencing technique. Consequently, these improvements have tremendously affected genetics and molecular biology as academic fields. The advent of NGS has created a new order that makes it possible for an in-depth analysis of genetic materials [12].

- **Whole Genome Sequencing (WGS):** The DNA test provides a complete genetic profile of a person, which helps identify inherited tendencies and sicknesses.
- **Targeted Sequencing:** This approach targets specific genes or areas, enhancing the identification of mutations associated with illnesses like cancer.

NGS is a potent technique that enables the sequencing of multiple DNA molecules, covering a range from thousands to billions. The comprehensive NGS process has four distinct stages, as shown in Figure 3.3: Sample preparation steps, Library Prep steps, Sequencing steps, and Data Analysis steps.

NGS, classified into different generations, has successfully addressed the limitations of traditional sequencing methods of DNA and is widely utilized in

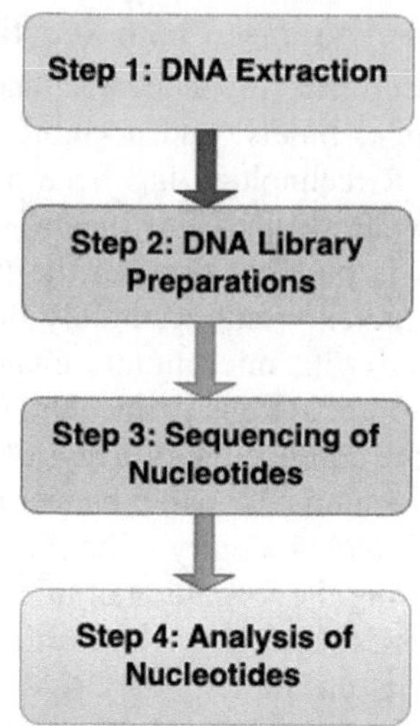

FIGURE 3.3 Next-Generation Sequencing Methodology.

TABLE 3.1
Generations of NSG

NGS Generations	Examples
1st GS	• Sanger
2nd GS	• Pyrosequencing, sequencing by ligation • Sequencing by reversible terminator chemistry
3rd GS	• Fluorescent sequencing of single molecule • Real-time sequencing of single molecule • Nanopore sequencing • Semiconductor sequencing
4th GS	• Conduct genomic analysis directly on cells

various areas of molecular biology [13]. Further, NGS generations are classified as shown in Table 3.1.

Applications: NGS is a very efficient technique for detecting genetic changes in an individual's genome.

3.2.4 Microarrays

Microarrays provide a way to search the entire genome in small, manageable pieces quickly. They generate a messenger RNA (mRNA) or a complementary DNA (cDNA) from DNA that is then hybridized into a gene array. After data is collected from the gene array, it is reviewed to see which genes are of interest or to find those upregulated in some way. The data can then be analyzed to look at the pathway or function of gene regulation using a pathway gene set or a gene ontology gene set.

3.3 IMAGING TECHNOLOGIES

Advancements have considerably improved diagnostic skills in clinical medicine and imaging technologies. These technologies comprehensively visualize internal structures and functions, facilitating the diagnosis and monitoring of disorders.

3.3.1 Computed Tomography and Magnetic Resonance Imaging

CT and MRI are the main imaging modalities for the best detailed cross-sectional images. CT emphasizes using X-rays for image generation in a loop, while MRI emphasizes magnets and radio waves. Both technologies are the backbone of detecting tumors, evaluating the conditions of vessels (vascular pathologies) caused by blood clots, and many types of abnormal processes, like weighing out what part of the function of the nerves/brain is working or not abnormal. The key element to remember is that the rapid growth of MRI technology has eliminated ionizing radiation while providing high-quality images ideal for soft tissue applications. Some recent advancements are as follows:

- **Functional MRI (fMRI):** Brain activities are observed by detecting alterations in blood flow, facilitating the investigation of neurological illnesses.
- **Diffusion Tensor Imaging (DTI):** Utilizes imaging techniques to track the spread of water in bodily tissues, providing valuable insights into the condition of the brain's white matter and identifying irregularities such as traumatic brain injuries and strokes.

CT scans have had improvements in speed and level of detail as a result of technologies such as:

- **Dual-Energy CT:** Classifies materials according to their energy absorption characteristics, enhancing the assessment of tissues and identification of illnesses.
- **Iterative Reconstruction Techniques:** Minimize radiation dose while preserving image quality, improving safety for patients requiring multiple scans.

3.3.2 Positron Emission Tomography

Positron emission tomography (PET) scans are a technique that gives functional images by showing the metabolic activity in various body organs. Oncology takes significant advantage of this technique to locate the position of malignant tissues and their borders, know the extent of cancerous spread, and confirm the effectiveness of the treatment.

3.3.3 Ultrasound

"Ultrasounds," an innovation in medical imaging, use high-frequency sound waves to produce images of internal organ structures of the body; they are particularly used in obstetrics, cardiology, abdominal imaging, and other fields. The advent and provision of high-resolution and three-dimensional/four-dimensional (3D/4D) ultrasound imaging have improved the diagnosis capability. The revolution of ultrasound technique has been processed due to improvements in imaging as an inert tool and in terms of physiological values.

- **3D and 4D Ultrasound:** Provide live three-dimensional imaging, which is advantageous in obstetrics and cardiology.
- **Elastography:** Utilizes a technique to assess the rigidity of tissues, facilitating the identification of liver fibrosis, tumors, and other medical disorders.

3.4 DIGITAL PATHOLOGY AND ARTIFICIAL INTELLIGENCE

Integrating digital pathology with AI is significantly changing diagnostics solutions as pathology analyses have become more precise and efficient. Digital pathology can be described as the process of scanning histological slides so that it becomes possible to analyze them remotely and interface them with AI algorithms. Patients, doctors, and pathologists can share detailed images with the assistance of this app as it connects to pathologists worldwide, making it simple to request second opinions and assist in diagnosis. AI integrated into digital pathology enhances the analysis of tissues through counting cells, recognition of patterns, and anomaly detection (AD).

3.4.1 Point-of-Care Testing (POCT)

POCT is diagnostics testing administered close to or at the patient care delivery site. These diagnostics give quick solutions that help with clinical choices and improve the patient's results. Technological advancement has seen the expansion of POCT due to increased diagnoses of various diseases by portable and easy-to-use devices. POCT devices have become important in clinical practices as they can provide fast results at patients' bedsides.

- **Biosensors and Lab-on-a-Chip Technologies:** Downsize complex laboratory procedures to form more efficient and portable diabetes, heart attack, and infectious disease diagnosis kits.
- **Wearable Devices:** This is true because patients' biochemical markers and vital signs should be monitored more frequently due to chronic diseases.

Examples of POCT equipment include glucometers that measure blood glucose, portable blood pressure analyzers, and fast antigen tests that check for infectious disorders such as COVID-19. With these devices providing correct and rapid results, the consumer does not have to go to a lab to be tested and can start therapy promptly.

3.4.2 Artificial Intelligence in Diagnostics

ML and DL are AI systems that can be deployed for big data analytics, pattern, and diagnosis identification. More and more techniques are being applied to imaging analysis and diagnostics, especially concerning detecting anomalies and diseases and predicting near-perfect outcomes [14–16]. For instance, AI algorithms in radiological scans to detect cancerous tissues are usually accurate, even surpassing the human expert's capabilities. AI and ML have revolutionized diagnostics because they make complicated data easier to understand. Because they make complicated data easier to understand, AI and ML have revolutionized diagnostics.

- **Image Analysis:** AI in diagnostics increases the solidity and specificity of detecting disorders and patterns in radiographs, MRI, or CT scans.
- **Predictive Analytics:** To allow for the formulation of tailor-made treatments, ML algorithms have the ability to analyze large amounts of patients' data to find correlations as to how a disease progresses or responds to a particular therapy.
- **Personalized Medicine:** AI can assess patient characteristics such as genetics, provide proper therapy, and enhance success.
- **Cost Effectiveness**: This is true because, by improving the current processes and decreasing unnecessary tests, AI has the potential to lower healthcare costs.
- **Enhanced Access**: By providing reliable diagnostics in areas with limited access to medical professionals, AI-powered diagnostic tools can cover the field of healthcare delivery.
- **Epidemiology and Public Health:** AI can analyze population-level data to analyze disease outbreaks, predict how diseases spread, and determine how to allocate resources during public health emergencies.

However, challenges arise when integrating AI tools into standard practice and guaranteeing data privacy and open systems. AI in diagnosis can improve patient outcomes and health delivery despite significant challenges.

3.4.2.1 Applications

AI is rapidly revolutionizing personalized therapeutic care and medical research. AI in health care and related research has been profoundly affected by the availability of big datasets and improvements in ML and DL models and algorithms. There is hope that AI can aid in detecting and treating large disease categories. Here are some of the major ways that AI has improved medical diagnosis and prognosis:

- **Cancer:** In recent years, clinical cancer research has increasingly included AI, particularly ML and deep learning, with unprecedented success in cancer prediction. AI is used for early detection and diagnosis of various categories of cancer, such as breast, lung, skin, and more. It assists in analyzing medical imaging (like mammograms, CT scans, and pathology slides) to detect tumors, analyzing the molecular makeup of tumors and their surrounding environment, developing new drugs and finding alternative uses for existing ones, and forecasting the effectiveness of treatments for patients [17–21].

- **Cardiovascular Disease (CVD):** AI is promising to improve the accuracy and speed of CVD therapy and diagnosis [22]. By detecting biomarkers, AI can help in the early identification and management of CVD and even forecast when a patient may die from heart disease [23–25]. Research suggests that AI could greatly benefit cardiovascular care through early biomarker discovery, illness outcome and progression prediction, and other similar applications. These AI-powered solutions can significantly speed up the detection and therapy of cardiovascular illness, as shown in Figure 3.4. Part of this is ensuring patient data is stored and analyzed properly so that diseases can be better diagnosed and managed [26].
- **Neurological Disorders:** Neurological disorders are a broad category of conditions that affect the spinal cord, brain, and nervous system. AI has been increasingly utilized in the diagnosis and management of various neurological conditions, including Parkinson's disease, Alzheimer's disease, stroke, and epilepsy [22–24]. AI-based algorithms can now interpret brain data, viz., MRI and CT scans, to help diagnose neurological diseases at an early stage. [21, 23–24] Additionally, AI can help doctors make more accurate decisions by identifying neurological symptoms and patterns [21–24]. AI can improve diagnostic procedures and patient outcomes in neurology by using advanced data analysis techniques. AI and ML technologies have shown potential in early diagnosis and monitoring of Parkinson's disease. By analyzing various data types, such as physical symptoms, voice/speech, and neurological patterns, AI models can identify patterns that may indicate an early diagnosis of Parkinson's disease. This suggests that AI could detect respiratory symptoms at night, as respiratory changes can be an early indicator of Parkinson's disease [24].

It is well known that Parkinson's disease affects breathing, including breathing during sleep. As shown in Figure 3.5, Parkinson's disease patients experience sleep problems, breathing difficulties, and changes in respiratory muscle control. The unique breathing characteristics during sleep can provide valuable information for AI-based Parkinson's disease diagnostic models [26].

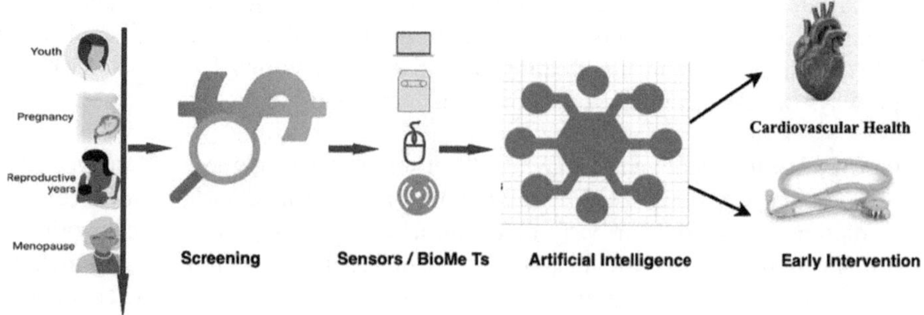

FIGURE 3.4 Cardiovascular Disease Detection and Therapy.

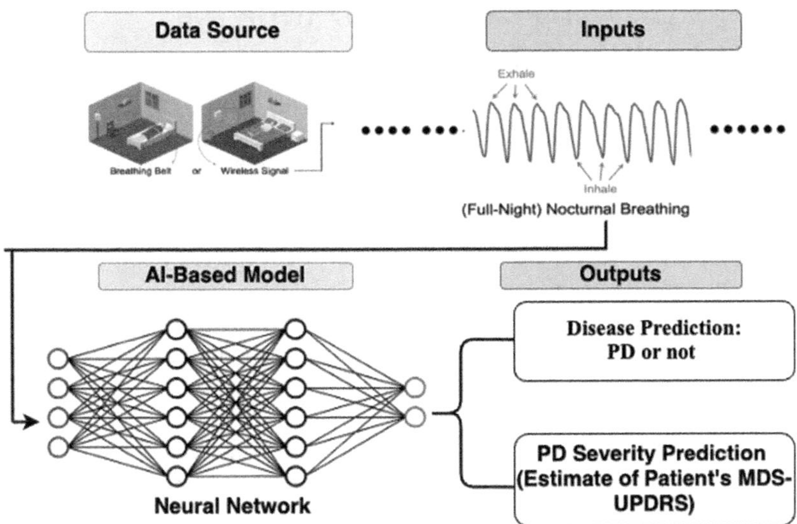

FIGURE 3.5 Monitoring Nocturnal Breathing Patterns for Detecting and Assessing Parkinson's Disease.

- **Diabetes and Endocrine Disorders**: By analyzing data from continuous glucose monitors and making predictions about blood glucose levels, AI helps with diabetes management. Endocrine diseases, including thyroid and adrenal issues, can be better diagnosed and treated with its help.
- **Infectious Diseases**: Infectious illness diagnostics and management use AI to optimize antimicrobial treatment algorithms, forecast disease outbreaks, and detect pathogens from genomic data.
- **Rare Diseases**: AI has the potential to shorten diagnostic times for uncommon diseases by evaluating patient symptoms, genetic data, and medical literature to provide possible diagnoses and treatment alternatives.
- **Mental Health Disorders**: By analyzing voice patterns, text data, and behavioral clues, new AI applications are appearing in the mental health field to aid in the diagnosis of illnesses, like anxiety disorders, schizophrenia, depression, and other similar conditions.
- **Ophthalmology**: Through the analysis of retinal pictures and other ophthalmic data, AI is utilized in the diagnosis and management of eye illnesses, including diabetic retinopathy, glaucoma, and age-related macular degeneration.
- **Respiratory Diseases**: By evaluating lung function tests, imaging investigations, and symptoms, AI aids in diagnosing respiratory disorders like asthma, chronic obstructive pulmonary disease, and pneumonia.

The examples provided here demonstrate how AI is being utilized to improve diagnostic accuracy, treatment strategies, and patient outcomes for various medical ailments and diseases.

3.5 GENOMICS AND PERSONALIZED MEDICINE

Genomic research has now been an active area of research that has opened the door to individualized medicine, which uses a patient's unique genetic composition to inform diagnostic and therapeutic decisions. Discoveries of disease-associated genetic variations have guided personalized treatment strategies, made possible by technological breakthroughs in genomics [27]. These innovations are as follows:

- **Pharmacogenomics:** The field known as pharmacogenomics investigates the role of genes in medication response. Healthcare practitioners can minimize side effects and optimize treatment outcomes by selecting the most appropriate drugs and dosages for each patient based on identified genetic differences influencing drug metabolism and efficacy.
- **Cancer Genomics:** Cancer genomics focuses on understanding the genetic mutations driving cancer development. Advanced sequencing technologies allow for identifying actionable mutations, guiding the selection of targeted therapies and immunotherapies. This approach has significantly improved many cancer patients' prognosis and treatment outcomes.

3.6 ADVANCEMENTS IN CLINICAL MEDICINE

The future of diagnostics in clinical medicine is poised for further advancements, driven by ongoing research and technological innovations. Emerging fields such as liquid biopsy (LB), wearable health technology, and advanced AI algorithms hold promise for even more precise and non-invasive diagnostic methods.

3.6.1 Liquid Biopsy

The term "liquid biopsy" describes a technique used to identify particular molecular indicators of disease in liquid samples, such as saliva, blood, urine, and other types of minimally invasive biological samples, as shown in Figure 3.6. LB involves the analyses of circulating tumor DNA (ctDNA) and other biomarkers in body fluids such as blood. This non-invasive approach offers a real-time snapshot of the genetic landscape of tumors, enabling treatment response monitoring, early detection, and minimal residual disease detection.

3.6.1.1 Applications

LBs have proven to be highly beneficial in identifying and characterizing solid tumors, providing a comprehensive understanding of tumor progression. They also have significant implications for diagnosis, prognosis, treatment selection, and long-term monitoring [28].

3.6.1.2 Challenges

The use of LBs in cancer diagnosis has shown encouraging results. However, LBs have a long way to go before they can be considered a legitimate alternative to more traditional diagnostic tools. Before their widespread adoption, more obstacles must be

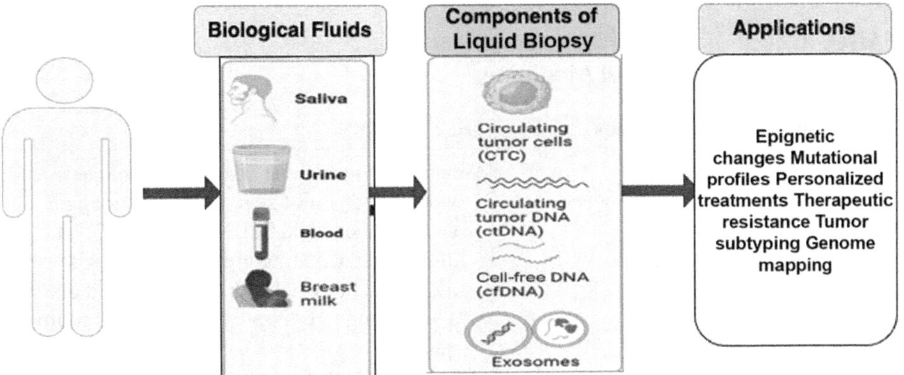

FIGURE 3.6 LB Components and Their Applications.

overcome. Examples of obstacles include evaluating therapy efficacy, finding minimal residual disease or resistance-causing mutations, dealing with microenvironmental factors, dealing with heterogeneity and circulating tumor cell counts, and possibly needing an initial histological examination through tissue biopsy. Researchers are currently trying to determine how well they work as a cancer diagnosis tool [29]. The expense also poses a major limitation. Some healthcare systems may not offer LBs because of the increased expense compared to traditional tissue biopsies or because patients need more insurance to afford the cost.

3.6.2 Wearable Health Technology

Continuous monitoring is done by wearable sensors of physiological parameters like blood pressure heart rate, and glucose levels [30]. Real-time data is provided by these devices enabling early detection of abnormalities and proactive monitoring of chronic conditions. The adoption of telemedicine and remote diagnostic technologies has accelerated in the COVID-19 pandemic.

- **Teleconsultations:** Enable remote diagnosis and management of patients, reducing in-person visits need.
- **Remote Monitoring Devices:** The ability to continuously monitor chronic illnesses and intervene early when needed is made possible by collecting and transmitting patient data to healthcare practitioners.

3.6.3 Advanced Artificial Intelligence Algorithms

New developments in explainable AI, reinforcement learning, and natural language processing show that AI is constantly progressing [31]. Improved analysis of complicated datasets, prediction of illness trajectories, and customization of treatment regimens are all outcomes of these advancements in the incorporation of AI in diagnostics. Some other developments in clinical medicine are shown in Table 3.2.

TABLE 3.2
Advancements in Clinical Medicine

Advancements	Techniques	Description
Diagnostic technologies	Imaging technologies	Diagnostics have been taken to a whole new level with the advent of state-of-the-art imaging technologies including MRI, CT, PET, and ultrasound. Creating high-resolution pictures of the inside body helps doctors treat and diagnose a wide range of diseases and ailments more quickly.
	Genetic testing	Advances in genetic testing enable personalized medicine, early diagnosis, and diagnosis of genetic diseases. Techniques such as NGS can be used for genomic research.
	Point-of-care testing	Healthcare workers can use portable diagnostic equipment and rapid tests to perform tests at the point of care or in remote locations. This will speed up diagnosis and treatment.
Therapeutic advances	Targeted therapies	Advances in molecular biology have made it possible to develop personalized medicine that targets diseased cells, such as cancer cells, while avoiding healthy tissue. Monoclonal antibodies and small-molecule antibodies are two examples.
	Immunotherapy	Cancer patients in particular can benefit from immunotherapy, which helps in fighting the disease by the body's immune system. There are encouraging advances in cancer treatments and therapies, including anticancer drugs, CAR-T-cell therapies, and investigational inhibitors.
	Regenerative medicine	There are now more options than ever to treat disease and tissue damage through stem cell therapy and tissue engineering. This technique can help treat problems such as spinal cord injury, heart disease, and neurodegenerative disease.
Surgical innovations	Minimally invasive surgery	These are just two examples of how surgical procedures are changing in the field. The results of these treatments include shorter hospital stays, less pain, and faster recovery times.
	Image-guided surgery	By providing real-time visualization during surgery, advanced imaging technologies like intraoperative MRI and CT improve precision and results.
	3D printing	Anatomical models, surgical implants, and prostheses are all made using this technology. It is also utilized for preoperative planning and education.

(*continued*)

TABLE 3.2 (Continued)
Advancements in Clinical Medicine

Advancements	Techniques	Description
Digital health and telemedicine	Telemedicine	Patients can now consult a doctor remotely because of its use, which improves access to care. Those who live in neglected or rural areas will benefit the most from this.
	Wearable devices	Health monitoring devices such as smartwatches and health monitors record vital parameters in real time. This information can be useful in the treatment of chronic diseases.
	Electronic health records (EHR)	The system provides more accurate and efficient management of patient data, enabling better care coordination and data-driven decisions.
Precision medicine	Personalized treatment plans	It tailors a treatment program based on a person's unique combination of genetic, environmental, and lifestyle variables. This method minimizes side effects and at the same time increases the chances of successful treatment.
	Pharmacogenomics	To choose the safest and most effective medications for each patient, researchers are studying how genes influence drug responses.
AI and ML	AI in diagnostics	Medical images, pathology slides, and other diagnostic data can be accurately analyzed by AI algorithms.
	Predictive analytics	Healthcare may now be more proactive and preventative because of ML models that can forecast disease outbreaks, patient outcomes, and treatment responses.

Improvements in patient outcomes and quality of life have resulted from expanding clinical medicine's capacity to detect, treat, and manage illnesses. Furthering these breakthroughs and resolving the growing issues in clinical medicine require continuous research, technological innovation, and collaboration among healthcare experts.

3.7 CHALLENGES AND FUTURE DIRECTIONS

The use of technology in clinical diagnostics still faces several obstacles despite major progress:

- **Data Privacy and Security:** The privacy and security of patients' information are of utmost importance [32, 33].
- **Interoperability:** The delivery of comprehensive patient care relies on smoothly integrating many data sources and technologies.

- **Accessibility:** A united effort will be needed to make technologies accessible and inexpensive if we close the gap between disadvantaged communities and advanced diagnostics.

Future directions in diagnostic technology may include:

- **Personalized Medicine:** Developing ever-more-specific diagnostic and therapeutic tools based on patients' unique genetic and molecular profiles.
- **Integration of Multi-Omics Data:** Integrating data from many omics sources to gain a comprehensive understanding of disease causes, including genomes, proteomics, metabolomics, and more.
- **Advancements in AI:** The ongoing improvement of AI algorithms to aid in clinical decision-making, decrease the likelihood of human mistakes, and increase the precision of diagnoses [34].

3.8 CONCLUSION

Implementing cutting-edge diagnostic technologies has revolutionized clinical care by enabling the detection and management of diseases with unparalleled speed, precision, and breadth. Progress toward more efficient, more accessible, and individually tailored healthcare is assured in the years to come because of developments made in diagnostics. Both diagnostic tools and treatment methods have been considerably improved by technological advancements, which have had a dramatic impact on clinical practice. Advancements in imaging technology, genetic testing, and point-of-care diagnostics have completely transformed the way how diseases are detected and diagnosed, allowing for more accurate and timely diagnoses. Therapeutic innovations like immunotherapy, regenerative medicine, and targeted medicines have enhanced survival rates and treatment efficacy. Surgical advancements, such as less invasive and image-guided procedures, have shortened healing periods and increased surgical accuracy. Because of innovations in digital health, telemedicine, and wearable technology, more people can access the healthcare they need, and doctors can track their patients' vitals in real time. With precision medicine, individualized treatment programs and medical procedures are now more effective and safer. Even more so, clinical decision-making and patient care have been improved by incorporating AI and ML into diagnostics and predictive analytics. Clinical results and general health are expected to improve due to these technological innovations, which together work toward a better healthcare system that is efficient, effective, and patient-focused.

REFERENCES

[1] Pulumati, A., Dwarakanath, B.S., Verma, A. and Papineni, R.V., 2023. Technological advancements in cancer diagnostics: Improvements and limitations. *Cancer Reports*, 6(2), p.e1764.

[2] Reddy, P., Singh, P., Kuril, S.R., Priyadarshini, A., Gosipatala, S.B., Chand, G., Kaur, T., Thakur, M. and Sobti, R.C., 2024. Technological Advancements in Cancer Diagnosis

and Prognosis. In *Handbook of Oncobiology: From Basic to Clinical Sciences* (pp. 111–126). Singapore: Springer Nature Singapore.

[3] Rahman, M.T., Uddin, M.S., Sultana, R., Moue, A. and Setu, M., 2013. Polymerase chain reaction (PCR): A short review. *Anwer Khan Modern Medical College Journal*, 4(1), pp.30–36.

[4] Millon, L., Caillot, D., Berceanu, A., Bretagne, S., Lanternier, F., Morio, F., Letscher-Bru, V., Dalle, F., Denis, B., Alanio, A. and Boutoille, D., 2022. Evaluation of serum Mucorales polymerase chain reaction (PCR) for the diagnosis of mucormycoses: The MODIMUCOR prospective trial. *Clinical Infectious Diseases*, *75*(5), pp.777–785.

[5] Kang, B.H., Lee, Y., Yu, E.S., Na, H., Kang, M., Huh, H.J. and Jeong, K.H., 2021. Ultrafast and real-time nanoplasmonic on-chip polymerase chain reaction for rapid and quantitative molecular diagnostics. *ACS Nano*, *15*(6), pp.10194–10202.

[6] Zhu, H., Zhang, H., Xu, Y., Laššáková, S., Korabečná, M. and Neužil, P., 2020. PCR past, present and future. *Biotechniques*, *69*(4), pp.317–325.

[7] Hu, T., Chitnis, N., Monos, D. and Dinh, A., 2021. Next-generation sequencing technologies: An overview. *Human Immunology*, *82*(11), pp.801–811.

[8] Kchouk, M., Gibrat, J.F. and Elloumi, M., 2017. Generations of sequencing technologies: From first to next generation. *Biology and Medicine*, *9*(3).

[9] Hu, T., Chitnis, N., Monos, D. and Dinh, A., 2021. Next-generation sequencing technologies: An overview. *Human Immunology*, *82*(11), pp.801–811.

[10] Yin, Y., Butler, C. and Zhang, Q., 2021. Challenges in the application of NGS in the clinical laboratory. *Human Immunology*, *82*(11), pp.812–819.

[11] Sisodiya, S., Kasherwal, V., Khan, A., Roy, B., Goel, A., Kumar, S., Arif, N., Tanwar, P. and Hussain, S., 2023. Liquid biopsies: Emerging role and clinical applications in solid tumours. *Translational Oncology*, *35*, p.101716.

[12] Lohmann, K. and Klein, C., 2014. Next generation sequencing and the future of genetic diagnosis. *Neurotherapeutics*, *11*(4), pp.699–707.

[13] Palmirotta, R., Lovero, D., Cafforio, P., Felici, C., Mannavola, F., Pellè, E., Quaresmini, D., Tucci, M. and Silvestris, F., 2018. Liquid biopsy of cancer: A multimodal diagnostic tool in clinical oncology. *Therapeutic Advances in Medical Oncology*, *10*, p.1758835918794630.

[14] Noor, J., Chaudhry, A., Noor, R. and Batool, S., 2023. Advancements and applications of liquid biopsies in oncology: A narrative review. *Cureus*, *15*(7). https://doi.org/10.7759/cureus.42731

[15] Mirbabaie, M., Stieglitz, S. and Frick, N.R., 2021. Artificial intelligence in disease diagnostics: A critical review and classification on the current state of research guiding future direction. *Health and Technology*, *11*(4), pp.693–731.

[16] Dias, R. and Torkamani, A., 2019. Artificial intelligence in clinical and genomic diagnostics. *Genome Medicine*, *11*(1), p.70.

[17] Savage, N., 2020. How AI is improving cancer diagnostics. *Nature*, *579*(7800), pp.S14–S14.

[18] Bhinder, B., Gilvary, C., Madhukar, N.S. and Elemento, O., 2021. Artificial intelligence in cancer research and precision medicine. *Cancer Discovery*, *11*(4), pp.900–915.

[19] Romiti, S., Vinciguerra, M., Saade, W., Anso Cortajarena, I. and Greco, E., 2020. Artificial intelligence (AI) and cardiovascular diseases: An unexpected alliance. *Cardiology Research and Practice*, *2020*(1), p.4972346.

[20] Stehlik, J., Schmalfuss, C., Bozkurt, B., Nativi-Nicolau, J., Wohlfahrt, P., Wegerich, S., Rose, K., Ray, R., Schofield, R., Deswal, A. and Sekaric, J., 2020. Continuous wearable monitoring analytics predict heart failure hospitalization: The LINK-HF multicenter study. *Circulation: Heart Failure*, *13*(3), p.e006513.

[21] Huang, S., Yang, J., Fong, S. and Zhao, Q., 2020. Artificial intelligence in cancer diagnosis and prognosis: Opportunities and challenges. *Cancer Letters, 471*, pp.61–71.

[22] Vinny, P.W., Vishnu, V.Y. and Srivastava, M.P., 2021. Artificial intelligence shaping the future of neurology practice. *Medical Journal Armed Forces India, 77*(3), pp.276–282.

[23] Jha, K. and Kumar, A., 2024. Role of artificial intelligence in detecting neurological disorders. *International Research Journal on Advanced Engineering Hub (IRJAEH), 2*(02), pp.73–79.

[24] Reddy, S., Giri, D. and Patel, R., 2024. Artificial intelligence diagnosis of Parkinson's disease from MRI scans. *Cureus, 16*(4). https://doi.org/10.7759/cureus.58841

[25] Yang, Y., Yuan, Y., Zhang, G., Wang, H., Chen, Y.C., Liu, Y., Tarolli, C.G., Crepeau, D., Bukartyk, J., Junna, M.R. and Videnovic, A., 2022. Artificial intelligence-enabled detection and assessment of Parkinson's disease using nocturnal breathing signals. *Nature Medicine, 28*(10), pp.2207–2215.

[26] Sun, X., Yin, Y., Yang, Q. and Huo, T., 2023. Artificial intelligence in cardiovascular diseases: Diagnostic and therapeutic perspectives. *European Journal of Medical Research, 28*(1), p.242.

[27] Yan, Y., Zhang, J.W., Zang, G.Y. and Pu, J., 2019. The primary use of artificial intelligence in cardiovascular diseases: What kind of potential role does artificial intelligence play in future medicine? *Journal of Geriatric Cardiology (JGC), 16*(8), p.585.

[28] Singh, M., Kumar, A., Khanna, N.N., Laird, J.R., Nicolaides, A., Faa, G., Johri, A.M., Mantella, L.E., Fernandes, J.F.E., Teji, J.S. and Singh, N., 2024. Artificial intelligence for cardiovascular disease risk assessment in personalised framework: A scoping review. *EClinicalMedicine, 73*.

[29] Namasivayam, V., Senguttuvan, N., Saravanan, V., Palaniappan, S. and Kathiravan, M.K., 2022. Artificial Intelligence and Its Application in Cardiovascular Disease Management. In: *Machine Learning and Systems Biology in Genomics and Health* (pp. 189–236). Singapore: Springer Nature Singapore.

[30] Gupta, S. and Prabha, C., 2021. Voting Regression Model for Covid-19 Time Series Data Analysis. In: *3rd International Conference on Advances in Computing, Communication Control and Networking (ICAC3N)* (pp. 2041–2046). IEEE. doi:10.1109/ICAC3N53548.2021.9725524.

[31] Sharma, G. and Prabha, C. et al., 2022. A Systematic Review for Detecting Cancer using Machine Learning Techniques. In: *Innovations in Computational and Computer Techniques: ICACCT-2021*. AIP Publishing. https://doi.org/10.1063/5.0108888

[32] Kaur, G., Prabha, C., Chhabra, D., Kaur, N., Veeramanickam, M. R. M. and Gill, S. K., 2022. A Systematic Approach to Machine Learning for Cancer Classification. In: *5th International Conference on Contemporary Computing and Informatics (IC3I), Uttar Pradesh, India* (pp. 134–138). IEEE. doi:10.1109/IC3I56241.2022.10072474

[33] Sharma, D. and Prabha, C., 2023. Security and Privacy Aspects of Electronic Health Records: A Review. In: *International Conference on Advancement in Computation & Computer Technologies (InCACCT), Gharuan, India* (pp. 815–820). IEEE. doi:10.1109/InCACCT57535.2023.10141814

[34] Mittal, P., Gahlot, K., Phul, V., Singh, Y., Verma, C., & Zoltán, I. (2023). Smart Healthcare System Based on AIoT Emerging Technologies: A Brief Review. In J. K. Singh (Ed.), *Proceedings of International Conference on Recent Innovations in Computing. ICRIC 2022*. DOI: 10.1007/978-981-99-0601-7_23.

4 Digital Health Records

Enhancing Data-Driven Clinical Decisions

Palvi Sharma, Rakesh Kumar, and Meenu Gupta

4.1 INTRODUCTION

Digital Health Records (DHRs) have considerably influenced the management and use of patient healthcare information. These include Electronic Health Records (EHRs), Electronic Medical Records (EMRs), and Personal Health Records (PHRs), which help in collecting, storing, and disseminating all information regarding a patient in an integral way [1]. The main aim of implementing DHR is to enable medical records to be more accessible, accurate, and efficient so that there can be better coordination between the providers of healthcare and improve the delivery of healthcare overall. In the business of healthcare, speedy access to correct patient information is critical for proper diagnosis, treatment, and patient outcomes as depicted in Figure 4.1 [2]. Traditional paper-based record-keeping has been highly time-consuming, error-prone, and ultimately compromises the safety and quality of patient care. The rise of digital transformation in the health sector has compelled the sector to engage in data-centric practices with the purpose of improving both patient care as well as management practices. As such, patients' records have been increasingly managed using Patient Record Management System (PRMS), driven by technological innovations that aim to streamline decision-making processes, optimize workflow, and provide easier data access [3, 4]. This analysis assesses the efficacy of PRMS in investigating the meaning and implications of data-driven healthcare. Skilful decision-making is an important part of standard healthcare, and the capacity to make knowledgeable decisions can greatly improve patient health outcomes [5]. Based on the latest and best evidence based on systematic research like Randomized Controlled Trial (RCTs), the concept known as Evidence-Based Practice (EBP) provides a basis for these decisions. Nevertheless, the confidence of healthcare providers in applying EBP has been eroded due to weaknesses in both the amount and the quality of the research output from RCTs [6, 7]. A different model that holds paramount significance for evidence coming from the actual world is known as Practical-Based Evidence. EHRs use health information technology to store applicable evidence that arises from clinical practice. Data-driven healthcare collects data from different sources – social media, wearable devices, and EHRs – to make appropriate decisions concerning treatment of the patient. The ability to identify patterns, predict outcomes, and personalize

DOI: 10.1201/9781003516163-4

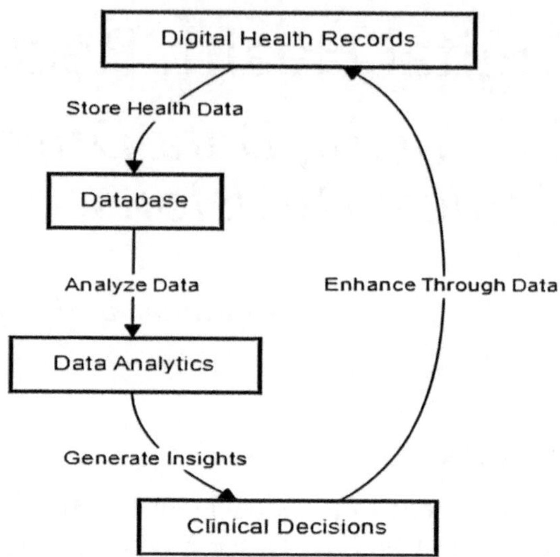

FIGURE 4.1 Digital Health Records.

interventions based on data analysis has changed the modern manifestations of healthcare providers' approaches to health and medicine [8, 9].

The healthcare industry has always used data in different forms since time immemorial. Medical doctors used to maintain quite detailed chronicles of their patients and disseminated medical information through the production of books and journals [10]. From analysing patient charts, symptoms, treatments, and outcomes, doctors are benefited from informed decisions [11]. EHRs make history mark a new chapter where records become electronic and can be digitally retrieved. Some of the latest innovations that define intelligent automation of healthcare include machine learning (ML) and artificial intelligence (AI). They process and analyse vast amounts of data much faster and with more accuracy than any human user. For example, an AI system can view medical images and detect early signs of diseases such as cancer long before a clinician can see them [12]. In summary, such a shift toward DHR together with the integration of sophisticated data analysis technologies fundamentally altered the healthcare landscape. This review explores the implications of changes like this in relation to data-driven clinical decision-making. The paper is divided into the following sections: Section 4.2 discusses the contextual and foundational understanding constituting background work. Section 4.3 describes the history of health records from the traditional paper-based record-keeping systems to the modern digital record. Section 4.4 explains the core components of DHR, including their form and working. Section 4.5 describes the protection of data security and privacy, with the importance of protecting sensitive patient data. Section 4.6 delves into the benefits of DHR and shows the impact on healthcare delivery. Section 4.7 explores the recent trends and advancements in DHR, which are related to the new and latest progress and prospective avenues within this field. In conclusion, Section 4.8 summarizes the study by encapsulating its key findings and implications.

4.2 BACKGROUND STUDY

To improve DHRs for data-driven clinical decision-making, this section examines research done by different researchers using A) and deep learning (DL) technologies.

In reference [13], Chakraborty et al. emphasized recent developments in data science in medicine, underscoring the use of ML and DL in the interpretation of EMR/EHR data, big data in personalized medicine, dataset changes in AI, and medical image data. With medical data, ML techniques developed into DL approaches that were more effective, necessitating a shift in handling numerous data sources. This study examined the value and challenges of ML and DL in the healthcare industry, emphasizing the need for cooperation and scalability among engineers, doctors, data scientists, computer scientists, and healthcare providers. Multidisciplinary cooperation, the implementation of standards and legal frameworks pertinent to AI in healthcare, stringent validation procedures, and thorough instruction and training are all necessary for the effective integration of these technologies. In reference [14], Shastry and Shastry examined the rate at which digital health technologies are being adopted. This leads to the development of massive volumes of health data, which may be used for advanced data analytics and cognitive computing to improve healthcare outcomes. This work presented an integrated DL and NLP approach for continuous remote monitoring, using DL algorithms such as convolutional neural networks (CNNs) and recurrent neural networks (RNNs) to analyse wearable device data and natural language processing (NLP) to interpret patient comments and EMRs. The authors contrasted this method with previous research and addressed the flaws and recommended remedies. The study looked at the promise and challenges of using data analytics and cognitive computing in healthcare and suggested future research topics. The method improved remote patient monitoring in real time, anticipated unfavourable situations, yielded better results, reduced costs, and raised the standard of care. In reference [15], Cai et al. examined the multimodal data-driven method that has become important for intelligent healthcare systems, influencing the diagnosis, treatment, triage, and analysis of diseases. Due to the enhanced data management and decision-making requirements of these systems, the healthcare industry is undergoing rapid changes and the development of AI-driven medical services. With an emphasis on decision-making processes, this study examined current methodologies, including cutting-edge approaches and current trends. Key areas included multimodal association mining with fine-grained data semantics, multimodal association mining with panoramic decision frameworks, multimodal data fusion, and intelligent decision support systems. This work illustrated how data-centred, comprehensive, whole-process decision-making can replace in-hospital linear management when cross-sectoral and cross-regional data resources are combined. In addition to highlighting the necessity for continued research and development, this study emphasizes the revolutionary potential of multimodal data-driven methodologies in smart healthcare. In reference [16], Zhang et al. focused on developing practice-based pathways for treatment using a data-driven methodology applied to 1,576 patients with acute kidney injury (AKI) and chronic kidney disease (CKD) as per EHRs between 2009 and 2013. Finding the best treatment plans that fit patient requirements and clinical workflows is the goal of putting evidence into practice. Thirteen unique patient categories were identified by clustering the one-dimensional sequences of purposes, procedures, drugs, and diagnoses that were created from patient visit data. This work extracted and visualized important clinical route transitions across these subgroups using Markov chain modelling, providing new information on patient health outcomes, guideline adherence, and disease development. In addition to addressing issues like patient diversity and data accuracy, the methodology intends to facilitate effective practice reviews and patient–provider collaborative decision-making, which could improve treatment quality and save costs in hospitals along with various contexts. In reference [17], Ruaya et al. investigated the revolutionary effects of putting the PRMS into place at RHU-Del Carmen, emphasizing how it improved data accessibility, streamlined healthcare processes, and supported evidence-based decision-making. The PRMS optimizes care coordination, improves patient care, and offers useful clinical information, earning it an overall evaluation score of 4.4 out of 5. It emphasizes the value of adopting data-driven healthcare practices and the advantages of using patient data to improve healthcare results.

In reference [18], Enticott et al. conducted a systematic review that investigated Learning Health Systems (LHS) and how data-driven methods could enhance healthcare from 2014 to 2019. Overall, 43 studies from 23 different LHS contexts were listed, most of them from the US but also from Canada, the UK, Sweden, Australia, and New Zealand. Results showed that longitudinal benchmarking and patient tracking lead to quantifiable improvements in clinical services, patient self-management, clinician care, and system-level performance. In reference [19], Rieke et al. discussed how data-driven ML potentially could be applied in healthcare, mentioning the current limitations due to data silos and the issues of privacy. Their study pointed out that ML in practice was still limited without access to all the comprehensive medical data available. To address these challenges, federated learning (FL) was proposed as a new approach to cooperatively train ML models between multiple institutions without moving the clients' private data. With FL, global data distributions were approximated, which should improve model robustness, security, and accuracy. Improving medical image analysis, facilitating precision medicine, and accelerating drug discovery will have sizeable effects on digital healthcare. In reference [20], Parker et al. studied EHRs, which have revolutionized healthcare by leading to data-driven decision-making and better patient outcomes. Unfortunately, there are some limitations of EHRs related to issues in data security, interoperability, and training that limit their full usage. Thus, these constraints need to be removed to unlock the full potential of EHRs for revolutionizing healthcare. Though there has been progress, harnessing EHRs to drive healthcare innovation and inform public health decisions still requires achieving seamless interoperability and guaranteeing strong data security. Recent work by Khalifa et al. [21] discusses how AI is revolutionizing Clinical Decision Support Systems (CDSSs) within the healthcare domain with the use of large datasets that further help patients in respect of a wide range of activities involving both administrative efficiency and individualized treatment, diagnostic accuracy, and predictive analytics among others. Collaboration between technologists, healthcare practitioners, and politicians was necessary due to challenges pertaining to data protection, ethical considerations, and system integration. AI has the potential to significantly improve patient-centred care, efficiency, and efficacy in healthcare, but only when combined with human expertise, ethical AI development, and ongoing professional training are prioritized.

In reference [22], Evans et al. observed the growing acceptance of data-driven CDSS by healthcare professionals (HCPs) and the critical role that trust plays in this process. Few researchers have delved thoroughly into stakeholder perceptions, especially with regard to trustworthiness, despite the abundance of studies in this area. Just a small percentage ($n = 85$) of the included research focused on measuring trust directly; the rest included topics like explainability, transparency, and supporting evidence that affect trust in data-driven CDSS. The wide variety of methodological methods brought to light the need for focused research on HCP uptake as well as the requirements for transparency and interpretability in these systems. In reference [23], Tsoukalas et al. used EHRs of 1,492 patients to enhance clinical decisions in sepsis treatment using a data-driven method based on a Partially Observable Markov Decision Process (POMDP). It demonstrated better patient outcomes than competing methodologies by accurately predicting the length of stay, appropriate antibiotic dosing, and mortality. The method showed promise for improving clinical decision-making as it remains stable as model parameters and data quality change. In reference [24], Ross et al. examined that EHR systems, which record copious amounts of clinical data, were becoming increasingly popular around the globe. With a focus on advanced analytics like NLP and data mining (pharmacovigilance, phenotyping, etc.), the paper reviewed recent research on "big data" applications in EHRs. Important aspects include personal monitoring, privacy and security challenges, and clinical decision support improvement. In reference [25], Chen et al. discussed the function that CDSSs offer in the healthcare industry by providing doctors with evidence-based recommendations at the point of care in an effort to increase clinical effectiveness, reduce errors, and enhance patient outcomes. Integration with current systems, clinician acceptability, and data privacy were some of the obstacles that CDSSs must overcome before they can be fully implemented and optimized, despite their potential advantages. The effectiveness of CDSS can be increased by connecting it with EHRs, utilising AI and ML, making sure the interfaces are user-friendly, and putting strong assessment procedures in place. By tackling these obstacles and possibilities, CDSS can have maximum impact on improving patient care and overall health outcomes.

In reference [26], Epizitone et al. explored how the adoption of Health Information Systems (HIS) has accelerated because of pandemics and the Fourth Industrial Revolution, driven by the digitalization of healthcare data. This study introduced a data-driven paradigm to enhance HIS, focusing on data sources, actions, decisions, data science techniques, and implementation. Emphasizing the need for integrating these elements, the study highlights their importance in improving healthcare outcomes and ensuring sustainable HIS. In reference [27], Wu et al. discussed the massive volumes of omic and EHR data that were produced as a result of the adoption of EHRs and advancements in high-throughput technology. These data are essential for precision medicine. This study covered modelling, mining, and pre-processing strategies for data as well as the characteristics and problems of omic and EHR data. This work discussed the characteristics and challenges of omic and EHR data, along with data pre-processing, mining, and modelling techniques. In reference [28], Mo et al. proposed a computable Phenotype Representation Model (PheRM) with 10 desired characteristics. These included the following: defining temporal relations, utilizing standardized terminologies, supporting text searching and NLP, utilizing a common data model, supporting both human-readable and computable forms, implementing set operations, representing criteria with structured rules, and structuring clinical data. Enhancing the phenotypic' dependability and portability between various EHR systems was the goal of PheRM. To evolve these requirements, users and developers worked together. Phenotyping emphasizes positive predictive value and frequently makes use of data corroboration and NLP. The goal of the proposed PheRM was to improve healthcare applications through the incorporation of data analytics, effective delivery, and medical knowledge. In reference [29], Garcelon et al. discussed that the reuse of clinical data from EHRs offers new opportunities for diagnosing and managing rare diseases but faces challenges. Developing decision support systems requires patient recruitment, data extraction and integration, data mining and stratification, and embedding algorithms into patient care, necessitating adaptable EHRs. Solutions include structured EHRs, free-text search engines, data warehouses, NLP, ML for patient classification, and similarity metrics for diagnosis. Ethical considerations are crucial for the appropriate use of health data. AI for diagnosing rare diseases via EHRs was underdeveloped. Key challenges include analysing free text efficiently and integrating research algorithms into clinical systems. Bridging the gap between care and research is essential to meet the high expectations of patients and clinicians.

In reference [30], Berros et al. explored the application of big data in digital health, discussing health data characteristics, tools, and recent research. It emphasizes the necessity for all medical organizations, from large institutions to individual clinics, to adopt big data technologies to optimize resource management and enhance treatment accuracy. Significant investments in big data analytics are anticipated due to its potential for vastly improved health services. Despite its benefits, healthcare faces unique challenges requiring further research. Future work will propose a methodology and flexible architecture for developing big data analysis in healthcare to address these challenges. In reference [31], Chen et al. quantified the "decay rate" of clinical data relevance and ascertained how past training data affected the forecast of upcoming clinical decisions. With different subsets of historical data (2009–2012), it projected 2013 admission orders using a clinical order recommender system using EHR data from a hospital. According to the results, a month's worth of data from 2012 was able to predict 2013 orders with a higher degree of accuracy than a year's worth of data from 2009 (ROC AUC 0.91 vs. 0.88). Existing human-authored order sets were not as good as older (2009) data models (ROC AUC 0.81). Only the most recent data was preferable to further longitudinal data (2009–2012), unless a declining weighting technique with a "half-life" of around 4 months was used. The study found that smaller amounts of recent data were more useful than greater amounts of older data for making clinical predictions in the future. In reference [32], Shalom et al. designed, implemented, and evaluated PICARD, a novel architecture for continuous guideline-based decision support that supports several tasks, continuous care, and both data-driven and user-driven modes. The evaluation included technical, functional, and clinical assessments using various scenarios and decision points. Results showed that PICARD significantly improved decision completeness (from 41% manually to 93%) and reduced redundant actions (from 68% manually to 3%), while maintaining a high level of correctness (~94.5%). The architecture was validated by domain experts and demonstrated technical feasibility and functional validity, making it potentially beneficial for managing chronic patients and enhancing clinical decision-making quality.

4.3 EVOLUTION OF HEALTH RECORDS

The delivery of healthcare services has changed due to the transition of medical records from outdated paperwork to advanced digital technologies (as shown in Figure 4.2). This change has been made possible by continuous technological advances and government support. The result is more efficient, accurate, and accessible health information that improves patient outcomes.

4.3.1 Health Information from a Historical Perspective

The origin of health records dates back to ancient times when doctors and healers documented patient information on scrolls made of papyrus and tablets crafted from clay. The majority of early records comprised observations, diagnoses, and treatment results of patients' conditions. With the advancement of medical understanding, the complexity of these records increased. Throughout the Middle Ages and Renaissance, patient histories were meticulously recorded in detailed casebooks and journals, serving as medical records and instructional resources.

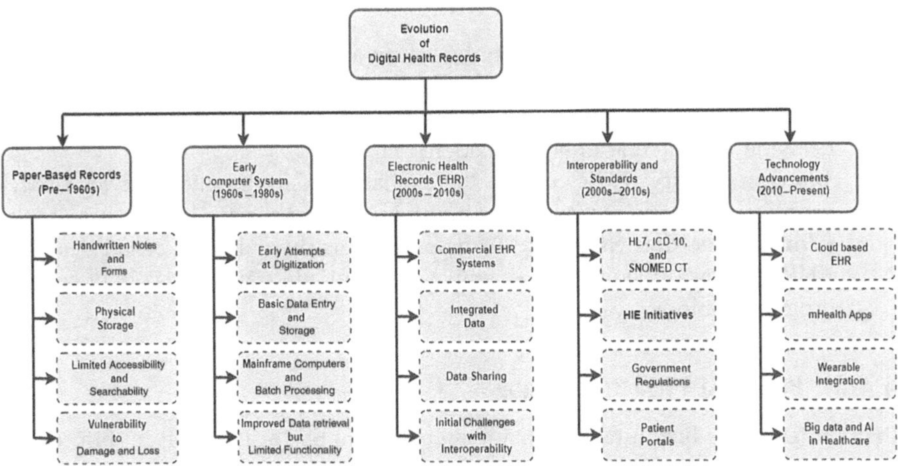

FIGURE 4.2 Evolution of Digital Health Records.

4.3.2 Transition from Paper to Digital Records

For most of the 20th century, the healthcare industry relied heavily on paper records. Managing and using these documents required significant manual labour because they were stored in physical files. The need for a better system arose due to the limitations of paper records, including the risk of loss or damage and the difficulty of transferring data between different healthcare systems. Digital records replaced paper during the mid-20th century, with the advent of computers. Initially, early electronic systems were mainly used for managing schedules and billing administrative tasks. However, as technology advanced, clinical information became integrated into the scope of EHRs.

4.4 COMPONENTS OF DIGITAL HEALTH RECORDS

DHRs have become quite popular in the healthcare industry for their ability to offer managed storage of patient information in a digital form. Their main purpose is to ensure greater security, efficiency, and accuracy in patient records but still allow HCPs easy access to and sharing of such information. Some of these features of DHR are explained below with the help of Figure 4.3.

4.4.1 Electronics Health Records

EHRs serve as the digital counterpart to traditional paper-based medical records. In addition to personal information, diagnoses, prescriptions, allergic reactions, lab results, and other information, they provide an enormous amount of information regarding a patient's prior medical experiences. Additionally, EHRs encompass historical medical information, encompassing medication schedules, healthcare provider notes, and the results of medical tests. Some of the key features of EHR are discussed below:

- **Comprehensive Data:** By merging information from multiple sources, EHRs can exhibit the overall health status of a patient.
- **Real-Time Access:** Real-time access to EHR data by HCPs facilitates rapid decision-making and improves patient outcomes.
- **Interoperability:** EHRs enable the exchange of information between HCPs, enabling data to be shared across multiple healthcare settings.
- **Clinical Decision Support:** To help HCPs make evidence-based decisions, EHR systems often offer preventative care reminders and alerts about potential drug interactions.

4.4.2 Personal Health Records

PHRs refer to the health records that patients maintain for themselves. Information about one's health is gathered into a PHR. An essential component of a basic PHR is having a vaccination record or a collection of medical documentation. The inconvenience of paper records becomes evident when paper records are rarely available when

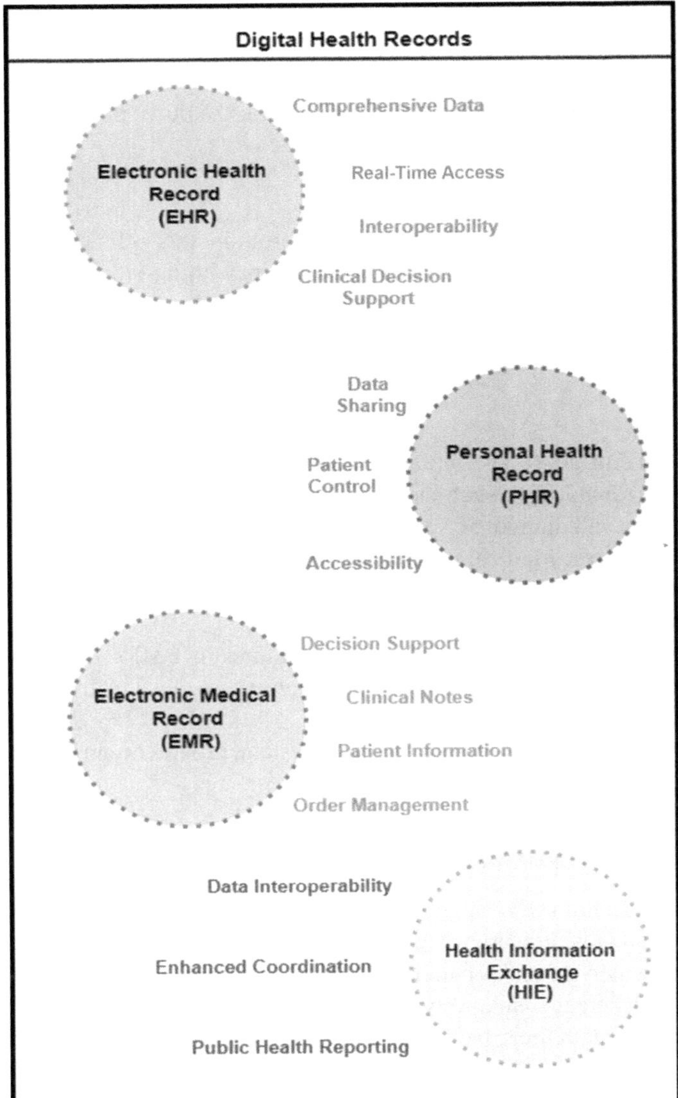

FIGURE 4.3 Components of Digital Health Records.

needed. This difficulty is effectively resolved by electronic PHRs, which allow access to information from any web-enabled device, including computers, cell phones, and tablets, at any time. These records enable patients to oversee and manage their own health data, such as lab results, prescriptions, medical histories, and allergies. Some of the key features of PHR are discussed below:

- **Data Sharing:** HCPs have the ability to retrieve PHRs, ensuring that everyone can access the latest information.

- **Patient Control:** Through PHRs, patients can take an active part in their care and have control over their health information.
- **Accessibility:** Using mobile apps or web portals, individuals can conveniently handle their health information even while on the move to access their PHRs.

4.4.3 Electronic Medical Records

Systems for EMRs are highly advantageous for doctors, clinics, and healthcare institutions. Only authorized clinicians and workers within a single healthcare organization can access these systems, which hold electronic health information about specific persons. EMR systems can improve process efficiency while simultaneously improving patient safety and care quality. Some of the key features of EMR are discussed below:

- **Decision Support:** The integration of EMRs often includes clinical decision support technologies such as medication interaction alerts, preventative care reminders, and diagnostic support.
- **Clinical Notes:** Medical professionals generate thorough clinical notes during patient visits, comprising observations, diagnosis, treatment plans, and progress notes.
- **Patient Information:** The information found in EMRs includes diagnoses, prescribed medications, date of immunizations, medical history, allergies, radiology images, and results of lab tests.
- **Order Management:** Within the EMR system, providers can order and monitor tests, prescriptions, and other services.

4.4.4 Health Information Exchange

A Health Information Exchange (HIE) makes it easier for physicians, nurses, chemists, and other healthcare workers to electronically access and share vital patient medical data, which enhances patient care in terms of speed, quality, safety, and cost. Despite the widespread availability of safe electronic data transmission, the majority of Americans maintain their medical records on paper, either in boxes and files at their homes or at multiple doctor's offices. The exchange of medical information between providers is usually done by mail, fax, or, in most cases, during transport from patient to patient, as patients often bring their own information with them. Electronic HIE can dramatically enhance the completeness of patient records, which can have a considerable impact on treatment. This includes historical history, current prescriptions, and more. However, it cannot completely replace provider–patient communication. Some of the key features of HIE are discussed below:

- **Data Interoperability:** HIE ensures the sharing and understanding of health information between different healthcare platforms and systems.
- **Enhanced Coordination:** HIE enables the transfer of patient information between various healthcare providers, thereby reducing unnecessary tests and procedures and improving care coordination.

- **Public Health Reporting:** HIE provides information on disease surveillance, epidemic control, and health trend analysis to support public health efforts.

4.5 DATA SECURITY AND PRIVACY

Ensuring the privacy and security of DHRs is essential for maintaining patient confidence and protecting sensitive health information as shown in Figure 4.4. This section covers data privacy and confidentiality, security best practices and precautions, as well as legal and regulatory issues.

4.5.1 Privacy Measures

- **Confidentiality:** It ensures that only authorized people have access to health information. Thus, the primary intent is patient data privacy and confidentiality and the prevention of unauthorized access to limit data security breaches. Therefore, it is essential to implement strong access controls, such as role-based access and user authentication. Authentication technologies rely on mechanisms like passwords, biometrics, and smart cards to authenticate user identities. Position Authorization Healthcare Organization grants the users access to only specific information that they are permitted to see, be it the doctors, nurses, or even administrative staff.

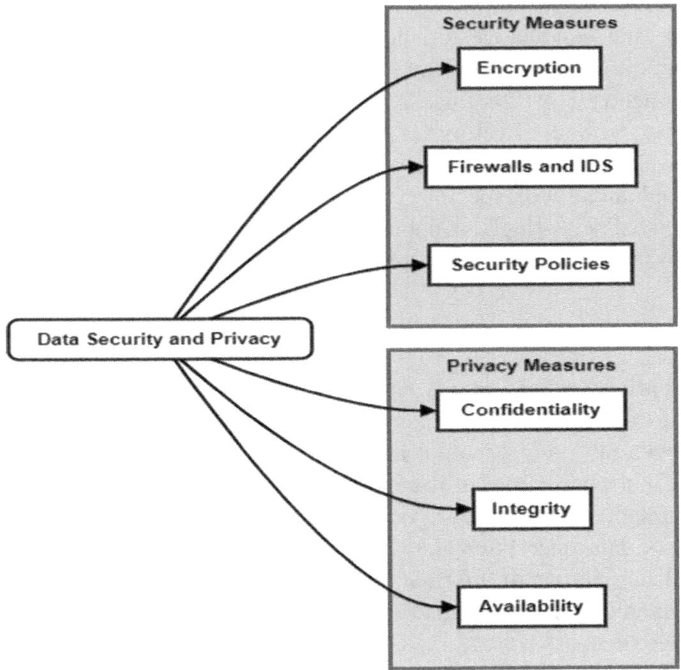

FIGURE 4.4 Privacy and Security Measures.

- **Integrity:** It confirms that information pertaining to health are accurate, consistent, and permanent. The accuracy and relevance of the information on health would be guaranteed in ensuring relevant patient care delivery and informed decision-making. Data validation tests should be conducted to ascertain that such information is accurately inputted into the system and retained in stipulated formats, like a correct patient identifier and date of birth. This is one of the fundamental steps in guaranteeing data integrity. The significance of audit trails lies in the tracing and detection of unauthorized changes to health information, which can be on authorship, content, reporting, and timing. Cryptographic hashing algorithms further protect data by creating different fixed-length strings of data inputs. Should there be a modification to the data, it would obviously change its hash value, which could indicate manipulation. The preservation of health information through backup devices is very essential as these ensure integrity and accuracy in case loss and damage of that information have occurred. Collectively, therefore, these strategies cultivate the sustained consistency and precision of health records, hence ensuring they remain a source of reliable information for practitioners in healthcare.
- **Availability:** It is important that authorized users have access to the DHR without interruption and in a uniform manner so that timely and accurate provision of critical health information can be ensured. This ensures healthcare providers offer care promptly and make decisions based on updated information. Its key strategies include designing strong disaster recovery plans to speedily recover data in case of a disaster, incorporating redundant systems and failover strategies so that any potential downtime can be kept to the minimum, and conducting routine system performance evaluations to identify probable problems before they happen. Data access is limited to authorized personnel as the system has access control that is scalable; it may be used at any time without affecting performance. Based on specific standards listed in service level agreements (SLAs), defined availability requirements are further clarified, along with specific response time determinations for availability and response times. A high availability focus is critical for healthcare organizations in improving the quality of care while maintaining operational efficiency.

4.5.2 Security Measures

- **Encryption:** Patient data is encrypted to prevent any unauthorized access to the information. Encrypted data is converted into a new format that no one can read without a key or code. Due to additional security measures, encrypted data cannot be read even if stolen. To meet Health Insurance Portability and Accountability Act (HIPAA) compliance requirements, the healthcare industry requires data encryption that can cipher in to protect against cyber-attacks and electronic health information. If electronic protected health (ePHI) is not safeguarded, then costly data breaches and illegal disclosure of patient information can occur.

- **Firewalls and Intrusion Detection System (IDS):** Firewalls and IDS play a crucial role in the protection of digital health information, necessitating their implementation. Firewalls act as barriers between secure internal networks and unsecured external networks by screening incoming and outgoing traffic in accordance with established information security standards. This functionality safeguards against unauthorized access and effectively blocks malicious traffic, including viruses and denial of service attacks. All types of firewalls, including packet filtering, stateful inspection, and application layer firewalls, need a security policy to be established. IDS, on the other hand, scrutinizes system or network activity for malicious behaviour or policy violations, alerting when that behaviour is detected.
- **Security Policies and Procedures:** Healthcare organizations are expected to develop security policies and procedures that ensure compliance with regulations and guard sensitive data such as health information. Sensitive data require that authentication protocols, encryption techniques, and access controls be used, so this framework establishes constant monitoring of system activities, regular vulnerability assessments, and a plan for incident response to effectively deal with breaches. Other important aspects include guidance on measures for physical security and on training employees in best practices for information security. These policies help prevent breaches of data, unauthorized access, sustain patient trust, and therefore improve the general robustness of HIS by clearly outlining these security practices and responsibilities.
- **Risk Assessments:** In the DHR arena, risk assessment is the systematic process aimed at understanding threats towards patient data confidentiality. It entails, first and foremost, identifying assets – network infrastructure, for instance, and such EHRs – and second, identifying potential risks associated with it, for instance, cyber-attacks, and system failure among others. Lastly, there is determining the vulnerabilities, including outdated software and lack of adequate access control. The likely impact and chance of each threat are also evaluated, and risks are categorized by their damage potential; then strategies to deal with the most critical threats are devised. Ongoing monitoring and regular assessments are essential to effectively address new threats and organizational changes. For example, healthcare organizations can enhance their security, adhere to regulations, protect patient privacy, and uphold trust.

4.6 BENEFITS OF DIGITAL HEALTH RECORDS

Digital healthcare is transforming the delivery and administration of health services, offering numerous advantages. Some of the primary benefits (as shown in Figure 4.5) are discussed below:

- **Enhancing the Standard of Care:** The ability for HCPs to access a patient's whole medical history in one location makes DHRs essential for enhancing the quality of patient care. A patient's DHR, for instance, can be viewed by a new physician to see what prescriptions the patient is taking, what allergies

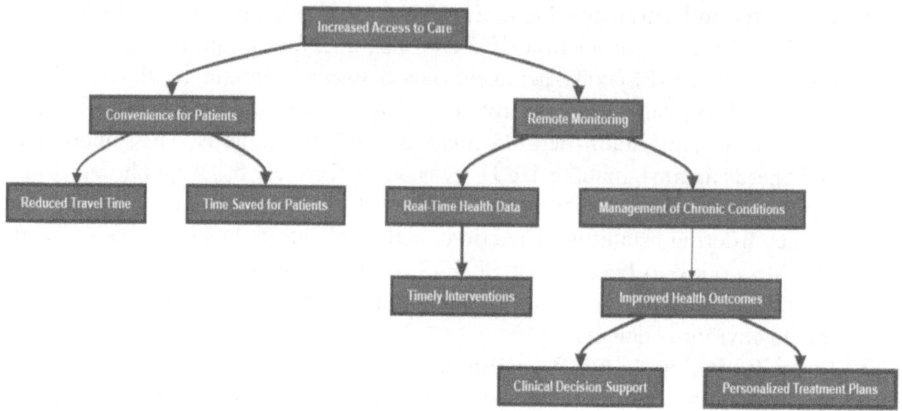

FIGURE 4.5 Benefits of Digital Health Care.

the patient has, and what illnesses the patient has been diagnosed with. This can assist the physician in making better-informed choices regarding the patient's care.

- **Reducing Medical Errors:** DHRs decrease the chances of medical errors. For instance, doctors avoid prescribing drugs to which patients are allergic by storing such knowledge in their patients' EHRs. Moreover, access to a patient's list of medications through EHRs reduces the chances of adverse drug interactions and medication errors.
- **Information Exchanged between Care Providers:** EHRs are also an important functionality to be used by many HCPs. People with chronic diseases should see several doctors in today's world. The cardiologist and primary physician can access the EHR containing all test completion, lab results, and medicines that have been prescribed to him. This allows for a consistent approach towards patient care and develops agreement among all HCPs involved.
- **Population Health Management:** EHRs can be used to analyse the data for many patients to identify a pattern or trend, thus providing better access and delivery of healthcare to the community. It may include a track record of infectious diseases' transmission, identification of persons at risk of certain illnesses, and study of the efficacy of treatment for all persons.
- **Lowering Healthcare Costs:** DHRs also lead to lower healthcare costs due to the ability of healthcare providers to avoid unnecessary tests and treatments when they have single-point access to a patient's medical history. Furthermore, by automating various tasks such as insurance claims, medication renewals, and appointment scheduling, DHRs can help reduce administrative expenses.

4.7 EMERGING TRENDS AND INNOVATIONS

As illustrated in Figure 4.6, the advancement of EHRs is transforming the healthcare sector by enhancing the security, usability, and effectiveness of patient data. The most important developments and trends are:

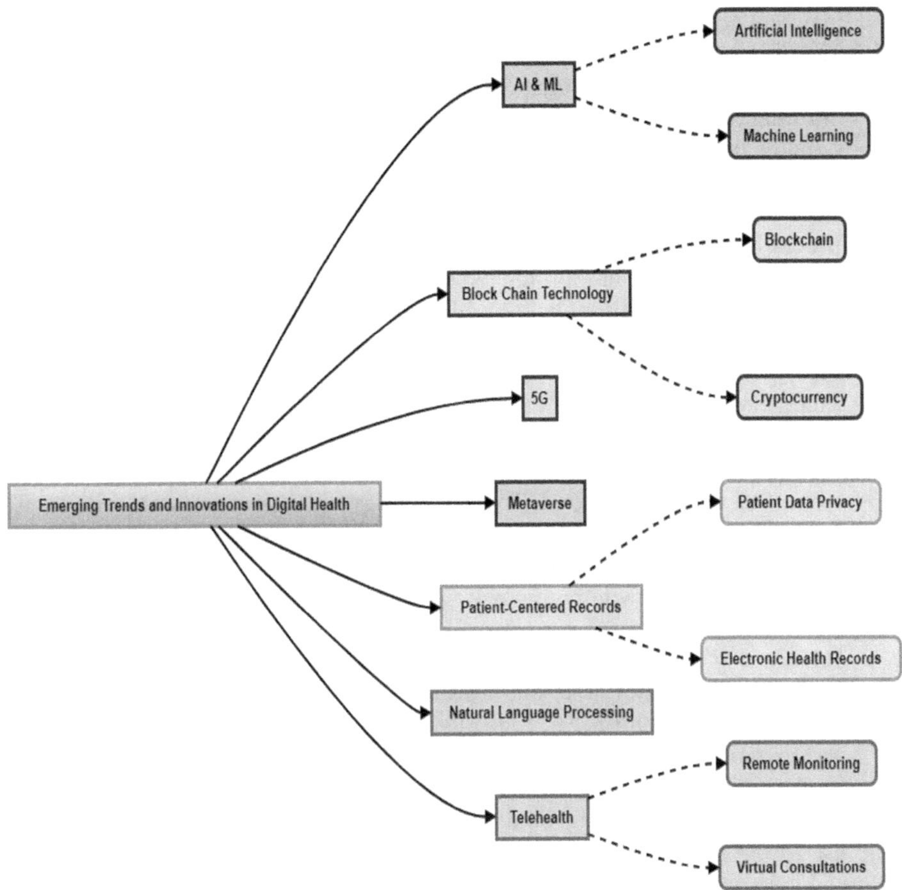

FIGURE 4.6 Innovations in Digital Health Care.

- **Artificial Intelligence and Machine Learning:** Healthcare is one of the sectors where AI and ML have generated much interest and usage. While a part of AI, the term "ML" refers specifically to algorithms and models that learn from data and make predictions or estimates about any phenomenon. AI refers to the development of intelligent computers, which can carry out a task that human beings have also been necessitated to do. By integrating AI and ML into the healthcare industry, large amounts of medical data can be analysed and the outcomes help better understand and improve the care of patients. Knowledge-based insights are crucial to medical practice because they represent evidence-based information that is part of its decision-making, and through AI and ML techniques, HCPs are able to perform extensive data analysis about trends, patterns, and relationships that could not be found using other means. This may lead to a higher diagnostic rate, treatment-specific plans, better patient results, and advancements in medical practice. AI and ML algorithms process patient data to make predictions about health outcomes. This allows for timely intervention and individualized treatment strategies. Because of their ability to identify and generate predictions or estimates independently, algorithms that use ML are a significant element in healthcare analysis. For example, clinical information, genetic information, medical imaging, and sensor-derived data are some of the complex medical data. With complex models of ML that require large datasets, the provider can derive hidden insights, predict outcomes, and make necessary decisions.

- **Blockchain Technology:** EHR improvement with blockchain technology improves security and promotes interoperability of EHRs, enhances the effectiveness of health policies, and empowers patients. This is done through the development of a decentralized ledger based on chains of blocks of encrypted data. The framework reduces the dangers of breached healthcare data as health information can be shared safely among different nodes. The addition of data blocks in the blockchain is transparent and coupled with verification through algorithms of consensus that trace a history of all alterations that cannot be altered. This technology will therefore enable the coordination of care and the proper integration of patient data that can smoothly be transferred from one EHR to another. Blockchain allows proper management access, thereby allowing patients to have more control over their health information.
- **5G:** Cutting-edge 5G wireless network technology has brought about unparalleled opportunities for the development of healthcare and improved treatment accessibilities. Specifically engineered to support next-generation user experiences and services, 5G is a robust, high-cohesion air interface. Implementing 5G technology is a must for the digitization of society and the integration of all elements contained in smart healthcare. The integration and use of 5G smart healthcare can create significant breakthroughs in medicine and help optimize resource allocation.
- **Metaverse:** The metaverse, a multidisciplinary ecosystem, was established through the addition of various technologies to its overall architecture at different levels. As its three-dimensional version in the online world, many things combine to help bring together the real and virtual worlds within the metaverse: Users are one of them. Using HMD and other augmented reality/virtual reality (AR/VR) glasses, users can thus interact with this virtual world through which the possibility of digital expression of such communications is availed and then, after that, the performance of multiple tasks is possible. Broad modules of Virtual Service Provider (VSP), Physical Service Provider (PSP), and Internet of Things (IoT) network modules enhance communication between physical and virtual environments while digital twins, as part of the IoT system, are derived from the information gathered from IoT and sensor networks. It is usually the VSPs and PSPs who will primarily be responsible for maintaining both the physical and virtual metaverse ecosystems.
- **Patient-Centred Records:** The patient-centred records should enable access to and management of health information about patients. With the clinical record, the patient can share the information easily with different providers, thus becoming a client-specific and more coordinated approach to care. The

involvement of the patient in clinical decision-making is associated with the satisfaction and overall outcomes of the patient.

- **Natural Language Processing:** NLP technology adds the ability to extract vital clinical information from unstructured data, such as patient histories and clinical documentation. This results in not just more accurate and detailed patient information, but also improved decisions made by caregivers. Additionally, NLP enables the development of prediction models targeted to disease detection in advanced stages and towards more personalized treatment plans.
- **Telehealth Integration:** Remote patient monitoring and virtual consultation allow remote health services to integrate with electronic health information. All telehealth interactions are documented, ensuring the patient's medical history is easily accessible and enabling informed decisions based on comprehensive knowledge of their condition and ongoing care.

4.8 CONCLUSION

Integration of electronic health data along with modern technology is transforming the healthcare sector and further improving patient outcomes. This study assesses how 5G, information society, metaverse, speech recognition, telemedicine, NLP, and patient records influence the usability, precision, effectiveness, and other perspectives of communication and technology integration in DHRs. It highlights the importance of interoperability standards for smooth data sharing and the function of blockchains in guaranteeing security, privacy, and legal compliance. Improved data collection and analysis of patients' early detection result in more effective and individualized therapy. Examples and trends from real-world uses, such as genetics and AI, show how continued improvements can improve health outcomes even more and create a system that is more patient-centred and responsive.

REFERENCES

[1] A. Dagliati, A. Malovini, V. Tibollo, and R. Bellazzi, "Health informatics and EHR to support clinical research in the COVID-19 pandemic: An overview," *Brief. Bioinform.*, vol. 22, no. 2, pp. 812–822, 2021, doi: 10.1093/bib/bbaa418.

[2] A. Abernethy et al., "The promise of digital health: Then, now, and the future," *NAM Perspect.*, vol. 6, no. 22, 2022, doi: 10.31478/202206e.

[3] K. Koochakpour et al., "Success factors of an early EHR system for Child and Adolescent Mental Health: Lessons learned for future practice data-driven decision aids," *Stud. Health Technol. Inform.*, vol. 290, pp. 182–186, 2022, doi: 10.3233/SHTI220057.

[4] M. Pikoula, J. K. Quint, F. Nissen, H. Hemingway, L. Smeeth, and S. Denaxas, "Identifying clinically important COPD sub-types using data-driven approaches in primary care population based electronic health records," *BMC Med. Inform. Decis. Mak.*, vol. 19, no. 1, pp. 1–14, 2019, doi: 10.1186/s12911-019-0805-0.

[5] R. C. Free et al., "A data-driven framework for clinical decision support applied to pneumonia management," *Front. Digit. Health*, vol. 5, no. October, 2023, doi: 10.3389/fdgth.2023.1237146.

[6] S. Arabia, "Critical Analysis of Harnessing Health Informatics Technology," *Chelonian Conservation and Biology*, vol. 17, pp. 930–944, 2022.

[7] C. Giordano, M. Brennan, B. Mohamed, P. Rashidi, F. Modave, and P. Tighe, "Accessing artificial intelligence for clinical decision-making," *Front. Digit. Health.*, vol. 3, no. June, pp. 1–9, 2021, doi: 10.3389/fdgth.2021.645232.

[8] F. Cascini, F. Santaroni, R. Lanzetti, G. Failla, A. Gentili, and W. Ricciardi, "Developing a data-driven approach in order to improve the safety and quality of patient care," *Front. Public Health.*, vol. 9, no. May, pp. 1–7, 2021, doi: 10.3389/fpubh.2021.667819.

[9] A. Black, T. Sahama, and R. Gajanayake, *eHealth-as-a-Service (eHaaS): A data-driven decision making approach in Australian context*, Studies in Health Technology and Informatics, Volume 205: e-Health – For Continuity of Care (pp. 915–919), 2014, doi: 10.3233/978-1-61499-432-9-915.

[10] A. L. Buczak, S. Babin, and L. Moniz, "Data-driven approach for creating synthetic electronic medical records," *BMC Med. Inform. Decis. Mak.*, vol. 10, no. 59, 2010, https://doi.org/10.1186/1472-6947-10-59.

[11] C. G. Macias, K. E. Remy, and A. J. Barda, "Utilizing big data from electronic health records in pediatric clinical care," *Pediatr. Res.*, vol. 93, no. 2, pp. 382–389, 2023, doi: 10.1038/s41390-022-02343-x.

[12] J. Sun et al., "Combining knowledge and data driven insights for identifying risk factors using electronic health records," *AMIA Annu. Symp. Proc.*, vol. 2012, pp. 901–910, 2012.

[13] C. Chakraborty, M. Bhattacharya, S. Pal, and S. S. Lee, "From machine learning to deep learning: Advances of the recent data-driven paradigm shift in medicine and healthcare," *Curr. Res. Biotechnol.*, vol. 7, no. November, p. 100164, 2024, doi: 10.1016/j.crbiot.2023.100164.

[14] K. A. Shastry and A. Shastry, "An integrated deep learning and natural language processing approach for continuous remote monitoring in digital health," *Decis. Anal. J.*, vol. 8, no. August, p. 100301, 2023, doi: 10.1016/j.dajour.2023.100301.

[15] Q. Cai, H. Wang, Z. Li, and X. Liu, "A survey on multimodal data-driven smart healthcare systems: Approaches and applications," *IEEE Access*, vol. 7, pp. 133583–133599, 2019, doi: 10.1109/ACCESS.2019.2941419.

[16] Y. Zhang, R. Padman, and N. Patel, "Paving the COWpath: Learning and visualizing clinical pathways from electronic health record data," *J. Biomed. Inform.*, vol. 58, pp. 186–197, 2015, doi: 10.1016/j.jbi.2015.09.009.

[17] Perfecto R. Ruaya Jr., "Data-driven healthcare: Evaluating the effectiveness of the Patient Record Management System at RHU-Del Carmen," *Int. J. Adv. Res. Sci. Commun. Technol.*, vol. 3, no. 2, pp. 552–561, 2023, doi: 10.48175/ijarsct-12178.

[18] J. Enticott, A. Johnson, and H. Teede, "Learning health systems using data to drive healthcare improvement and impact: A systematic review," *BMC Health Serv. Res.*, vol. 21, no. 1, pp. 1–16, 2021, doi: 10.1186/s12913-021-06215-8.

[19] N. Rieke et al., "The future of digital health with federated learning," *NPJ Digit. Med.*, vol. 3, no. 1, pp. 1–7, 2020, doi: 10.1038/s41746-020-00323-1.

[20] G. Parker and C. Parker, "Future of electronic health records: A challenge to maximize their utility," *SSRN Electron. J.*, p. 16, 2023, doi: 10.2139/ssrn.4457214.

[21] M. Khalifa, M. Albadawy, and U. Iqbal, "Advancing clinical decision support: The role of artificial intelligence across six domains," *Comput. Methods Programs Biomed. Updat.*, vol. 5, no. February, p. 100142, 2024, doi: 10.1016/j.cmpbup.2024.100142.

[22] R. P. Evans, L. D. Bryant, G. Russell, and K. Absolom, "Trust and acceptability of data-driven clinical recommendations in everyday practice: A scoping review," *Int. J. Med. Inform.*, vol. 183, p. 105342, 2024, doi: 10.1016/j.ijmedinf.2024.105342.

[23] A. Tsoukalas, T. Albertson, and I. Tagkopoulos, "From data to optimal decision making: A data-driven, probabilistic machine learning approach to decision support for patients with sepsis," *JMIR Med. Inform.*, vol. 3, no. 1, pp. 1–15, 2015, doi: 10.2196/medinform.3445.

[24] M. K. Ross, W. Wei, and L. Ohno-Machado, "'Big data' and the electronic health record," *Yearb. Med. Inform.*, vol. 23, pp. 97–104, 2014, doi: 10.15265/IY-2014-0003.

[25] Z. Chen et al., "Harnessing the power of clinical decision support systems: Challenges and opportunities," *Open Hear.*, vol. 10, no. 2, 2023, doi: 10.1136/openhrt-2023-002432.

[26] A. Epizitone, S. P. Moyane, and I. E. Agbehadji, "A data-driven paradigm for a resilient and sustainable integrated health information systems for health care applications," *J. Multidiscip. Healthc.*, vol. 16, pp. 4015–4025, 2023, doi: 10.2147/JMDH.S433299.

[27] P. Y. Wu, C. W. Cheng, C. D. Kaddi, J. Venugopalan, R. Hoffman, and M. D. Wang, "–Omic and electronic health record big data analytics for precision medicine," *IEEE Trans. Biomed. Eng.*, vol. 64, no. 2, pp. 263–273, 2017, doi: 10.1109/TBME.2016.2573285.

[28] H. Mo et al., "Desiderata for computable representations of electronic health records-driven phenotype algorithms," *J. Am. Med. Inform. Assoc.*, vol. 22, no. 6, pp. 1220–1230, 2015, doi: 10.1093/jamia/ocv112.

[29] N. Garcelon, A. Burgun, R. Salomon, and A. Neuraz, "Electronic health records for the diagnosis of rare diseases," *Kidney Int.*, vol. 97, no. 4, pp. 676–686, 2020, doi: 10.1016/j.kint.2019.11.037.

[30] N. Berros, F. El Mendili, Y. Filaly, and Y. El Bouzekri El Idrissi, "Enhancing Digital Health Services with Big Data Analytics," *Big Data Cogn. Comput.*, vol. 7, no. 2, pp. 64, 2023, doi: 10.3390/bdcc7020064.

[31] J. H. Chen, M. Alagappan, M. K. Goldstein, S. M. Asch, and R. B. Altman, "Decaying relevance of clinical data towards future decisions in data-driven inpatient clinical order sets," *Int. J. Med. Inform.*, vol. 102, pp. 71–79, 2017, doi: 10.1016/j.ijmedinf.2017.03.006.

[32] E. Shalom, Y. Shahar, and E. Lunenfeld, "An architecture for a continuous, user-driven, and data-driven application of clinical guidelines and its evaluation," *J. Biomed. Inform.*, vol. 59, pp. 130–148, 2016, doi: 10.1016/j.jbi.2015.11.006.

5 Telemedicine and Remote Monitoring
Expanding Access to Care

Fathimathul Rajeena P.P. and Shakeel Ahmed

5.1 INTRODUCTION

The advancement of technology has indeed affected almost all fields of work, with the healthcare sector being the main beneficiary. Telemedicine and mobile health (mHealth) have emerged as innovative technologies that can change the way people access and use healthcare services [1]. These state-of-the-art services use information and communication technology to overcome the problems of inequitable distribution of healthcare services in underdeveloped rural areas.

Telemedicine [2] and remote monitoring improve healthcare recordings by utilizing communication technologies at a distance. The term "telehealth" refers to remote consultations conducted using video-enabled devices and components. Remote monitoring means aggregating and analyzing patient health information through appliances and sensors at their homes, as well as periodic reporting to medical providers.

Telemedicine and remote monitoring have completely transformed health service delivery, making it easier for patients to reach out for services. They have made the linkage between patients and healthcare practitioners more effective than ever and are changing the traditional practice of healthcare. The integration of artificial intelligence (AI) into telehealthcare services and mobile healthcare is poised to fundamentally transform the healthcare landscape. This chapter delves into the problems and advancements in telehealth and remote monitoring under the influence of AI, further providing a conceptual framework that enables telehealth and remote monitoring.

5.2 TELEMEDICINE: A REVOLUTION IN HEALTHCARE DELIVERY

Telemedicine has expanded over the years and today it is offered through various technologies. Initially, telemedicine included phone calls whereby patients would engage with a health and wellness practitioner over the phone. However, with evolution, there is a significant increase in technology usage that centers on video calls, some apps and even devices which can be used to care for patients remotely.

For years, telemedicine has been a solution that some people used, even in the 1960s with different initiatives developed, to seek care, notably in far-off and

DOI: 10.1201/9781003516163-5

neglected areas. Although such technology-driven practices took a long time to be acknowledged, it was the growth of the internet together with digital technologies in the 21st century that encouraged the acceptance and use of telemedicine in the health sector. The 1990s and the early 21st century were such a period of a technological revolution where a lot of modernization took place with the advent of the use of the internet and digital technology. Telemedicine emerged from how a patient and a doctor interact through the telephone in a complicated network with video communication systems, intensive care unit upon hospital's electronic health system, and mobile applications for healthcare. The advent of broadband connections and smartphones also helped expedite the development of telemedicine. In the 2010s, telemedicine started to garner increased attention and even become a part of normal practices resulting from a unique mix of technological changes and sociological changes which provided easier healthcare [3].

5.2.1 Types of Telemedicine

Telemedicine can be classified as:

- **Synchronous Telemedicine:** Synchronous telemedicine defines the interaction that occurs between a patient and a healthcare provider in real time, most commonly over the phone or through a video link. This type of telemedicine allows for instant communication and the capacity to conduct real-time assessments and offer treatment. Examples of this platform include seeing the doctor through video link, engaging in teletherapy, or having specialty consultations with a doctor over the internet [4].
- **Asynchronous Telemedicine:** This involves the transmission of medical information, such as images or test results, without real-time interaction. The health data is sent by the patients, which is later reviewed by healthcare providers. This method is used in consultations where immediate feedback is not required, such as in dermatology or radiology [5].
- **Remote Monitoring:** Remote monitoring implies using technology to assess health parameters while away from the clinical environment. This encompasses the use of mobile phones with diagnostic capabilities, passive monitoring systems for patients in their homes and fitness gadgets. For the treatment of patients with chronic conditions such as diabetes, remote monitoring helps by allowing healthcare professionals to receive the information required to manage their patients better remotely [6].
- **Store-and-Forward:** Store-and-forward telemedicine sends clinical data electronically for review. This method comprises health professionals collecting and sending data via desktop or mobile devices. Better waiting times, faster second opinions, freed-up outpatient appointments, and fewer unnecessary medications and surgeries. The specialist may not examine the patient immediately, requiring an in-person or video appointment. Teleradiology,

teledermatology, retina screening, and patient–general practitioner portals are store-and-forward processes [7].

5.2.2 Benefits of Telemedicine

Important benefits of telemedicine are:

- **Improved Accessibility to Healthcare:** The main advantage of telemedicine is its approach to providing access to healthcare for people in remote and rural areas. Because telemedicine means no travel (and consultations can be provided remotely), patients can receive the medical expertise they may not find locally.
- **Convenience:** One simplest benefit of telemedicine is that the patient can see the doctor without necessarily having to leave the comfort of the house. This eliminates the requirement of time-consuming journeys and makes it easy for the patients to schedule their appointments. It also increases accessibility for those who are mobility-challenged or live in regions where transport options are limited.
- **Cost Savings:** Telemedicine cuts down on the costs of in-house visits by allowing broad consultations to be done at home, thus reducing healthcare expenses. This reduces the level of hospitalization rates by ensuring that the patients get their consultations and treatments before the health deterioration occurs.
- **Continuity of Care:** It is only when patients come back for chronic disease management and follow-ups, that the "culture" of continuity of care is fully realized. Patients may contact healthcare providers for appointment scheduling, medication refills, routine evaluations, as well as treatment adjustments as required.

5.2.3 Challenges and Limitations

Telemedicine also experiences some technological challenges, such as:

- **Technology Barriers:** High-speed internet and digital devices are the main aspects of telemedicine. The lack of these resources in rural areas can adversely affect providing the required treatment. So, it is a necessity to solve the technical issues to provide an equitable telemedicine service.
- **Regulatory and Reimbursement Issues:** Criteria for the use of telemedicine differ universally between countries, regions, and within individual healthcare systems. So, the conflicting policies that create hurdles in telemedicine adoption should be avoided as they may cause challenges for healthcare providers in obtaining compensation for their services.
- **Privacy and Security Concerns:** The use of telemedicine also has developed concerns about the privacy and security issues on patient's data. They must also secure telemedicine platforms as per privacy regulations – like the Health Insurance Portability and Accountability Act (HIPAA) in the United States – or else sensitive health information will be at risk and with it goes patient trust.

- **Quality of Care:** One of the concerns both patients and providers have is regarding the quality of care in a remote setting. Tele consultations are likely to miss out on the physical components associated with in-office appointments which may lead to increased diagnostic errors and treatment failure. Telemedicine services must be of high quality if they are to succeed and gain acceptance.

5.3 REMOTE MONITORING: ENHANCING PATIENT MANAGEMENT

Remote monitoring is the technology used to perform remote patient monitoring. Using an array of tools and devices, this provides health data gathered for analysis by healthcare providers to effectively manage conditions, timely intervene when necessary, and ultimately improve patient outcomes. The main aim of remote monitoring is better patient management and the provision of real-time data that can be used, for instance in personalized care. It is precisely in scenarios such as dealing with chronic diseases and delivering post-acute care to preventive health, that this approach can have a fundamental role. These data by electronic means, to gather and analyze, are clinically referred to as remote monitoring.

5.3.1 Importance in Modern Healthcare

In modern healthcare, remote monitoring has become increasingly important due to several factors:

- **Increase in Chronic Diseases:** As chronic diseases such as diabetes, cardiac, and respiratory conditions become very common, remote monitoring can be used to manage those proactively.
- **Healthcare Accessibility:** By overcoming the barriers related to distance and time, remote monitoring extends healthcare services to patients in underserved areas, thereby reducing the access inequity among populations.
- **Cost-Effectiveness:** This can reduce the cost of care without influencing the nature of healthcare or increasing it, providing efficient data transmission for patient monitoring, and reducing the need for frequent in-person visits and hospital admissions.
- **Empowering Patients:** With remote monitoring, patients have more assistance in controlling their health, increasing the likelihood that they will adhere to their treatment plans, and ultimately boost health results.

5.3.2 Historical Context and Evolution

The historical antecedent of remote monitoring is grounded in the early days of telemedicine and has leveraged base-level technologies such as telephone consultations and a few data-sharing medical devices for distant patient care, respectively. Early examples include the telegraph and telephone when they first started to be mentioned as a method of contacting healthcare workers across distances (patient care). As early as the 1960s and 1970s, rudimentary remote monitoring devices (such as electrocardiograms (ECGs)) existed that could wirelessly communicate back data over traditional telephone lines. Many of those first-generation devices were designed for very narrow use cases and came out of a research perspective. Progress in remote monitoring took place because of the digital transformation. The real transformation happened in the 1980s and 1990s when digital technology, specifically with the advent of the internet, marched into every sphere of life. The ability to be more robust with digital health records, better data transmission ability, and the creation of some early wearable devices were indeed key considerations in remote monitoring. Wearable technology has grown in popularity after 2000, with the introduction of consumer-grade wearable devices like fitness trackers and heart rate monitors. These devices evolved and became more tech-enabled to work along with mobile applications and healthcare platforms. mHealth came in the 2010s when smartphones and mobile apps started gaining popularity, changing remote monitoring once again by giving individuals the means to engage with providers on health measurement information that could be sent from one phone to another. Remote monitoring technologies have matured rapidly due to increased connectivity in a growing digital age. Key impacts include increased communication and advanced analytics. The growth of high-speed internet and cellular technology has made it much easier to send data from remote monitoring devices to healthcare professionals. The incorporation of advanced analytics and machine learning algorithms has improved the ability to analyze and act upon remote monitoring data which allows for more actionable, accurate insights. Increased consumer awareness and patient demands for health management lead to innovations in remote monitoring technologies, diverse devices, and applications [8].

5.3.3 Types of Remote Monitoring Technologies

Different types of remote monitoring technologies available are:

- **Wearable Devices:** Wearable devices are one of the most common remote monitoring technologies. They include fitness trackers such as Fitbit and Garmin, which monitor physical activity (steps), sleep patterns, and heart rate. They track how physically active you are every day and your overall health. Smartwatches like the Apple Watch and Samsung Galaxy Watch offer ECG monitoring, fall detection, and even blood oxygen level tracking. Wearable biosensors, like continuous glucose monitors for diabetes management, offer real-time data on specific health metrics which allows for personalized treatment adaptations.
- **Home-Based Monitoring Tools**: Home-based monitoring tools are specifically made for patients at home. This group includes blood pressure monitors, to measure patients' blood pressure and send data to healthcare providers for acute or chronic hypertension tracking and management. Pulse oximeters check the oxygen-carrying blood level of the body and are useful for monitoring respirational status and detecting treatment outcomes.

- **mHealth Apps:** mHealth apps are applications assisting in the supervision and communication of health issues. Health tracking apps allow users to keep track of diet, exercise, and sleep habits among other health metrics. Medication management apps give you reminders to take your medications and allow you to follow your medication schedule. Telehealth apps are software that assists in having virtual meetings along with conversations with medical consultants.
- **Advanced Monitoring Systems:** Advanced monitoring systems bring together an array of technology and can deliver complete solutions. This includes integrated health platforms, that aggregate data from various channels such as monitoring devices, EHRs, and analytics to present a complete picture of patient health, remote monitoring systems, that allow healthcare providers to monitor and manage many patients at the same time (real-time alerts, data visualization, etc.), and TeleICU Systems, that facilitate monitoring of critically ill patients in intensive care units, aggregating data from different sensors and devices and remotely managing the patient.

5.3.4 Applications and Benefits

Remote monitoring is used in a variety of areas such as:

- **Chronic Disease Management:** Remote monitoring is effective in managing chronic diseases like cardiovascular disease, diabetes, and respiratory conditions like chronic obstructive pulmonary disease and asthma [9, 10].
- **Post-Acute and Post-Surgical Care**: Post-surgical monitoring for patients recovering from surgery using remote monitoring tools is helpful to track vital signs, manage pain, and report any complications to the respective healthcare providers. Virtual follow-up appointments allow healthcare providers to assess the progress of their recovery, adjust treatments, and address any concerns without requiring in-person visits [11, 12].
- **Preventive Health and Wellness:** Wearable devices and health apps encourage users to adopt healthy behaviors, such as regular exercise and balanced nutrition, by providing feedback and setting goals. Continuous monitoring of health indicators can lead to the early discovery of possible health problems, which in turn enables prompt action and the prevention of more severe disorders [13, 14].
- **Elderly and Disability Care**: Wearable devices, along with accelerometers and gyroscopes, detect falls and immediately alert the caregivers or emergency services. Remote monitoring systems track daily activities and routines, helping in managing care for the elderly or disabled individuals and detecting any changes in health status [15, 16].

5.3.5 Challenges and Limitations

A few limitations of remote monitoring are:

- **Reliability and Validity of Data:** The verification and validation of remotely gathered information pose a major problem. Regular maintenance and

calibration of monitoring equipment should be exercised to avoid compromising the quality of the information collected. Differences in the quality of data can be attributed to user error, equipment failure, or changes in environmental conditions [17, 18].
- **Patient Adherence and Engagement:** One of the main goals in effective care provision is to ensure patients follow the inner and outer boundaries of remote monitoring systems. Some of the relevant encouraging methods for patient adherence and participation in clinical remote monitoring programs include educating the patient, reminders, and encouragement. Information and support that are directed toward the patients for the usage of monitoring devices and applications can also help them take control of their health [19].
- **Privacy and Security Concerns:** A common concern when it comes to remote monitoring is ensuring the confidentiality and security of health information. There should be precautions taken to ensure that such telehealth systems respect laws protecting private health information, for instance, compliance with HIPAA. These can mostly be carried out through the organization of strong internet security measures including encryption and secure access of data to prevent unapproved data entry and other forms of data compromise [20, 21].
- **Integration and System Compatibility:** Ensuring that remote monitoring systems integrate effortlessly with existing healthcare systems and workflows is important for efficient data management and care delivery. Addressing interoperability challenges requires the adoption of standardized protocols and collaboration between device manufacturers, healthcare providers, and technology developers [22, 23].

5.3.6 Integration with Healthcare Systems

- **EHRs**: These are well-established records to include remote monitoring data with patient health to enable coordinated care and informed decisions. EHR systems should have the ability to integrate remote monitoring data to help guide clinical decisions (e.g., changing the course of treatments based on real-time data) [24, 25].
- **Interoperability and Data Integration:** Data from various monitoring devices/systems can be easily integrated comprising standardized data topology with Health Level 7 Fast Healthcare Interoperability Resource (HL7 & FHIR) to standard definition sets. Healthcare providers, patients, and monitoring systems can share data securely with each other, leading to improved care collaboration and continuity [26].

5.4 FUTURE DIRECTIONS AND INNOVATIONS

In the future of telemedicine, technology is likely to keep getting better. AI and machine learning are currently becoming a very important part of telemedicine. These technologies can improve the accuracy of diagnoses, make treatment suggestions more relevant to each person, and make routine chores easier. For example, AI algorithms help healthcare workers to make decisions by suggesting alternatives. The range of services telemedicine provides is growing systematically. As part of this, telemedicine could be combined with other health services, like telepsychiatry or remote medical appointments. Telemedicine will work better and reach more people if it is connected to bigger healthcare networks and systems. For telemedicine to keep growing, ongoing work must be done to solve problems with regulations and policies. Standardizing telemedicine rules, making reimbursement policies better, and making sure data security are all things that can help make the setting more favorable for telemedicine use and acceptance [27, 28].

5.5 INTEGRATING ARTIFICIAL INTELLIGENCE TO TELEHEALTH AND REMOTE MONITORING

AI is revolutionizing patient care through telemedicine and remote monitoring, enabling healthcare providers to monitor patients' vital signs in real time, intervene when needed, and provide timely, effective treatment to prevent complications. AI uses in healthcare are shown in Figure 5.1.

Several healthcare fields use AI to increase patient engagement and education. AI-powered chatbots [29] have been used to answer patients' enquiries and provide them

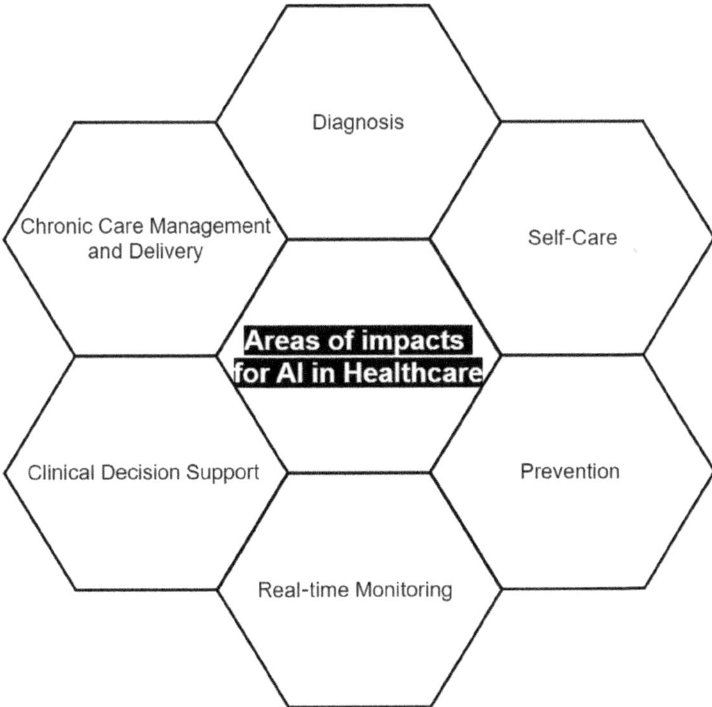

FIGURE 5.1 Areas of the Impact of AI on Healthcare.

with regularly updated information on their health status, treatment alternatives, and health-related advances. This increases patients' basic health knowledge and helps them understand their health situation, making them more likely to take charge of their self-care.

As healthcare AI improves, it may be used to improve operations. AI's future is limitless with AI-powered medical gadgets and clever algorithms that can understand massive datasets. Deep learning (DL)-based AI is being utilized to diagnose diseases faster, provide customized treatments, automate drug discovery, and enhance disease diagnostics [30]. It improves treatment outcomes, safety, and pricing for effective healthcare delivery. WHO defines telehealth as utilizing information and communication technology (ICT) to deliver healthcare. It promotes individual and community health via diagnosis, treatment, prevention, research, and education. This real-time or store-and-forward method improves accessibility, cost-effectiveness, time savings, and infection risk. Telemedicine surged during the COVID-19 pandemic, with many healthcare institutions switching to virtual visits for chronically ill patients [31]. Telemedicine services like forward triage, decreasing needless emergency department visits, and minimizing exposure helped control the illness. Telemedicine, with AI integration, reduced physician burnout post pandemic. AI algorithms improve image analysis, remote monitoring, and patient care via smartphones and wearable devices [32].

Telemedicine, patient screening, triage, test results notification, and medical guidance use AI-driven chatbots. AI-based solutions may detect particular diseases or make differential diagnoses based on patient data, helping physicians make accurate diagnoses and streamline workflow [33]. Technology reluctance, lack of access, privacy concerns, usability challenges, and inadequate accuracy hinder AI-based telemedicine adoption. To improve patient care, initiatives should provide user-friendly interfaces, fund technological access, protect data, increase compatibility, and monitor AI applications by physicians. Research should improve telemedicine and AI to better serve all patients.

AI in healthcare might lead to innovation. It might transform patient care and enhance health. As we progress toward a more connected digital environment, AI will benefit healthcare. Many healthcare services offer virtual medical consultations via video conferencing. However, AI diagnostic technologies might improve telemedicine by offering accurate diagnoses without physical consultations. AI algorithms might evaluate patients using medical imaging, test findings, and vital signs. This breakthrough might make telehealth services more accessible and effective, especially in areas with few healthcare practitioners.

Uniform data gathering and analysis are also important for telehealth AI. AI algorithms must be trained on large, high-quality data to work well. However, healthcare data quality might vary; therefore, AI systems may be trained on biased, incomplete datasets. Such issues can be rectified using standardized procedures for collecting and analyzing data as this ensures the consistency and reliability of data collected and that the datasets involve a cross-section of the patient base. The next steps will involve the ethics of AI in telemedicine. Extending and refining the existing literature AI bias issues are ethical issues concerning discrimination within AI systems and images or data used to train AI systems. To inform clinicians and patients about telehealth systems with integrated AI components, future work should aim at developing AI systems that are explainable in both functionality and capability. AI telemedicine systems may also relieve some of the health inequities. AI systems may be less successful in determining the health conditions of minorities. Future studies should seek to fill such gaps and support the development of AI algorithms by carrying out studies that include diverse populations within the study that will feed into the AI algorithms [34].

Telehealth systems that incorporate AI technologies prove useful. AI is expected to bring changes to the healthcare system by increasing the quality of care, and effectiveness, and reducing costs also. In the future, telehealth systems that incorporate AI should be studied concerning how they impact healthcare services, healthcare costs, and the satisfaction of healthcare providers. Researchers may hope to concentrate on predicting models empowered by AI systems. These predictive models will be used to find individuals who are likely to develop certain diseases so that doctors can manage these individuals with the hope of preventing the disease from occurring. Possibly, the data mining systems can use behavioral patterns, medical, and genetic data to locate individuals likely to develop diabetes, heart disease, or cancer. Early intervention measures by healthcare practitioners can aid in disease prevention and also enhance patient outcomes by pointing out populations at risk of various catastrophes. The possibility of advanced virtual assistants to enhance patient experience during telehealth consultations should be encouraging in formulating telehealth policies. Virtual assistants are programmed to field queries from patients, offer them medically related guidance, and set up appointments. Unquestionably, these assistants may use AI technology to optimize and expedite care for patients and on-board staff attending to routine tasks. With the design of virtual assistants, the major concern should be the protection and confidentiality of the patient's data.

5.5.1 Challenges with Artificial Intelligence-Powered Wearable Devices

AI-powered wearable gadgets also present challenges such as

- **Data Privacy and Security:** One of the most critical aspects that we need to keep safe is the patient data collected by smart devices. This health data gathered by AI devices is potentially crucial and should be treated with the utmost care.
- **Regulatory Compliance:** Designing and utilizing smart technology based on AI can become problematic when it comes to crossing the limits of healthcare legislation such as HIPAA. The rules for data privacy and medical devices are both key to follow, yet tricky to get right.
- **Accuracy and Reliability of Data**: AI systems require information that is needed to track patients well. In the "real world," it is very difficult to maintain real-time accuracy and reliability of statistics from wearables.
- **User Acceptance and Engagement:** It is a challenge to drive consistent use or interaction of the AI-powered wearable health trackers. A holistic view of the user experience and the safety implications of how smart technologies integrate into life are also encouraged.

- **Interoperability and Integration:** Portable AI devices have a challenging time connecting to the systems of hospitals or EHRs. For patient monitoring data to ever be useful, it has to be easy for end users and hospital IT systems to exchange and use.
- **Ethical and Legal:** It is challenging to address ethical dilemmas in monitoring patients with AI, such as obtaining informed consent from them, being transparent on how decisions are made by algorithms, and using the findings that AI offers wisely.
- **Longer-term Sustainability:** It is not easy to determine the long-term sustainability of AI-enabled wearable technology, as such aspects as battery life, the tendency to break, reliability, support, and maintenance need to be considered.

5.6 ARTIFICIAL INTELLIGENCE-ENHANCED HEALTH CARE SYSTEM – A CONCEPTUAL FRAMEWORK

Here we discuss a conceptual framework of an AI-enhanced smart healthcare system for making healthcare decisions. A sophisticated healthcare network links individuals, resources, and healthcare institutions, adeptly overseeing and intelligently adapting to the needs of the medical environment. This is accomplished by employing technologies like wearables, the Internet of Things, and mobile internet to gain real-time access to information. The main goal of this smart system is to make healthcare services available to patients whenever and wherever they need them. It also makes sure that the smart system network is secure to prevent malicious attacks on patient security and privacy. Here, three design artefacts are suggested as shown in Figure 5.2.

A shared screen is first (for access). By facilitating patient involvement in decision-making and honoring their choices and preferences, this shared-screen feature improves the provision of patient-centered care.

Second, the inclusion of voice recognition abilities is crucial for communication purposes. This technology alleviates the need for manual input by interpreting spoken commands, transcribing them, and offering selectable options to users. By streamlining system usage, this feature accelerates interactions and treatments, allowing physicians to focus more on patients, and ultimately enhancing patient-centered care.

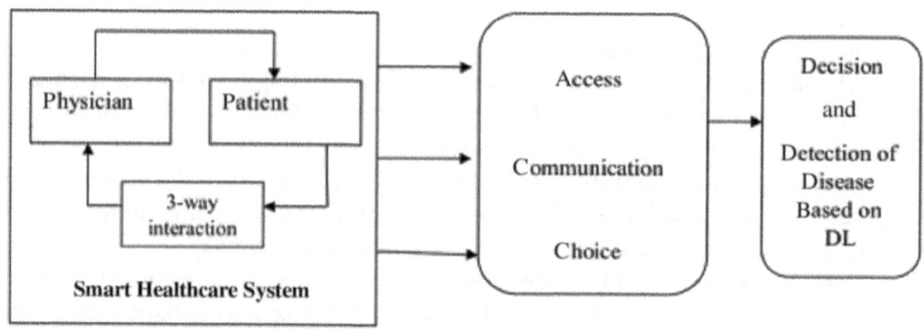

FIGURE 5.2 Conceptual Framework for a Smart Health Care System.

The third element comprises choices or decisions. With their wants and preferences considered, the patient is empowered to engage in the treatment process because of the choice option in this design. Because of the way this artefact is designed, the system can offer several options based on user triggers. Questions could be used as triggers.

HIPAA, overseeing the handling of patient health data to ensure privacy and security, stands as an illustration of regulations that systems must comply with. In a hospital setting, the architectural layout supports the smooth transfer and processing of information, aiding both patients and physicians.

As in Figure 5.3, the healthcare system, driven by DL, operates as a pathway that processes data to assess vital signs in patients for diagnosis and treatment. A model for collecting device data acquires information from sophisticated medical devices that reflect a patient's vital signs and condition, transferring it to a data preprocessing model. Utilizing suitable sampling frequencies, this preprocessing model captures and stores the data within a specified range. Machine learning, trained with this data, enables real-time disease monitoring and detection. The training data contains labeled information on various illnesses and healthy conditions to comprehend data patterns across scenarios. Physiological data collected during testing will be analyzed using the previously trained machine learning model to identify diseases or patient conditions. This data processing pipeline forms the context for delineating our assault strategy a competitive endeavor aimed at altering the original DL model through data processing or collection.

Foundational learning enables machines to analyze diverse data types, including audio, video, and images, which can significantly enhance medical diagnostics and patient care by facilitating timely and accurate disease detection.

To achieve effective machine learning outcomes, a comprehensive system must be designed and developed, emphasizing the importance of proper planning in the abstract design phase. This underscores the critical role of data pre-processing, which involves cleaning and validating real-life data to eliminate inaccuracies such as missing values or out-of-range entries. Failure to address these issues can lead to erroneous outputs, potentially resulting in serious medical errors.

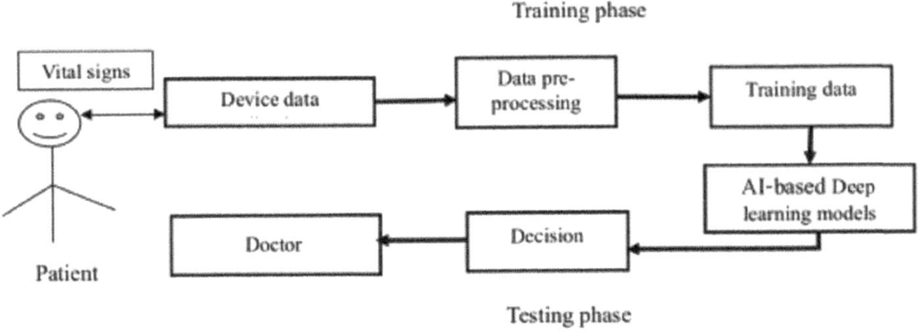

FIGURE 5.3 DL Driven Healthcare System.

Furthermore, the process where data from various sources are merged and corrected is essential for ensuring the integrity of the information used in machine learning models. Pre-processing algorithms are employed to refine this data, applying machine learning or DL techniques to create predictive models. These models undergo rigorous testing with separate test data to ensure their reliability before being deployed in real-world applications [35].

5.7 USE CASES: ARTIFICIAL INTELLIGENCE IN TELEMEDICINE AND REMOTE MONITORING

AI integration in remote monitoring is improving healthcare by enhancing patient care and efficiency. Remote monitoring uses technology to monitor patients remotely, reducing in-person visits. AI algorithms analyze patient data to detect trends and anomalies, improving early intervention.

Let's examine some use cases where AI is becoming the future in telehealth and remote monitoring.

5.7.1 Early Detection of Health Deterioration

Early detection of health deterioration through AI-enabled remote monitoring is very important for people with serious long-term conditions or who are healing from short-term illnesses. It allows for timely treatment, fewer hospitalizations, better patient results, and data-driven insights for healthcare workers. AI systems gather information from gadgets and patient reports to set personalized criteria and thus identify the changes in real time. Pattern recognition, anomaly detection, and prediction analysis are some of the important aspects. AI has become an essential part of healthcare, as it helps find health problems earlier, which improves patient results and saves money for healthcare systems [36]. Monitoring and analyzing patient data all the time allow doctors act quickly, which lowers the risk of problems and raises patients' quality of life. However, problems like algorithm accuracy, data security, and getting patients to participate must be solved in order for the AI-enabled remote tracking systems to be used successfully.

5.7.1.1 Essential Elements in Early Detection Enhanced by Artificial Intelligence

The essential elements in early detection using AI include,

- **Real-Time Continuous Monitoring:** Wearable gadgets and sensors are consistently monitoring and collecting patient data. AI systems with real-time tracking and data-collecting capabilities can accurately identify or detect minute variations from previous measurements.
- **Pattern Recognition:** AI models can interpret and recognize patterns accurately. The analysis of data patterns, such as irregular heart rhythms, unexpected spikes or declines in vital signs, and abrupt changes in activity levels, enables AI to identify possible indicators of health deterioration that may otherwise go unnoticed.

- **Anomaly Detection:** The field of anomaly detection involves training AI systems to identify deviations from the normal range. Upon detecting an anomaly, the AI system promptly alerts healthcare professionals, enabling them to take immediate action and initiate an intervention.
- **Predictive Analysis**: AI systems can detect present anomalies and determine future health issues from past data trends. For example, when a patient's heart rate decreases or increases gradually, AI can alert the healthcare professionals.

5.7.1.2 Advantages and Challenges of Utilizing Artificial Intelligence in Early Detection

- Allows fast response actions due to early detection of changes in health.
- Able to stop the progression of health problems and their severity.
- This could decrease the likelihood of hospitalization.
- Performs proper care on the patients at their homes, hence reducing costs.
- Increases patient satisfaction for early prevention of any health complications and improved quality of life.
- Daily analysis of the patient's information helps in making changes in the treatment plan, dosage, and lifestyle adopted by the patient.
- The accuracy of the algorithms is important to reduce the occurrence of false-positive and false-negative rates.
- Better security measures are required to protect patient data.
- Active user engagement is important for successful early detection in remote monitoring.
- Patients should regularly be wearing the devices for better and steady monitoring.

5.7.2 Personalized Treatment and Predictive Analytics for High-Risk Patients

Personalized treatment plans are extremely important for managing chronic conditions and complex medical scenarios. Remote monitoring with AI is also reshaping the way physicians develop personalized treatment plans. AI can incorporate information, such as a patient's medical history, genetic makeup, and lifestyle choices to generate personalized care plans. Critical aspects of personalized treatment plans powered by AI include data aggregation, predictive analytics, risk stratification, and suggestions for when to act. Benefits associated with AI-supported personalized treatment plans include that they can be consistently personalized, facilitate better decision-making, are amended in real time, foster patient engagement, and promote efficiency of resource utilization [37].

However, challenges related to unreliable data and data integration, ethical considerations, and limitations in the physician–patient relationship must be resolved. Successful implementation of predictive analytics reflecting AI in a patient-centered personalized treatment system relies on ensuring that data is accurate and comprehensive, navigating potential data privacy breaches and problems with the AI system integrity, and emphasizing the significance of the provider–patient relationship.

AI and remote monitoring offer predictive analytics to identify high-risk patients, anticipate healthcare crises, and prompt healthcare staff to conduct pre-emptive care once these events are predicted. AI is designed to efficiently analyze large data sources and identify trends to predict individuals about potential future health statuses. The following components contribute to AI-supported predictive analytics: data capturing, machine learning algorithms, risk stratification, and alerts for potential health decline. The implementation of predictive analytics is highly contingent on data access, algorithmic transparency, and what is most salient in addressing the ethical delivery of care to patients [38].

The use of AI in oncology has been developed largely in the area of personalized cancer treatment, particularly in breast cancer [39]. AI systems can evaluate multi-data, medical imaging, and EHRs to develop personalized treatment plans. Predictive modeling evaluates how patients will respond to treatment and, within that, what is the most efficient treatment in terms of chemotherapy or targeted therapy. Other systems and predictive models suggest which targeted therapies should be used or what chemotherapy to include. Systems built on AI can also execute real-time monitoring and determine when treatments should be changed.

AI can be used in real time to manage cancer treatment response and to manage side effects. It is capable of evaluating the tumor size and biomarkers to ensure that the treatment is working or provide alternative strategies. AI is used to predict and manage many of the side effects often lowering dosages of chemotherapeutical agents or managing side effects to improve the quality of life. AI can empower a repository of personalized therapy plans based on genomic profiles, a more efficient reasonable allocation of resources, improved patient outcomes, and possibly increased patient satisfaction due to a legible transparent treatment plan [39].

5.7.3 Enhanced Medication Adherence

Non-adherence to medication is one of the most common problems in healthcare. The result of this is higher treatment costs and bad outcomes. This can be greatly improved by integrating AI in remote monitoring so that the patients are under continuous and personalized intervention. AI checks the activity from the patient behavior, individual help updates, and potential challenges in adherence. AI humanizes adherence by following along with patients and providing real-time feedback so that they remain within their medication schedules to improve treatment outcomes, lower mortality, and health risks, as well as reducing costs. Further, AI helps in maintaining the health of patients with some insights for healthcare providers. Nevertheless, for a successful adoption of AI-driven medication adherence solutions, several obstacles like patient privacy trust and access to the technology, user acceptance, and cultural considerations will need to be overcome [40].

Poor medication adherence can result in poor health outcomes and increased hospitalizations (and therefore healthcare costs). AI technologies are stepping up to the great challenge of medication adherence and its many fronts.

5.7.3.1 How Artificial Intelligence Enhances Medication Adherence?

AI applications provide reminders and notifications to patients, considering their medication schedules, preferences, and behaviors. For instance, applications such as Medisafe [41] employ machine learning algorithms to examine patient data and forecast reminders to enhance the probability of adherence. AI-powered voice assistants, available as incorporated components of smart speakers, can deliver immediate reminders and address enquiries regarding medicine, therefore facilitating patients in maintaining their drug regimens.

Behavioral patterns refer to the statistical analysis of medication-taking behavior by AI systems, including instances of skipped doses or inconsistent scheduling. Through the identification of these patterns, AI may forecast and notify healthcare professionals of possible non-adherence, therefore enabling early intervention. AdhereTech [42] uses AI to examine patient data and pinpoint those with a high likelihood of not adhering to treatment. This allows focused interventions, such as further assistance or counseling, to tackle particular difficulties in adherence.

Automated dispensing using smart pill dispensers that incorporate AI, like the one from MediSprout [43], can monitor the timing of drug intake and offer feedback. Furthermore, these devices can alert carers or healthcare professionals in the event of missing or wrongly administered dosages. Wearables integrated with AI can track physiological reactions and drug consumption. For example, Proteus Digital Health [44] has created a system in which ingestible sensors and wearable patches collaborate to evaluate compliance and offer immediate feedback.

Behavioral adaptation refers to the ability of AI systems to modify their reminders and suggestions by considering patient input and changes in adherence habits. For instance, if a patient does not care for the reminders, the system may modify the time or mode of communication to enhance involvement. Adaptive learning facilitates customization to suit individual requirements. AI with EHRs can provide a far more comprehensive perspective on patient health and treatment adherence. This enables enhanced care coordination and helps healthcare practitioners to make better decisions.

5.7.3.2 Benefits of Artificial Intelligence in Medication Adherence

Personalized and timely reminders have shown an increase in medication compliance rates, which leads to improved health outcomes and fewer hospitalizations. Through predictive analytics and behavioral monitoring, these tools can help detect adherence challenges so that healthcare providers and patients can recognize the issue early and act in advance. Immediate response among the patient is improved. AI can give deep data-driven insights related to the factors that influence medication-taking behaviors, and also help in developing innovative tools and interventions for supporting adherence. Over time, as the technology landscape changes, we believe that AI-powered solutions will become increasingly important in driving better patient outcomes and improving medication management.

5.7.4 Generative Artificial Intelligence and Healthcare Use Cases

Generative AI (GenAI) like ChatGPT is changing healthcare analytics by using DL algorithms to detect unstructured datasets like clinical recordings, diagnostic images, and so on. Some of the key applications ofthis potential technology include extracting vital clinical data, automating tasks, and functioning as a revolutionizer system in healthcare. However, it must be done carefully – within the parameters of existing data strategy and AI journey including critical elements of data security and regulatory compliance that determine patient benefit. Although there are possible risks and biases, GenAI experiences are something you cannot ignore.

Industry leaders and practitioners should evaluate the landscape, use data to anticipate challenges, correct for risks and biases, and emphasize people and partnerships to guide GenAI through the era of healthcare that lies ahead. Strategic assessment and ethical employment of GenAI at a systemic level in health systems can drive better patient experiences, superior levels of equity, and an unparalleled level of effectiveness. So, by promoting responsible adoption, healthcare can start to change for the better [45].

5.7.4.1 Key Roles and Benefits of Generative Artificial Intelligence in Revolutionizing Telemedicine

The essential roles and advantages of GenAI in the healthcare sector, especially concerning telemedicine, include [46]:

- **Virtual Consultation and Improved Patient Engagement:** GenAI consultations enhanced patient engagement and communication by providing a more authentic and engaging experience.
- **Improvements to the Telehealth Infrastructure:** GenAI-enhanced virtual assistants and chatbots can complete routine tasks, set appointments, and communicate information contributing to an effective telehealth infrastructure that flows seamlessly.
- **Patient Monitoring:** GenAI can monitor patient health with remote sensor systems to assure patient health and send alerts, notifications, and updates to caregivers.
- **Diagnostic Accuracy:** Diagnosing patients, particularly through imaging studies and examination of health data, is among the areas GenAI will excel and improve operationalization to diagnostic accuracy, with health professionals contributing to optimal diagnosis.
- **Patient Education and Support:** Interactive health platforms that integrate GenAI could automate the development of individualized patient education content and follow-up conversations.
- **Scalability and Flexibility:** The introduction of GenAI-based services to the telemedicine platform makes scaling the service dependent on demand and enables flexibility in demand in health services.
- **Data Protection and Privacy:** It will enable the development of secure telehealth architecture to promote data protection and privacy of patients.
- **Cost Savings and Resource Utilization:** Patient utilization of health facilities supported by GenAI will be savings in health use for patients and resource utilization improvements and developments in health facilities.

5.7.4.2 Challenges with Generative Artificial Intelligence in Healthcare

Some of the challenges that arise, when we consider the integration of GenAI solutions with existing healthcare systems and workflows, are compatibility and interoperability. Today, healthcare systems have different formats, standards, and protocols for data, making it hard to implement AI solutions. Further, making certain that the AI technology will match up with current clinical workflows and practices is essential for successful deployment. On the other hand, health professionals have to be trained to use AI and believe in its recommendations. Healthcare is one of the many sectors in which such GenAI technologies can be transformational, from drug discovery to diagnostics to personalized medicine and data augmentation. Getting the full value of GenAI will require overcoming data quality, ethics, and system integration challenges. The GenAI integration into healthcare will further augment patient care, improve operations, and foster innovation in medical research and treatment.

5.8 CONCLUSION

Healthcare has completely changed with the revolution in telemedicine and remote monitoring, allowing greater access, increased patient engagement, and promoting care continuity. When AI is combined with any of these, it further increases its power and gives the way for new approaches to more personalized proactive healthcare. But corollary to the advancements in these areas is confronting their challenges and ethical implications as well; both of which are mandatory for a prospective global health advancement. The future of telemedicine and remote monitoring, fueled by AI, is likely to further revolutionize healthcare delivery, providing unimaginable access and personalization more cost-effectively. The path forward will require continued study, thoughtful regulations, and cautious adherence to ethical standards as we continue to evolve our understanding of the possibilities of these technologies in driving a better healthcare system for all. Telemedicine has now become an indispensable part of modern healthcare bringing immense advantages and progressive solutions to problems. Telemedicine is on track to be central in the future of healthcare as technology advances and the delivery of healthcare changes.

REFERENCES

[1] A. Haleem, M. Javaid, R. P. Singh, and R. Suman, "Telemedicine for healthcare: Capabilities, features, barriers, and applications," *Sensors International*, vol. 2, p. 100117, Jan. 2021, doi: 10.1016/j.sintl.2021.100117.

[2] "International Medical Center Hospital," *International Medical Center*. www.imc.med.sa/telemedicine (accessed Jul. 19, 2024).

[3] M. A. Hyder and J. Razzak, "Telemedicine in the United States: An introduction for students and residents," *Journal of Medical Internet Research*, vol. 22, no. 11, p. e20839, Nov. 2020, doi: 10.2196/20839.

[4] "Synchronous direct-to-consumer telehealth," *telehealth.hhs.gov*, Oct. 28, 2022. https://telehealth.hhs.gov/providers/best-practice-guides/direct-to-consumer/synchronous-direct-to-consumer-telehealth (accessed Jul. 20, 2024).

[5] "What is asynchronous telemedicine?," *Talking HealthTech*, Mar. 08, 2022. www.talkinghealthtech.com/glossary/asynchronous-telemedicine (accessed Jul. 20, 2024).

[6] C. Hood, N. Sikka, C. M. Van, and S. Mossburg, "Remote patient monitoring," *PSNet*, Mar. 15, 2023. https://psnet.ahrq.gov/perspective/remote-patient-monitoring (accessed Jun. 15, 2024).

[7] "Store and forward," *Telehealth.* www.telehealth.org.nz/health-provider/what-is-telehealth/store-and-forward/ (accessed Jun. 22, 2024).

[8] J. Murphy, "History of remote patient monitoring: 1800–2024," *Tenovi*, Sep. 23, 2024. www.tenovi.com/remote-patient-monitoring-telehealth-history-future/ (accessed Sep. 25, 2024).

[9] O. Tolu-Akinnawo, F. Ezekwueme, and T. Awoyemi, "Telemedicine in cardiology: Enhancing access to care and improving patient outcomes," *Cureus*, Jun. 2024, doi: 10.7759/cureus.62852.

[10] J. Dunn, A. Coravos, M. Fanarjian, G. S. Ginsburg, and S. R. Steinhubl, "Remote digital health technologies for improving the care of people with respiratory disorders," *The Lancet Digital Health*, vol. 6, no. 4, pp. e291–e298, Apr. 2024, doi: 10.1016/s2589-7500(23)00248-0.

[11] A. Spaulding et al., "Postsurgical remote patient monitoring outcomes and perceptions: A mixed-methods assessment," *Mayo Clinic Proceedings Innovations Quality & Outcomes*, vol. 6, no. 6, pp. 574–583, Dec. 2022, doi: 10.1016/j.mayocpiqo.2022.09.005.

[12] M. McGillion et al., "Postoperative remote automated monitoring and virtual hospital-to-home care system following cardiac and major vascular surgery: User testing study," *Journal of Medical Internet Research*, vol. 22, no. 3, p. e15548, Mar. 2020, doi: 10.2196/15548.

[13] A. Żarnowski, M. Jankowski, and M. Gujski, "Use of mobile apps and wearables to monitor diet, weight, and physical activity: A cross-sectional survey of adults in Poland," *Medical Science Monitor*, vol. 28, Aug. 2022, doi: 10.12659/msm.937948.

[14] Y. Liao, C. Thompson, S. Peterson, J. Mandrola, and M. S. Beg, "The future of wearable technologies and remote monitoring in health care," *American Society of Clinical Oncology Educational Book*, vol. 39, pp. 115–121, May 2019, doi: 10.1200/edbk_238919.

[15] P. Kulurkar, C. K. Dixit, V. C. Bharathi, A. Monikavishnuvarthini, A. Dhakne, and P. Preethi, "AI based elderly fall prediction system using wearable sensors: A smart home-care technology with IOT," *Measurement Sensors*, vol. 25, p. 100614, Feb. 2023, doi: 10.1016/j.measen.2022.100614.

[16] N. T. Newaz and E. Hanada, "The methods of fall detection: A literature review," *Sensors*, vol. 23, no. 11, p. 5212, May 2023, doi: 10.3390/s23115212.

[17] D. R. Bassett, A. Rowlands, and S. G. Trost, "Calibration and validation of wearable monitors," *Medicine & Science in Sports & Exercise*, vol. 44, no. 1S, pp. S32–S38, Jan. 2012, doi: 10.1249/mss.0b013e3182399cf7.

[18] "Insights | The Challenges with Remote Patient Monitoring (RPM) | General," *Doccla.* www.doccla.com/post/challenges-with-remote-patient-monitoring (accessed Jul. 25, 2024).

[19] T. L. Rotering, S. J. Hysong, K. E. Williams, M. H. Raitt, M. A. Whooley, and S. S. Dhruva, "Strategies to enhance remote monitoring adherence among patients with cardiovascular implantable electronic devices," *Heart Rhythm O2*, vol. 4, no. 12, pp. 794–804, Dec. 2023, doi: 10.1016/j.hroo.2023.11.002.

[20] B. L. Filkins et al., "Privacy and security in the era of digital health: What should translational researchers know and do about it?," *PubMed Central (PMC)*, 2016. www.ncbi.nlm.nih.gov/pmc/articles/PMC4859641

[21] S. H. Houser, C. A. Flite, and S. L. Foster, "Privacy and security risk factors related to telehealth services – A systematic review," *PubMed Central (PMC)*, Jan. 01, 2023. www.ncbi.nlm.nih.gov/pmc/articles/PMC9860467

[22] A. Torab-Miandoab, T. Samad-Soltani, A. Jodati, and P. Rezaei-Hachesu, "Interoperability of heterogeneous health information systems: A systematic literature review," *BMC Medical Informatics and Decision Making*, vol. 23, no. 1, Jan. 2023, doi: 10.1186/s12911-023-02115-5.

[23] X. Zhang and R. Saltman, "Impact of electronic health record interoperability on telehealth service outcomes," *JMIR Medical Informatics*, vol. 10, no. 1, p. e31837, Jan. 2022, doi: 10.2196/31837.

[24] J. Gandrup, S. M. Ali, J. McBeth, S. N. Van Der Veer, and W. G. Dixon, "Remote symptom monitoring integrated into electronic health records: A systematic review," *Journal of the American Medical Informatics Association*, vol. 27, no. 11, pp. 1752–1763, Sep. 2020, doi: 10.1093/jamia/ocaa177.

[25] E. Li, J. Clarke, H. Ashrafian, A. Darzi, and A. L. Neves, "The impact of electronic health record interoperability on safety and quality of care in high-income countries: Systematic review," *Journal of Medical Internet Research*, vol. 24, no. 9, p. e38144, Sep. 2022, doi: 10.2196/38144.

[26] S. Maxhelaku and A. Kika, "Improving interoperability in Healthcare using Hl7 FHIR," Jul. 30, 2019. www.iises.net/proceedings/iises-international-academic-conference-prague/table-of-content/detail?article=improving-interoperability-in-healthcare-using-hl7-fhir

[27] "Advancements in telehealth and its impact on public health – James Lind Institute Public Health School in Switzerland," *James Lind Institute Switzerland*. https://jliedu.ch/advancements-in-telehealth-and-its-impact-on-public-health (accessed Aug. 05, 2024).

[28] N. Tikhomirov, "Top telemedicine trends shaping the future of digital health | Beetroot," *Beetroot*, May 28, 2024. https://beetroot.co/healthcare/top-telemedicine-trends-shaping-the-future-of-digital-health/ (accessed Aug. 4, 2024).

[29] Authors, M. Clark, and S. Bailey, "Chatbots in health care: Connecting patients to information," *NCBI Bookshelf*, Jan. 1, 2024. www.ncbi.nlm.nih.gov/books/NBK602381

[30] A. A. Kuwaiti et al., "A review of the role of artificial intelligence in healthcare," *Journal of Personalized Medicine*, vol. 13, no. 6, p. 951, Jun. 2023, doi: 10.3390/jpm13060951.

[31] M. Tukur, G. Saad, F. M. AlShagathrh, M. Househ, and M. Agus, "Telehealth interventions during COVID-19 pandemic: A scoping review of applications, challenges, privacy and security issues," *BMJ Health & Care Informatics*, vol. 30, no. 1, p. e100676, Aug. 2023, doi: 10.1136/bmjhci-2022-100676.

[32] X. Liu et al., "A comparison of deep learning performance against health-care professionals in detecting diseases from medical imaging: A systematic review and meta-analysis," *The Lancet Digital Health*, vol. 1, no. 6, pp. e271–e297, Oct. 2019, doi: 10.1016/s2589-7500(19)30123-2.

[33] D. L. Labovitz, L. Shafner, M. R. Gil, D. Virmani, and A. Hanina, "Using artificial intelligence to reduce the risk of nonadherence in patients on anticoagulation therapy," *Stroke*, vol. 48, no. 5, pp. 1416–1419, May 2017, doi: 10.1161/strokeaha.116.016281.

[34] S. Yelne, M. Chaudhary, K. Dod, A. Sayyad, and R. Sharma, "Harnessing the power of AI: A comprehensive review of its impact and challenges in nursing science and healthcare," *Cureus*, Nov. 2023, doi: 10.7759/cureus.49252.

[35] A. Panesar, "Risks and ethical challenges of precision health," in *Precision Health and Artificial Intelligence : With Privacy, Ethics, Bias, Health Equity, Best Practices, and Case Studies,* 2023, pp. 87–104. Apress eBooks. doi: 10.1007/978-1-4842-9162-7_5.

[36] L. Lämmermann, P. Hofmann, and N. Urbach, "Managing artificial intelligence applications in healthcare: Promoting information processing among stakeholders," *International Journal of Information Management*, vol. 75, p. 102728, Apr. 2024, doi: 10.1016/j.ijinfomgt.2023.102728.

[37] S. S. Ahmad, A. Meehan, M. Crispin-Ortuzar, and N. E. Weckman, "Personalized, connected health enabled by AI and home-based diagnostics," *Trends in Biotechnology*, vol. 41, no. 7, pp. 982–983, Jul. 2023, doi: 10.1016/j.tibtech.2023.03.013.

[38] A. Shete, "Predictive analytics in remote patient monitoring (RPM) | eCareMD," *eCareMD Blog*, Jul. 03, 2024. www.ecaremd.com/blog/witnessing-the-future-predictive-analytics-in-remote-patient-monitoring-rpm-program/ (accessed Aug. 11, 2024).

[39] "The future of breast cancer treatment is personalized," *Breast Cancer Research Foundation*, Apr. 24, 2024. www.bcrf.org/blog/ai-predictive-analytics-precision-medicine-breast-cancer/ (accessed Aug. 11, 2024).

[40] A. Babel, R. Taneja, F. M. Malvestiti, A. Monaco, and S. Donde, "Artificial intelligence solutions to increase medication adherence in patients with non-communicable diseases," *Frontiers in Digital Health*, vol. 3, Jun. 2021, doi: 10.3389/fdgth.2021.669869.

[41] "Digital health • Platform • Adherence • Persistence • Solutions | Medisafe," *Medisafe*, Sep. 05, 2024. www.medisafe.com/ (accessed Sep. 07, 2024).

[42] "AdhereTech – Products, competitors, financials, employees, headquarters locations," *AdhereTech*. www.cbinsights.com/company/adheretech (accessed Aug. 12, 2024).

[43] "Hybrid practice management software," *MediSprout*, Apr. 30, 2024. https://medisprout.com/ (accessed Aug. 14, 2024).

[44] "Proteus-digital-health," *LinkedIn*. www.linkedin.com/company/proteus-digital-health-inc/people/ (accessed Aug. 28, 2024).

[45] S. Reddy, "Generative AI in healthcare: An implementation science informed translational path on application, integration and governance," *Implementation Science*, vol. 19, no. 1, Mar. 2024, doi: 10.1186/s13012-024-01357-9.

[46] P. Zhang and M. N. K. Boulos, "Generative AI in medicine and healthcare: Promises, opportunities and challenges," *Future Internet*, vol. 15, no. 9, p. 286, Aug. 2023, doi: 10.3390/fi15090286.

6 Artificial Intelligence and Machine Learning in Clinical Care

Revolutionizing Decision Support

Nagashruthi M.K. and Hemanth K.S.

6.1 INTRODUCTION

6.1.1 Overview of Artificial Intelligence in Medical Image Analysis: Purpose and Scope

Artificial intelligence (AI) in medical imaging undergoes extensive evaluation in finding patterns and analyzing using different techniques to help experts, which consequently helps identify tumors, lesions, segmenting regions, and so on. In the healthcare sector, it is necessary to use imaging techniques like radiography, computed tomography (CT) scan, ultrasound images, single photon emission computed tomography (SPECT), positron emission tomography (PET) scans, and histopathological images to help the radiologist make quick assessments. Medical images hold the richest information about the patient which is quite a challenging and time-consuming task for radiologists to do manually which is resolved by AI. Trained models can help in better and early predictions when new cases arise; it is also used to extract prominent regions or features from the given input images and are further used for classification. Deep learning (DL) models convert these images to output by finding features with the help of its hidden layers. DL can be used for classification, prediction, and so on. AI can be used to improve the visual quality of images and assist in precisely identifying locations, lesions, and segments. An automated process will reduce the time and effort needed by the specialists. Finding the abnormalities at the earliest can be achieved with the help of AI models, which also help in easy access and retrieval of patient data [1]. Models are trained with a large amount of data so that they will ensure quality output and help in diagnosis faster, which helps practitioners with easy primary analysis of the cases. AI models are useful in effectively allocating resources by prioritizing sensitive cases if the resources available are limited. The use of AI models must ensure quality, accuracy, and consistency, which is most needed in medical cases [2]. In critical cases like heart attacks, first few minutes are most crucial

DOI: 10.1201/9781003516163-6

to patients; in such cases, use of an AI model for analysis helps radiologists in quick decision-making and treatment planning, which ensures a lower error rate, thereby revolutionizing the healthcare sector.

An in-depth analysis of AI in medical image analysis is provided in this chapter using a variety of imaging modalities and models. Advanced AI techniques support practitioners' decision-making within specific parameters and are crucial for early diagnosis and treatment plans with improved overall patient care.

6.1.2 Fundamentals of Artificial Intelligence in Medical Image Analysis

AI models performed exceptionally well in identifying features from the images, identifying anomalies, and generating predictions. Sometimes early detection of the problem is very crucial in a patient's life [3]. AI is capable of processing huge quantities of data with remarkable efficiency. It can also process smaller amounts of data by employing augmentation techniques, which raises the sample count needed to train the models. Models can be used to analyze issues with internal organs of the human body which helps the radiologist in making decisions. AI in medical imaging encompasses a broad range of modalities, applications, and analytic approaches. A few of these are compiled into groupings with commonly used AI techniques, as illustrated in Figure 6.1. Figure 6.2 depicts a thorough subcategorization of Figure 6.1.

6.1.3 Background

Previously, radiologists analyzed medical images, manually interpreted the abnormalities, and later started treating the patients. Currently, development of DL and machine learning (ML) models helps automate the process of analyzing medical images, which makes the task easy for radiologists.

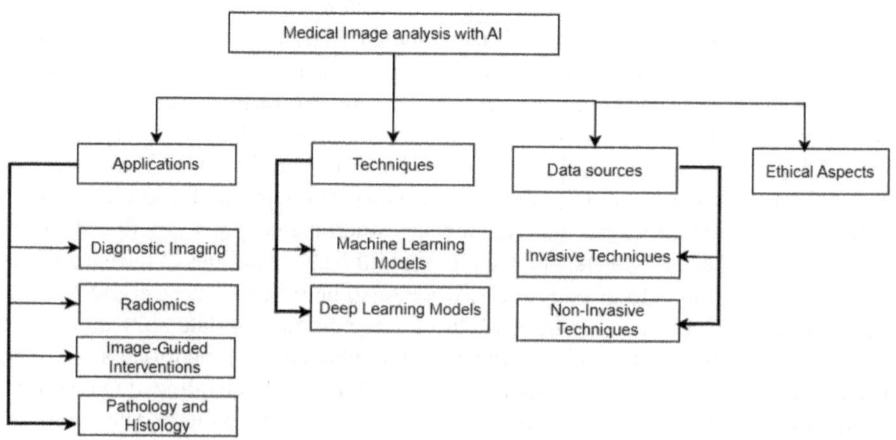

FIGURE 6.1 Overview of Medical Imaging AI Process.

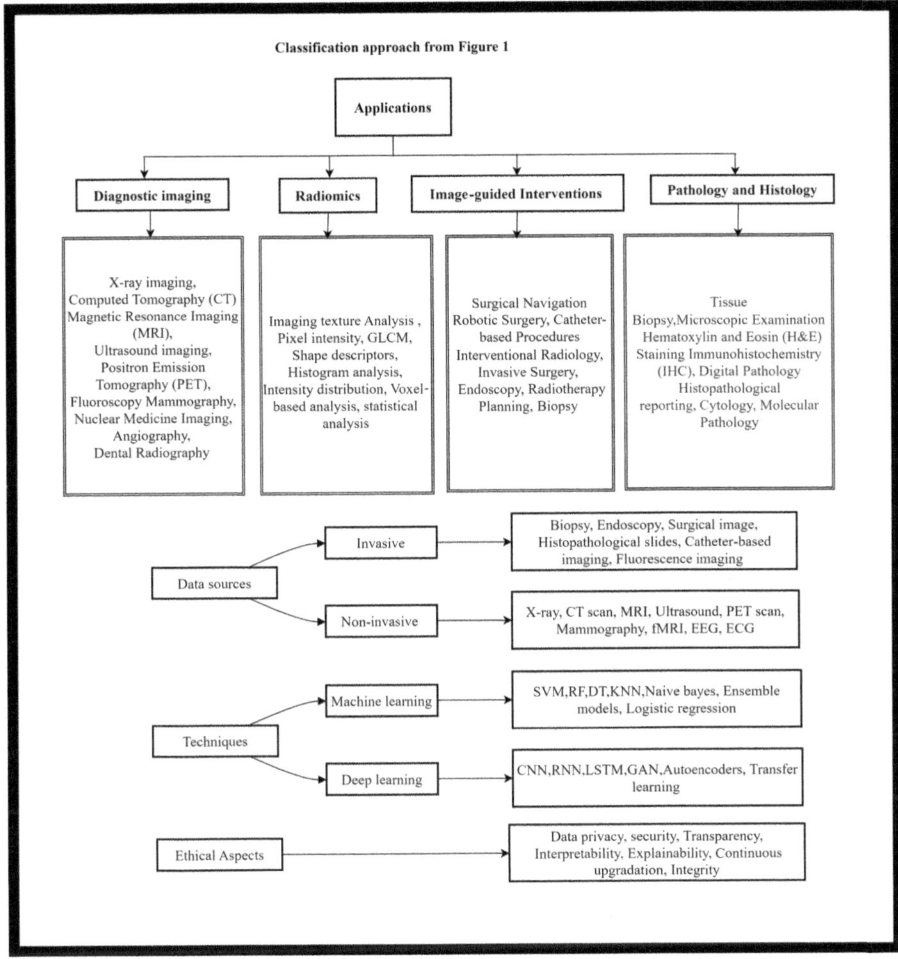

FIGURE 6.2 Detailed Grouping Information from Figure 6.1.

Models should handle complicated and variable types of medical data to help with decision-making [4]. The model should be capable of processing images, volumes, electronic health record (EHR) data, genomic data, and their integration. Variants of convoluted neural networks (CNNs) have been identified as an appropriate framework for processing this type of data with significant efficiency. Some models have employed supervised and unsupervised approaches, transfer learning methods, pre-trained models, and ensemble models on this sort of medical data [5]. Additionally, it has to handle three-dimensional (3D) and 4D data effectively [6], allowing the model to perform better with less annotated data. Natural language processing (NLP) models have been designed to handle EHR data, resulting in more accurate and improved diagnoses [7]. DL models improve the accurate and timely detection of microscopic malignant cells. Models assist with accurate medication using genomic data by identifying biomarkers that aid in personalized treatment [8]. Long short-term memory (LSTM) has been used to keep track of patient EHR and other records that are required for decision-making in follow-up cases. This enables practitioners to make the process simpler and smoother [9].

The increasing number of patients diagnosed every minute, driven by the modern lifestyle, has led to an overload of data, making manual assessment difficult and necessitating the usage of AI models. The integration of AI and medical image analysis considerably benefits practitioners. Models are capable of handling both minimal and huge quantities of data with equal effectiveness. In certain situations, medical image analysis suffers from a lack of accessible data. AI system works like the human brain in problem-solving; ML algorithms use features from data from which patterns are identified and decisions are made. DL models are models already trained by using inputs like image, audio, or video so that when new input arrives the model makes a decision based on previously learned data. Challenges lie in the reliability and generalizability of AI models. Sometimes the model has to handle data that has not been encountered during the training process. A situation may arise in which the model has to handle critical and sensitive cases.

6.2 MEDICAL IMAGING ANALYSIS

6.2.1 Overview of Models

Medical images represent images captured on organs or tissues of the human body using any imaging techniques. Imaging techniques help to find abnormalities in the internal structure of human organs. These help radiologists diagnose the problems. Medical imaging is a part of radiology where techniques are used in different modalities to capture images of internal body organs of the human body which helps in the analysis of the problem. These images help reveal the internal organ that suffers from the problem. Heatmap images of multiple DL models used on 11 organs using 8 radiology imaging modalities can be found in [3]. Imaging techniques help in understanding the structure and function of internal body organs and assist in finding abnormalities [10, 11]

They are mainly categorized as invasive and non-invasive processes of capturing images based on instrument intrusion level into the body. In a non-invasive process, images are captured using tools externally where it is not required to insert inside the body. X-ray imaging, CT scan, magnetic resonance imaging (MRI), and ultrasound all can be categorized into these processes. As an invasive process involves the insertion of instruments into a body like an angiograph, endoscopy, or biopsy, these techniques are usually used when it is required to have a detailed view of some part of an organ. It is quite a complex task with risk involvement compared to a non-invasive process. These techniques are also used during the surgical process.

6.2.2 Types of Imaging Techniques

In the medical field of radiology, radiation is used to create images of the body's internal organs, including bone structure and joint function. These imaging techniques can also be applied post treatment or post-surgery to monitor the body's response and determine how much complexity has been reduced.

Diagnostic radiology: It gives a detailed view of CT scans, MRI, X-ray, and PET images; doctors can identify issues with bones and tissues, and the structure of organs, and analyze the conditions. It helps in treatment planning and management.

Interventional radiology: This technique includes the insertion of tools, caterpillar valves, or implants inside the body. It helps in complex surgeries and involves angiography and biopsy, tests body fluids, tissue samples, and cell samples to assist in decision-making. It ranges from the most basic blood test procedure to the most intricate autopsy.

6.3 ROLE OF ARTIFICIAL INTELLIGENCE IN MEDICAL IMAGE ANALYSIS

6.3.1 X-Ray

Electromagnetic radiations are used to create X-rays. It is typically used to identify fractured bones as well as bone tumors and abnormalities in the heart's blood vessels on chest X-rays. It is also used in spotting fractures and wounds in ongoing complications. To detect pneumonia using chest X-ray imaging, feature extraction, and classification using deep CNN have been carried out with augmented and dropout layers in CNN. Techniques for data augmentation include rescaling, rotating, zooming, width and height shifting, and flipping [12]. CNN is primarily used in level 2 of the preprocessing of a chest X-ray to identify pneumonia infected with COVID-19. As there are not as many samples, CNN with transfer learning techniques is used. It is not possible to compare patterns within an image with patterns already in existence. As a result, the model is used to preprocess data at various levels by removing the diaphragm region and using filters to ensure that the input is appropriate for the Visual Geometry Group 16 (VGG16) model [13]. A combination of CNN and various transfer learning models is used to detect pediatric pneumonia. As most medical data are imbalanced, CNN was once used to supplement and balance the data before being fed into the model. A 3D image of the bone is created using front 2D X-ray images, which helps in the creation of surgical and treatment plans. The CNN model is created for this purpose using the bounding box technique, which makes use of feature points and ellipses [14]. With the aid of a backpropagation algorithm, fractured bones are automatically classified using X-rays. Before being used by CNN for classification, the fractured area is filtered and segmented [15]. CNN-based encoder model that uses panoramic X-ray images to segment the tooth areas. Segmentation is crucial in this situation because panoramic teeth X-rays capture a 2D image of the entire mouth, which contains many artifacts [16]. The use of computer vision techniques to improve fracture detection methods protects the patient from additional life-threatening situations. The Region-based Convolutional Neural Network (R-CNN) model was created to identify sternum fractures. Identification of bone fractures and their severity is crucial because bone protects most other organs from injury. Different types of bone fractures like transverse fracture, open fracture, simple fracture, spiral fracture, and comminuted fracture can be found in [17]. Using ante-posterior hand

X-ray images, R-CNN is designed to quickly identify distal radius fractures [18]. To identify and classify knee osteoarthritis early on, X-ray images are used to extract a local binary pattern and histogram of an oriented gradient. Combining complex and noticeable features from an X-ray and CNN produces excellent identification results [19]. Overall, CNN and its variants perform well when used with feature extraction techniques, segmentation techniques, and balancing techniques on X-ray images of various body organs.

CNN variants are often used to detect anomalies such as malignancies, fractures, and so on. The models learn patterns and perform tasks. Transfer learning can also be utilized when data availability is limited; models trained on little data may be overfitted or fail to deliver accurate predictions. They are additionally useful for automating processes to identify regions of interest (ROI), such as fracture locations and malignant areas. The U-Net architecture also functioned well in segmentations. Explainability can be achieved using Class Activation Mapping (CAM), Gradient-weighted Class Activation Mapping (Grad CAM), Local Interpretable Model-Agnostic Explanations (LIME), Shapley Additive Explanations (SHAP), and other methods.

In some circumstances, such as cancer and a few neurological conditions, it is essential to follow the progress before and after treatment, surgery, or therapy. Genomic data can be combined with imaging data and medical history to build a model that recommends timely treatment for improved medical care. Obtaining high-quality data and annotated data from specialists is difficult. Issues such as class imbalance problems, unusual cases that were not trained by the model throughout the training phase, and disorder identification with comparable symptoms should be handled carefully. Machine settings are also important during training. Because the equipment setup differs when data is collected from various devices, this bias should be minimized.

6.3.2 Computed Tomography Scan

A detailed 2D scan view is created by combining several X-ray images produced by the CT scanner as they travel around the body. Additionally, soft tissues and a few other parts can be seen which a standard X-ray cannot. The process takes between 10 and 20 minutes to complete. A CT scan is typically used to find lesions, injuries, and, in some cases, heart disorders. In situations like complex bone fractures and bone cancer, it will provide a detailed view. Using DL architecture, automatic tumor segmentation and classification are carried out on CT scan images. As it is a Digital Imaging and Communications in Medicine (DICOM) standard image, DICOM images are a unique format for storing medical data that includes meta-data as well as images from various modalities [20]. Using fully connected CNN, the regions of bone tumors are segmented [21]. U-Net is an effective framework for region segmentation and determining region boundaries in diseases such as cancer. These models assist in improving low-quality CT scans. CT scans only provide structural information. Handling 3D data is complex, as 2D data does not capture all of the region's structural features.

6.3.3 Magnetic Resonance Imaging

MRI can help detect tumors and injuries. It is a frequently employed non-invasive technique for imaging the joints and the brain. The most frequent type of injury suffered by athletes is an ankle sprain. Effusion in the tibiotalar and talocalcaneal joints increases the risk of severe ligament injuries, involving anterior talofibular ligament (ATFL) rupture and partial or complete syndesmotic ligament rupture. Cross-sectional connections were examined between the severity of injuries such as osteochondral lesions, syndesmotic injuries, and bone injuries, as well as the presence and volume of effusion in the tibiotalar and talocalcaneal joints. MRI is more effective than ultrasound in detecting deep soft tissue and osteochondral injuries responsible for ankle sprains. To determine the risk of suffering severe injuries, conditional logistic regression was used [22].

MRI is more technically advanced than X-rays because it gives 3D data. Handling a 3D volume or slice is a more complicated task that necessitates significant computational capacity. The model should be able to recognize the underlying anatomical and temporal patterns in brain-related data. Artifacts must be correctly detected and removed. Deep convolutional neural networks (DCNN), U-Net, and LSTM are useful for classification and segmentation applications. In the case of neurological disorders, it is essential to observe activation over time; functional magnetic resonance imaging (fMRI) can be utilized for this. When compared to MRI, fMRI produces lower-quality images; identifying patterns is challenging, and most conditions have identical symptoms. Time series data handling is more complicated because the model has to manage both temporal and spatial data.

Generative adversarial networks (GANs) can be used to augment and label brain patterns. Combining genomic data and clinical history with imaging modalities can aid in customized medicine, which is particularly essential in neurological disorders. Coupling with other modes, such as EEG and CT scans, may assist with diagnosis. Handling 3D and 4D data is difficult and necessitates expensive and complex architectures. Variations in instrument configurations make it difficult to generalize the model. It needs a robust machine with sufficient random-access memory (RAM), capable of handling a long training time, and complicated network topologies. Reducing data is challenging. Common methods include principal component analysis (PCA) and independent component analysis (ICA); however, latent spaces can also be employed depending on the data and task.

A brain tumor is considered one of the most serious types of cancer. According to WHO standards, Grade 1 tumors are classified as benign while Grade 4 tumors are classified as malignant. The work proposes a new 3D CNN and correlation along a feedforward neural network (FNN) -based automated approach for the detection and classification of brain tumors. CNN architecture is used to extract the brain tumor, VGG19 is used to extract deep features, and Pearson correlation features are chosen for the final classification. The database contains the ground-truth images for four different classes, including Flair, T1CE, T1, and T2. Both high-grade glioma (HGG) and low-grade glioma (LGG) -type images can be found in these datasets. All images have anisotropic resolutions that have been resampled to isotropic resolutions [23].

The central nervous system (CNS) consists of the brain and spinal cord, which are responsible for tasks like organizing, analyzing, making decisions, issuing commands, and integrating several biological processes. Without the help of imaging technique evaluation, diagnosis and the creation of effective treatments are very difficult for some CNS issues. Radiologists and neuropathologists have trouble identifying brain tumors produced by abnormal cell growth. The abnormal development of nerve cells in brain tumors, which can range from benign to malignant and from extremely rare to often occurring, serves as a warning sign. These cancers can start in the brain or migrate there from other body organs. Primary brain tumors are those that develop directly from the brain. Gliomas, meningiomas, and pituitary brain tumors can be recognized using MRI data and a YOLO v7 model with transfer learning fine-tuning. The results show that the Spatial Pyramid Pooling Fast+ (SPPF+), Bi-directional Feature Pyramid Network (BiFPN), and Decoupled Head (DP) modules improve the performance of the model. The model demonstrates successful outcomes in the diagnosis of brain cancers. To reduce mortality rates globally, early detection of brain cancers is crucial. Brain tumors can be difficult to diagnose due to their intricate architecture, wide range in size, and unusual shapes [24].

Life expectancy has increased because of medical advancements in all parts of the world. The DCGAN-based Augmentation and Classification (D-BAC) system divides dementia into different categories based on severity using a GAN-based data augmentation technique. Dementia begins in elderly patients with mild cognitive impairment (MCI) and gradually progresses to a more severe stage known as serious dementia. The early MCI stage itself is the only known way to diagnose and stop this disease [25]. Worldwide, prostate cancer (PCa), which accounts for more than one-fifth of all cancer diagnoses in men, is the second most prevalent malignancy. Surveillance sequential MRI changes that are explicable and diagnostically significant were detected by AI. The approach was able to reliably detect clinically significant prostate cancer (csPCa) in instances where sequential MRI features alone would not have been sufficient. U-Net correctly recognized every PCa in every scan, including small lesions. This approach differs from most other studies on the computer-aided diagnosis of PCa, in which DL models are trained to recognize only csPCa. An ML classifier was used for prediction. Serial MRI diagnostic performance may become more reliable by postponing unnecessary biopsies [26]. Brain tumors are categorized using magnetic resonance (MR) images. Early on in a tumor's development, a biopsy is not required. Morphological operations are used to precisely identify tumor pixels. Because an automatic technique is recommended for tumor detection at the image and lesion levels, a feature set consisting of texture, shape, and intensity is used. Brain tumors start as abnormally developing cells that multiply uncontrollably. When cells proliferate abnormally and out of control, a brain tumor develops. Tumor tissues are segmented using K-means clustering with fuzzy C-Means (FCM) techniques. Lesion candidates in an image are segmented based on threshold. Gaussian filter is used for removing noise and smoothing the image. For each lesion, a collection of features based on texture, shape, and intensity is applied. Support Vector Machine (SVM) is used in multiple cross-validation tasks [27].

6.3.4 Mammography

X-rays are used to create images of the breast tissue that aid in the early detection of cancer. The use of AI algorithms in screening mammography supports clinical practice and provides evidence of the procedure's effectiveness. To evaluate implementation of AI tools, three conditions must be met: the tool must function properly, the user must understand it, and the tool must be incorporated into the current workflow. Radiologists can investigate predictions and assess model performance in multiple cases. AI applications for mammography examination are gaining focus, including risk assessment, image processing, and lesion detection and diagnosis; AI algorithms are validated in the real-time clinical environment and are properly coupled to existing systems [28].

The development of computer-aided diagnosis (CAD) systems has been a recent development in the detection of breast cancer. There are several imaging methods mentioned, with mammography being particularly effective, including MRI, ultrasound, histopathology, and various imaging techniques. Radiologists can identify breast cancer at an early stage with the help of CAD systems, which combine computer analysis with diagnostic images. Images are improved using preprocessing techniques like polynomial curve fitting, cropping, augmentation, and contrast limited adaptive histogram equalization (CLAHE). CNN techniques are used to extract significant features [29].

AI-based computer-aided detection systems can detect cancer with accuracy levels that are comparable to multiple radiologists' average levels in standalone setups. The clinic's adoption of a reading protocol based on an AI system may enhance screening results and lower the number of mammograms that radiologists are required to read. A subgroup of mammograms from similar detection performances of the AI system would be read by radiologists. Radiologists would not read normal mammograms, and they would recall any suspicious ones. The Recall Threshold (RT) was fitted by matching the radiologist's sensitivity using a different independent cohort. Each BI-RADS density was then subjected to this protocol in turn. AI-based models can identify normal, low-risk, and high-risk mammograms, which helps in reducing the workload of the radiologist. Due to an increase in the incidence of breast cancer and widely used screening, there is an increasing need for specialized radiologists [30].

6.3.5 Angiography and Endoscopy

Angiography is a process of injecting a special dye into the blood and capturing an X-ray; this technique is typically used to find blockages. Normally, the process takes between one and two hours to complete. The diagnosis of cardiovascular problems becomes easier with this technique. It enables the diagnosis of blood vessel blockages and narrowing, helps in the decision-making process of surgical procedures like angioplasty, and the assessment of blood flow in tissues and organs.

Endoscopy is a process to examine issues with the digestive system, the respiratory system, or other issues, where a camera attached to a tube is inserted into the body. This camera takes pictures of the interior of the body. The process of taking pictures is complicated, and it can take anywhere between 20 and 30 minutes to complete. This process might involve watching a series of images one by one to identify the problem and occasionally result in a manual error. AI models greatly assist in this type of processing by identifying the problems associated with the tracks.

CNN-based segmentation is used to detect the boundaries of angiodysplastic lesions on capsule endoscopic images. ResNet-50 was used with global features and texture details to accurately segment the regions. This was also evaluated for clinical application with high precision and observed at a time of 0.6 seconds per image [31]. Automated detection of intracranial aneurysms using CT angiography images and a 3D CNN was used on the DeepMedic platform. Experiments were conducted to determine the size and location of aneurysms and classify them into >10 mm, 3–10 mm, and ≤3 mm. A sensitivity of 92.3% and a positive predictive value (PPV) of 100% were achieved. Sensitivity decreased to 66.7% for classes smaller than 3 mm. In addition, the segmentation task produced better results than manual labeling [32]. The endoscopic image classification model is designed to enhance accuracy while reducing runtime for usage in real-time applications using MobileNet V2, which employs preprocessing elements and a network-on-chip (NOC) to ensure minimal energy consumption and computing time. It achieved 4.56×10^9 multiplier–accumulator (MAC) energy usage and a runtime of 1.73×10^7 cycles. This study found that specialized integrated circuits can outperform general-purpose processors in terms of power efficiency and speed in real-time medical applications. They can also be used on X-ray and CT scan images using complex architectural models like ResNet and Inception V3 [33]. Active bleeding regions were identified using angiographic images of the mesenteric and celiac arteries and a pre-trained CNN (Efficient-Net B5) trained on the ImageNet dataset. A total of 587 digital subtraction angiography (DSA) images from 142 individuals are used. Normal and active bleeding regions in the upper gastro tract were classified with an average accuracy of 77.43% [34]. Table 6.1 summarizes a few commonly used DL models along with the datasets and techniques used.

6.4 ARTIFICIAL INTELLIGENCE-ENHANCED MEDICAL IMAGE ANALYSIS TECHNIQUES

The creation of gadolinium (Gd)-enhanced liver tumors on nonenhanced liver MR images will be crucial for the diagnosis and treatment of liver tumors. A pixel-level graph reinforcement learning method (Pix-GRL), which is a pixel-level graph reinforcement learning network that accepts regular, unextracted images of liver tumors, is developed. These results show the great potential of the Pix-GRL to develop a precise clinical substitute for contrast agents (CAs) in liver tumor imaging. The model successfully extracted liver tumors without the use of Gd, and the results were comparable to those of Gd-enhanced liver tumor imaging. Details can be found in case study 1 [43]. CAD systems act as a secondary opinion tool to support radiologists' evaluation. These systems use a variety of ML-based components, including image preprocessing, tumor feature extraction, and data classification. ML employs MRI to find breast lesions that are difficult to diagnose like non-mass enhancing (NME) lesions.

TABLE 6.1
An Overview of Methods and Strategies Utilized in Medical Imaging

	Model	Description	Dataset	Results	Conclusion
[35]	CCN-PR-Seg-net (cross channel normalization)	Automated segmentation of brain tumors	TCIA (The Cancer Imaging Archive)	Mean intersection over union = 98.86%, and boundary F1 score = 97.52%.	Resolve boundary loss issue from other methods like U-Net
[36]	Faster R CNN with VGG16	Detection and classification of brain tumors	MRI publicly available	Mean average = 77.60%	Class containing variation intensity and texture in the same class are considered
[37]	VGG19 with features extracted (LBP, HOG features) (histogram of oriented gradients)	Segmentation of glioma	BRATS (Brain Tumor Segmentation)	Achieved accuracy of more than 90% on various versions of the dataset with different models	The model is fused with texture and shape features
[38]	Enhanced CNN with BAT optimization	Segmentation of tumor	BRATS 2015	Accuracy = 92%	Segmentation of different regions with more precision
[39]	DCNN	Classification of the presence or absence of lesions in DBT images (Digital breast tomosynthesis)	DBT images from two hospitals	Accuracy = 90%	Also used Grad-CAM for explainability to help radiologists
[40]	U-Net, FCNN (Fully Connected Neural Network)	Segmentation of breast tumor using DCE-MRI	Forty-three patients' data after chemotherapy	Mean Intersection over Union = 76.14%	Automated segmentation with a small dataset

(continued)

TABLE 6.1 (Continued)
An Overview of Methods and Strategies Utilized in Medical Imaging

	Model	Description	Dataset	Results	Conclusion
[41]	AlexNet, ResNet18, ResNet34	Identify microcalcifications and classify them into benign or malignant.	Mammograms from patients annotated by experts	AlexNet classification, AUC = 94% (Area Under Curve)	Focus on microcalcifications with small data available
[42]	Ensemble models constructed with logistic regression, or neural network or using transfer learning	Classification of breast lesions as benign or malignant.	DDSM and CBIS-DDSM mammography dataset (Curated Breast Imaging Subset of Digital Database for Screening Mammography)	Greater than 95% for different ensemble models	Small dataset, imbalanced data

CNN-based models have been made to work directly with raw images in medical imaging. Applications used today are built on tried-and-true methods like enhancement curve extraction from dynamic contrast-enhanced (DCE)-MRI and feature engineering. It has been shown that ML-based CAD systems can improve the interpretation of breast imaging for the presence or absence of cancer and reduce interobserver variability. This calls for the use of more advanced radiomics features and additional MRI techniques, combining genetic and imaging data from medical sources to assess the risk of type 2 diabetes (T2D). Based on genetic and medical imaging data, the study uses AI to create T2D predictive models. The findings demonstrate that accurate T2D prediction using genetic information alone is not possible, but that accurate prediction using medical imaging data is significantly increased. The identification of high-risk subgroups for T2D risk assessment was made possible by the Polygenic Risk Score (PRS) and Multi-image Risk Score (MRS). The study employed PRSs as genetic elements to assess the hereditary risk of T2D. Overall, the findings highlight the potential of combining genetics and medical imaging data for better disease management and prevention [44].

6.5 CASE STUDIES

6.5.1 Case 1: Automated Detection and Classification of Oral Lesions Using Deep Learning for Early Detection of Oral Cancer

Oral cancer is one of the most common cancers in the world, with delayed detection, high mortality rates, and severity due to a lack of awareness. Working well for classifying oral lesions and early oral cancer detection are DL-based frameworks for object detection and image classification. The model can be useful in early detection and treatment planning for oral cancer. The mobile app called Mobile Mouth Screening Anywhere (MeMoSa) helps in communicating between multiple specialists and building of annotated library that contains images of oral lesions which further helps in the training of the model. Strategies are developed by grouping and combining bounding boxes which helps in identifying lesion regions further used for classification. Performance measures can be found in Table 6.2.

TABLE 6.2
Performance Metrics for the Tasks

Purpose	Task	F1 Score
Classification	Identifying images with lesions	87.07%
	Identifying images needing referral	78.30%
	Macro-average	50.57%
Object detection	Detecting lesions	41.35%
	Identifying lesions	41.18%
	Macro average	24.50%

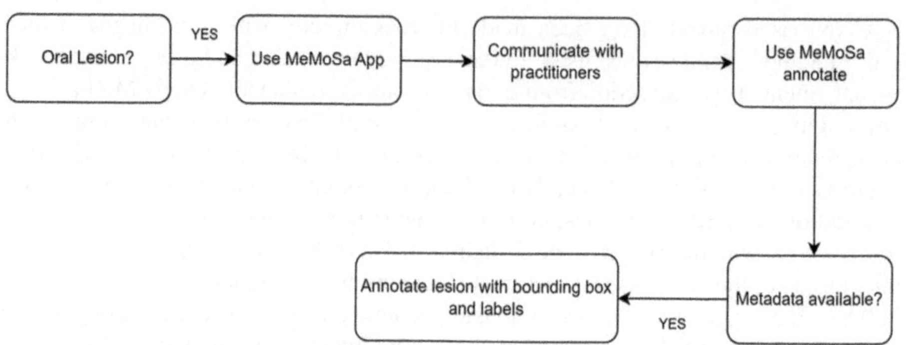

FIGURE 6.3 Flowchart of MeMoSa App for Annotating Bounding Box and Labeling the Lesions.

Figure 6.3 shows the flow while developing the MeMoSa app, after annotating lesions which are further used for classification with the use of a DL model. Images from the oral cavity are collected and captioned to automate the early diagnosis of oral cancer. The method employs bounding box annotations from several doctors, which are then evaluated against two distinct DL-based approaches.

6.5.2 Case 2: A Deep Neural Network for Early Detection and Prediction of Chronic Kidney Disease

Chronic renal disease reduces the kidney's functional capacity and lowers the quality of life for a patient [45]. Symptoms include excessive blood pressure, anemia, brittle bones, and nerve damage. A DL model for early diagnosis of chronic diseases was developed, which identifies the features that are important for prediction. The Recursive Feature Elimination approach was utilized to extract features, and the most important chronic kidney disease (CKD) characteristics identified were red blood cell count, albumin, cell volume, and serum creatinine and classified using these feature sets; a detailed process is depicted in Figure 6.4. In comparison to the other five classifiers (SVM, K-Nearest Neighbor (KNN), Logistic Regression, Random Forest, and Naive Bayes classifier), the proposed deep neural model performed well [46].

6.5.3 Case 3: A Deep Learning Algorithm for Automatic Detection and Classification of Acute Intracranial Hemorrhages in Head Computed Tomography Scans

Intracranial hemorrhage (ICH), or bleeding inside the skull, is a medical emergency that can leave a person seriously disabled or even result in death. The accurate classification of the types of acute intracranial hemorrhage from head CT scans is crucial for this disease's management. AI algorithm for non-contrast head CT scans for the automatic detection of acute ICH and classification of its subtypes. Figure 6.5 illustrates the three stages of processing that make up the algorithm. It is necessary for making decisions about surgical procedures and emergency conditions. The DL

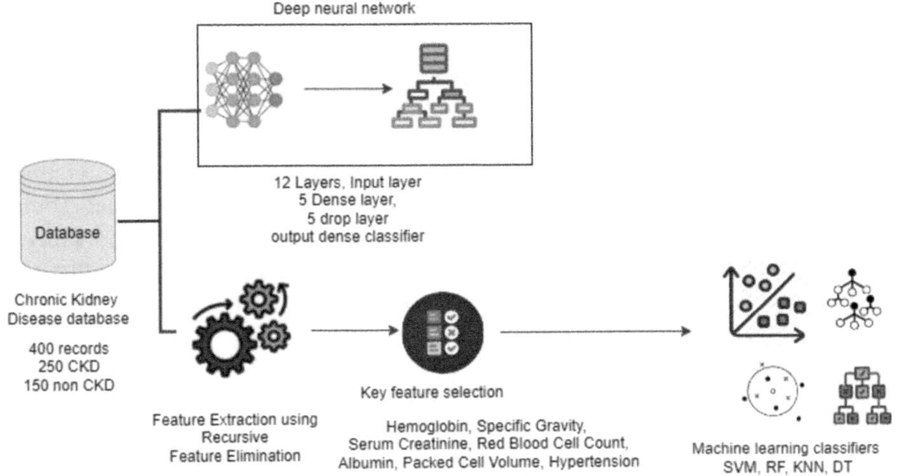

FIGURE 6.4 Overview of Comparison Analysis of Deep Neural Network (DNN) and ML Models Used.

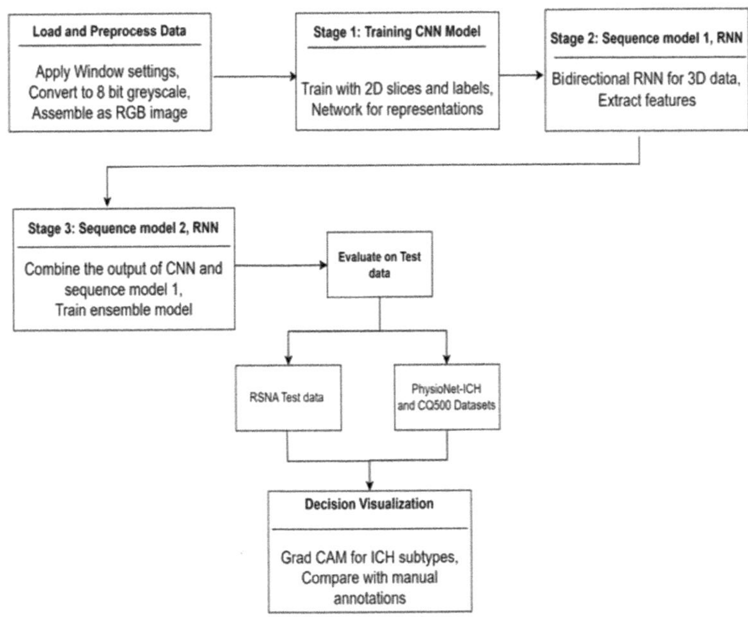

FIGURE 6.5 A Detailed View of the Three-Stage Algorithm.

method utilizes non-contrast 3D head CT images to automatically detect and classify acute ICH and its five variants.

A CNN classifier is utilized for each slice of a head scan to determine whether or not each ICH subtype exists. Using the first stage's feature outputs, the Sequence Model 1 stage uses a bidirectional RNN with the GRU unit to generate an enhanced subtype of the ICH for each slice. The final prediction of the ICH subtypes combines the classifier output for each slice of a 3D scan with the Sequence Model 1 output. The network parameters for the DL models at all stages are optimized using the Radiological Society of North America (RSNA) training data to reduce the difference between the model outputs and the ground-truth labeling [47].

6.6 ETHICAL CONCERNS AND DATA PRIVACY

The moral principles and criteria that affect people's behavior and decision-making are known as ethical concerns. It includes protecting people's rights to privacy and the use of their personal information. The main focus of data ethics is right and wrong. Addressing ethical issues may lead to better models with more accurate and transparent predictions [48, 49]. Table 6.3 shows a few ethical and privacy issues to be considered while developing a model for clinical use [50].

TABLE 6.3
Ethical and Privacy Aspects, Policies for Use of Artificial Intelligence in Medical Care

Ethical Concerns and Data Privacy	Technical Challenges	Integration and Reliability	Regulations and Policies
Patient privacy, data security, unauthorized access, transparency, and trust	Interpretability and explainability, handle multiple modalities, managing the visual quality of images, manage model training processes like avoiding overfitting and underfitting problems	Compatibility with techniques and devices available, continuous upgradation, validation	Food and Drug Administration (FDA) regulations, Health Insurance Portability and Accountability Act (HIPAA) compliance, International Organization for Standardization (ISO) standards, ethical guidelines, data security guidelines

6.7 DISCUSSION

Lack of information and ambiguity surround the use of AI in clinical settings. Additional challenges to acceptance include varying levels of trust in AI among patients, clinicians, and radiology professionals. Practical considerations include images to be formatted according to model requirements. Model suitability for methods and equipment and the amount of time and storage are needed. AI algorithms that automatically classify, identify, and describe issues, generate reports, and minimize the workload of screening exams by automatically reporting normal examinations could be useful to radiologists.

AI-assisted diagnosis lowers risk and helps in segmentation, identification, and disease prediction. A trend in the healthcare industry has been produced by the rapid growth of AI on clinical data. Classification, prediction, and segmentation tasks on various types of data are all part of medical image analysis. CNN is typically used for tumor detection. When treating cancer, it is crucial to pinpoint the location of the tumor and any areas where it has spread. Medical image analysis models are primarily affected by low-sampled data because DL models are data-hungry. AI can also be applied to improve the visual quality of images, and it learns the patterns of normal control and abnormalities and performs the task. In general, ML and DL models use algorithms to build expert systems that make predictions and classifications that help radiologists and practitioners make treatment decisions and diagnose patients.

6.7.1 Benefits

AI models can analyze large volumes of data quickly and accurately. It is possible to find patterns that, in some cases, the eyes cannot detect. Consistent models not subject to any constraints aid in quickly locating the issue, and assist experts in sensitive and complex cases. Data can be kept for a long time and made accessible through a network of hospitals, allowing other facilities to easily access it if a patient needs additional care. Multiple experts' assessments may occasionally not agree, but radiology images can help them reach a consensus. Multiple modalities can be combined, leading to real-time resolution of rare cases with ensured quality.

6.7.2 Challenges and Limitations

As DL models are data-hungry algorithms, they require sizable, diverse datasets. The performance of a model is decreased when there is a lack of real-time data to train it. The issue is whether or not one has confidence in the model because of trust issues in the model. Patients' privacy must be protected when it comes to their medical records. The evaluation system for the fully automated AI analysis model must be carefully defined. Safety measures for AI models should be put in place to prevent attacks; this is essential because even a small change in the input can lead to completely different predictions, which could have a negative impact on a diagnosis. Additionally, a patient's information can be lost. Managing complicated medical data is the most challenging task.

6.7.3 Opportunities

It encourages early detection, which is critical when detecting tumors and identifying their locations, combining the patient's medical history and the input image to develop a comprehensive diagnosis strategy. Development of dynamic and a report generating models. Model explicability helps to overcome the trust issue. When developing an interactive AI model to aid in the surgical process with minimal information, use a model that robustly enhances images from the original data. Create a global model that incorporates local models that can be accessed from multiple locations, thus allowing the model to learn from a large amount of data from numerous hospitals. In interventional radiology, more secure models are required. There is a need to create a model to help with therapy or drug combination suggestions.

6.8 CONCLUSION

AI and radiology integration changed the healthcare industry; significant advancements in AI have produced extremely accurate results when performing tasks like segmentation, forecasting, finding patterns, and identifying abnormalities in medical image analysis. This enables quicker and more accurate decision-making. The most important factor to take into consideration is maintaining privacy and being ethically transparent. The most popular and reliable model in the majority of image analysis is CNN. Using CNN, it has been possible to reliably identify tumor regions, track their spread, and segment that portion. However, it is necessary to have an ongoing training and validation process, the model must be reliable in spotting patterns, and it must be able to recognize occasionally seen data. The reliable and safe models help in eliminating bias. The model must be upgraded according to hardware advancements. AI should help doctors smoothly to make tasks easier.

REFERENCES

1. Wang, L., Wang, H., Huang, Y., Yan, B., Chang, Z., Liu, Z., ... & Li, F. "Trends in the application of deep learning networks in medical image analysis: Evolution between 2012 and 2020," *European Journal of Radiology*, vol. 146, p. 110069, 2021, doi: 10.1016/j.ejrad.2021.110069.
2. Meyer-Base, A., Morra, L., Tahmassebi, A., Lobbes, M., Meyer-Base, U., & Pinker, K. "AI-enhanced diagnosis of challenging lesions in breast MRI: A methodology and application primer," *Journal of Magnetic Resonance Imaging*, vol. 54, no. 3, pp. 686–702, 2021, doi: 10.1002/jmri.27332.
3. Heiliger, L., Sekuboyina, A., Menze, B., Egger, J., and Kleesiek, J. "Beyond medical imaging: A review of multimodal deep learning in radiology," *Frontiers in Artificial Intelligence*, 2021, doi: 10.3389/frai.2021.694584. www.researchgate.net/publication/358581125_Beyond_Medical_Imaging_A_Review_of_Multimodal_Deep_Learning_in_Radiology
4. Kitsios, F., Kamariotou, M., Syngelakis, A. I., and Talias, M. A. "Recent advances of artificial intelligence in healthcare: A systematic literature review," *Applied Sciences*, vol. 13, no. 13, p. 7479, 2023.

5. Miotto, R., Wang, F., Wang, S., Jiang, X., and Dudley, J. T. "Deep learning for healthcare: Review, opportunities and challenges," *Briefings in Bioinformatics*, vol. 19, no. 6, pp. 1236–1246, doi: 10.1093/bib/bbx044.
6. Siebra, C. A., Kurpicz-Briki, M., and Wac, K. "Transformers in health: A systematic review on architectures for longitudinal data analysis," *Artificial Intelligence Review*, vol. 57, p. 32, 2024, doi: 10.1007/s10462-023-10677-z.
7. Alowais, S. A., Alghamdi, S. S., Alsuhebany, N., Alqahtani, T., Alshaya, A. I., Almohareb, S. N., ... & Albekairy, A. M. "Revolutionizing healthcare: The role of artificial intelligence in clinical practice," *BMC Medical Education*, vol. 23, p. 689, 2023, doi: 10.1186/s12909-023-04698-z.
8. Sebastian, A. M., and Peter, D. "Artificial intelligence in cancer research: Trends, challenges and future directions," *Life (Basel)*, vol. 12, no. 12, p. 1991, 2022, doi: 10.3390/life12121991.
9. Harerimana, G., Kim, J. W., Yoo, H., and Jang, B. "Deep learning for electronic health records analytics," *IEEE Access*, vol. 7, pp. 101245–101259, 2019, doi: 10.1109/ACCESS.2019.2928363.
10. Zhou, S. K., Greenspan, H., Davatzikos, C., Duncan, J. S., Van Ginneken, B., Madabhushi, A., ... & Summers, R. M. "A review of deep learning in medical imaging: Imaging traits, technology trends, case studies with progress highlights, and future promises," *Proceedings of the IEEE*, vol. 109, no. 5, pp. 820–838, 2021.
11. Pesapane, F., Codari, M., and Sardanelli, F. "Artificial intelligence in medical imaging: Threat or opportunity? Radiologists are again at the forefront of innovation in medicine," *European Radiology Experimental*, vol. 2, no. 1, p. 35, 2018, doi: 10.1186/s41747-018-0061-6.
12. Sharma, H., Jain, J. S., Bansal, P., and Gupta, S. "Feature extraction and classification of chest X-ray images using CNN to detect pneumonia," in *10th International Conference on Cloud Computing, Data Science & Engineering*, 2020, IEEE, pp. 227–231, doi: 10.1109/Confluence47617.2020.9057809.
13. Heidari, M., Mirniaharikandehei, S., Khuzani, A. Z., Danala, G., Qiu, Y., & Zheng, "Improving the performance of CNN to predict the likelihood of COVID-19 using chest X-ray images with preprocessing algorithms," *International Journal of Medical Informatics*, vol. 144, p. 104284, 2020.
14. Kim, H., Lee, K., Lee, D., and Baek, N. "3D reconstruction of leg bones from X-ray images using CNN-based feature analysis," in *International Conference on Information and Communication Technology Convergence (ICTC)*, IEEE, 2019, pp. 669–672, doi: 10.1109/ICTC46691.2019.8939984.
15. Rao, L. J., Ramkumar, M., Kothapalli, C., Savarapu, P. R., and Basha, C. Z. "Advanced computerized classification of X-ray images using CNN," in *Third International Conference on Smart Systems and Inventive Technology (ICSSIT)*, IEEE, 2020, pp. 1247–1251, doi: 10.1109/ICSSIT48917.2020.9214136.
16. Arora, S., Tripathy, S. K., Gupta, R., and Srivastava, R. "Exploiting multimodal CNN architecture for automated teeth segmentation on dental panoramic X-ray images," *Proceedings of the Institution of Mechanical Engineers, Part H: Journal of Engineering in Medicine*, vol. 237, no. 3, pp. 395–405, 2023, doi: 10.1177/09544119231157137.
17. Bigham-Sadegh, A., and Oryan, A. "Basic concepts regarding fracture healing and the current options and future directions in managing bone fractures," *International Wound Journal*, vol. 12, no. 3, pp. 238–247, 2015, doi: 10.1111/iwj.12231.
18. Yahalomi, E., Chernofsky, M., and Werman, M. "Detection of distal radius fractures trained by a small set of X-ray images and faster R-CNN," in *Intelligent Computing: Proceedings*

of the 2019 Computing Conference, Vol. 1, Springer International Publishing, 2019, pp. 12–25, doi: 10.1007/978-3-030-22868-2_1.

19. Mahum, R., Rehman, S. U., Meraj, T., Rauf, H. T., Irtaza, A., El-Sherbeeny, A. M., & El-Meligy, M. A. "A novel hybrid approach based on deep CNN features to detect knee osteoarthritis," *Sensors*, vol. 21, no. 18, p. 6189, 2021.
20. Potter, I. Y., Yeritsyan, D., Mahar, S., Wu, J., Nazarian, A., Vaziri, A., & Vaziri, A. "Automated bone tumor segmentation and classification as benign or malignant using computed tomographic imaging," *Journal of Digital Imaging*, vol. 36, pp. 869–878, 2023, doi: 10.1007/s10278-022-00771-z.
21. Wu, S., Bai, X., Cai, L., Wang, L., Zhang, X., Ke, Q., & Huang, J. "Bone tumor examination based on FCNN-4s and CRF fine segmentation fusion algorithm," *Journal of Bone Oncology*, vol. 42, p. 100502, 2023.
22. Crema, M. D., et al. "MRI of ankle sprain: The association between joint effusion and structural injury severity in a large cohort of athletes," *European Radiology*, vol. 29, pp. 6336–6344, 2019.
23. Rehman, A., Khan, M. A., Saba, T., Mehmood, Z., Tariq, U., & Ayesha, N. (2021). Microscopic brain tumor detection and classification using 3D CNN and feature selection architecture. *Microscopy Research and Technique*, *84*(1), 133–149.
24. Abdusalomov, A. B., Mukhiddinov, M., and Whangbo, T. K. "Brain tumor detection based on deep learning approaches and magnetic resonance imaging," *Cancers*, vol. 15, no. 16, p. 4172, 2023, doi: 10.3390/cancers15164172.
25. Jain, V., Nankar, O., Jerrish, D. J., Gite, S., Patil, S., & Kotecha, K. "A novel AI-based system for detection and severity prediction of dementia using MRI," *IEEE Access*, vol. 9, pp. 154324–154346, 2021, doi: 10.1109/ACCESS.2021.3127394.
26. Roest, C., Kwee, T. C., Saha, A., Fütterer, J. J., Yakar, D., & Huisman, H. "AI-assisted biparametric MRI surveillance of prostate cancer: Feasibility study," *European Radiology*, vol. 33, no. 1, pp. 89–96, 2023.
27. Martis, R. J., Lin, H., Javadi, B., Fernandes, S. L., and Yasmin, M. "Editorial of the special issue DLHI: Deep learning in medical imaging and health informatics," 2020. *Pattern Recognition Letters*, vol. 140, December 2020, pp. 116–118
28. Lamb, L. R., Lehman, C. D., Gastounioti, A., Conant, E. F., & Bahl, M. "Artificial intelligence (AI) for screening mammography, from the AJR special series on AI applications," *American Journal of Roentgenology*, vol. 219, no. 3, pp. 369–380, 2022.
29. Karthiga, R., Narasimhan, K., and Amirtharajan, R. "Diagnosis of breast cancer for modern mammography using artificial intelligence," *Mathematics and Computers in Simulation*, vol. 202, pp. 316–330, 2022, doi: 10.1016/j.matcom.2022.04.008.
30. Lauritzen, A. D., Rodríguez-Ruiz, A., von Euler-Chelpin, M. C., Lynge, E., Vejborg, I., Nielsen, M., ... & Lillholm, M. "An artificial intelligence–based mammography screening protocol for breast cancer: Outcome and radiologist workload," *Radiology*, vol. 304, no. 1, pp. 41–49, 2022.
31. Chu, Y., Huang, F., Gao, M., Zou, D. W., Zhong, J., Wu, W., ... & Wang, L. F. "Convolutional neural network-based segmentation network applied to image recognition of angiodysplasias lesion under capsule endoscopy," *World Journal of Gastroenterology*, vol. 29, no. 5, pp. 879–889, 2023, doi: 10.3748/wjg.v29.i5.879.
32. Liu, X., Mao, J., Sun, N., Yu, X., Chai, L., Tian, Y., ... & Lu, L. "Deep learning for detection of intracranial aneurysms from computed tomography angiography images," *Journal of Digital Imaging*, vol. 36, pp. 114–123, 2023, doi: 10.1007/s10278-022-00698-5.
33. Bolhasani, H., Jassbi, S. J., and Sharifi, A. "DLA-E: A deep learning accelerator for endoscopic images classification," *Journal of Big Data*, vol. 10, p. 76, 2023, doi: 10.1186/s40537-023-00775-8.

34. Barash, Y., Livne, A., Klang, E., Sorin, V., Cohen, I., Khaitovich, B., & Raskin, D. "Artificial intelligence for identification of images with active bleeding in mesenteric and celiac arteries angiography," *CardioVascular and Interventional Radiology*, vol. 47, pp. 785–792, 2024, doi: 10.1007/s00270-024-03689-x.
35. Tripathi, S., Verma, A., and Sharma, N. "Automatic segmentation of brain tumour in MR images using an enhanced deep learning approach," *Computer Methods in Biomechanics and Biomedical Engineering: Imaging & Visualization*, 2021, vol. 9, no. 2, pp. 121–130, doi: 10.1080/21681163.2020.1818628.
36. Bhanothu, Y., Kamalakannan, A., and Rajamanickam, G. "Detection and classification of brain tumor in MRI images using deep convolutional network," IEEE 2020 6th International Conference on Advanced Computing and Communication Systems (ICACCS), Coimbatore, India, 2020, pp. 248–252, doi: 10.1109/ICACCS48705.2020.9074375.
37. Saba, T., Mohamed, A. S., El-Affendi, M., Amin, J., and Sharif, M. "Brain tumor detection using fusion of hand crafted and deep learning features," *Cognitive Systems Research*, vol. 59, pp. 221–230, 2020.
38. Thaha, M. M., Kumar, K. P. M., Murugan, B. S., Dhanasekeran, S., Vijayakarthick, P., & Selvi, A. S. "Brain tumor segmentation using convolutional neural networks in MRI images," *Journal of Medical Systems*, vol. 43, p. 294, 2019, doi: 10.1007/s10916-019-1416-0.
39. Ricciardi, R., Mettivier, G., Staffa, M., Sarno, A., Acampora, G., Minelli, S., ... & Russo, P. "A deep learning classifier for digital breast tomosynthesis," *Physica Medica*, vol. 83, 184–193, 2021.
40. Benjelloun, M., Adoui, M. E., Larhmam, M. A., and Mahmoudi, S. A. "Automated breast tumor segmentation in DCE-MRI using deep learning," IEEE, in 2018 4th International Conference on Cloud Computing Technologies and Applications (Cloudtech), Brussels, Belgium, 2018, pp. 1–6, doi: 10.1109/CloudTech.2018.8713352.
41. Pesapane, F., Trentin, C., Ferrari, F., Signorelli, G., Tantrige, P., Montesano, M., ... & Cassano, E. "Deep learning performance for detection and classification of microcalcifications on mammography," *European Radiology Experimental*, vol. 7, no. 69, 2023, doi: 10.1186/s41747-023-00384-3.
42. Nemade, V., Pathak, S., and Dubey, A. K. "Deep learning-based ensemble model for classification of breast cancer," *Microsystem Technologies*, vol. 30, pp. 513–527, 2024, doi: 10.1007/s00542-023-05469-y.
43. Xu, C., Zhang, D., Chong, J., Chen, B., & Li, S. "Synthesis of gadolinium-enhanced liver tumors on nonenhanced liver MR images using pixel-level graph reinforcement learning," *Medical Image Analysis*, vol. 69, p. 101976, 2021, doi: 10.1016/j.media.2020.101976.
44. Huang, Y. J., Chen, C. H., and Yang, H. C. "AI-enhanced integration of genetic and medical imaging data for risk assessment of type 2 diabetes," *medRxiv*, 2023, doi: 10.1101/2023.08.29.23293718.
45. Zhao, D., Wang, W., Tang, T., Zhang, Y. Y., and Yu, C. "Current progress in artificial intelligence-assisted medical image analysis for chronic kidney disease: A literature review," *Computational and Structural Biotechnology Journal*, vol. 21, pp. 3315–3326, 2023, doi: 10.1016/j.csbj.2023.05.029.
46. Singh, V., Asari, V. K., and Rajasekaran, R. "A deep neural network for early detection and prediction of chronic kidney disease," *Diagnostics*, vol. 12, no. 1, p. 116, 2022, doi: 10.3390/diagnostics12010116.
47. Wang, X., Shen, T., Yang, S., Lan, J., Xu, Y., Wang, M., ... & Han, X. "A deep learning algorithm for automatic detection and classification of acute intracranial hemorrhages in head CT scans," *NeuroImage: Clinical*, vol. 32, p. 102785, 2021.

48. Saw, S. N., & Ng, K. H. (2022). Current challenges of implementing artificial intelligence in medical imaging. Physica Medica, 100, 12–17.
49. Farhud, D. D., and Zokaei, S. "Ethical issues of artificial intelligence in medicine and healthcare," *Iranian Journal of Public Health*, vol. 50, no. 11, pp. i–v, 2021, doi: 10.18502/ijph.v50i11.7600.
50. Naik, N., Hameed, B. Z., Shetty, D. K., Swain, D., Shah, M., Paul, R., ... & Somani, B. K. "Legal and ethical consideration in artificial intelligence in healthcare: Who takes responsibility?" *Frontiers in Surgery*, vol. 9, p. 862322, 2022, doi: 10.3389/fsurg.2022.862322.

7 Wearable HealthTech
Empowering Patients and Preventive Care

Ushaa Eswaran, Vivek Eswaran, Keerthna Murali, and Vishal Eswaran

7.1 INTRODUCTION

The advancement in technology, under the change of focus from the disease-centered medical model to the patient-centered one due to the increasing importance of self-management and prevention, has some significant impact on the future healthcare. HealthTech, in simple terms, is wearable health technology or technology that helps people monitor and manage various facets of health and wellness or the process through which an individual reclaims control over his/her health. Wearable health technology is among the most dynamic fields that factors in the management of health and healthcare delivery [1]. Because of the fact that they provide data in real time, tailored and actionable, wearables that can span from wristbands and smartwatches to complex biosensors and distant perceptual systems are empowering citizens to be active players in their health.

As the current structure of healthcare delivery, we have seen that the majority of healthcare facilities have worked on the model that is known as the sickness model of healthcare. While this model is good at quick fixes, it does not work as effectively in addressing the increasing chronic diseases, rising costs, or the required primary prevention [2]. Better healthcare strategies focused on the prevention of diseases rather than treatment are rather scarce, as the rates of chronic diseases such as diabetes, hypertension, cardiovascular diseases, etc., are rising progressively. This is where the actual potential of wearable health technologies as transformational devices is found.

Wearable technology adds a new dimension to knowledge about a person's state of health by constantly recording pulse, activity levels, sleep quality, and other health indicators. These gadgets enhance these capabilities through big data analytics, and machine learning (ML) as well as artificial intelligence (AI)/ML technologies [3]. The data collected by these devices can be viewed on a massive scale for mass health recommendations, detection of vital health risks, and prevention using AI Boolean algorithms. Wearable technology, for instance, can monitor blood glucose, diagnose arrhythmia, or assess one's probability of having a stroke. It could also transmit such data to healthcare practitioners to improve the decisions they are making.

DOI: 10.1201/9781003516163-7

Outside of diet and exercise, the free movement of consumer health technologies is altering patient relations with doctors. Real-time monitoring devices enable medical personnel to monitor a patient's condition so that a patient can receive ongoing care without being admitted to the hospital regularly [4]. It makes treatment more timely and personalized, thus producing better patient outcomes while at the same time reducing the healthcare costs. Moreover, wearable technology is very useful in the treatment of continuous monitoring because people can be monitored continuously, thereby increasing their compliance with the prescribed treatment regimens.

Wearable health technology has impacts not only on health outcomes but also on broader society. Challenges faced in the healthcare sector across the globe, such as unequal distribution of healthcare gadgets, could be solved by these gadgets [5]. Wearable technology can help patients and their caregivers in underdeveloped areas by establishing connections with them through the use of telemedicine and basic health diagnosis. Furthermore, the concept of wearable technology is expected to integrate with ultimate advancements like telemedicine, virtual reality (VR), and augmented reality (AR) innovations. This way, the wearables will be more applicable not just to patients but also to teaching as well in the healthcare field.

Altogether, wearable health technology is quickly changing how people approach and engage in healthcare. HealthTech puts the shifting of power back into the hands of people so that many of those who need healthcare can take responsibility and avail more personalized and effective treatment from practitioners by shifting the focus from acute care to preventive one. They could in the future improve individual health and organizational healthcare system's accessibility, equity, and sustainability.

7.2 LITERATURE REVIEW

Wearable health technology or HealthTech which has emerged as the new era in healthcare is a revolutionary sector supporting empowered patient-centered preventive care. It presents a synthesis of current literature on wearable health technology, its use, and implications for practicing healthcare. Main outcomes, methods used in the studies, and contributions that have been made in the field will be discussed, as well as possible shortcomings or directions that have not been studied enough yet [6].

7.2.1 Wearable HealthTech: An Overview

Fit trackers, smartwatches, and other types of customized health monitoring instruments such as medical devices are incorporated into wearable technologies to record health indicators [7]. Such gadgets can detect blood sugar levels, pulse, sleep, activity, and other things and provide the users as well as physicians with information within a short time.

This section employs a pie chart in Figure 7.1 to illustrate the several applications of wearable health technology (HealthTech). The graphic focuses on how wearable technology impacts health management by covering important topics that include medication reminders and compliance, sleep, heart rate, chronic illness, exercise, patient control, and health prevention.

Figure 7.1 shows the applications of wearable health technology.

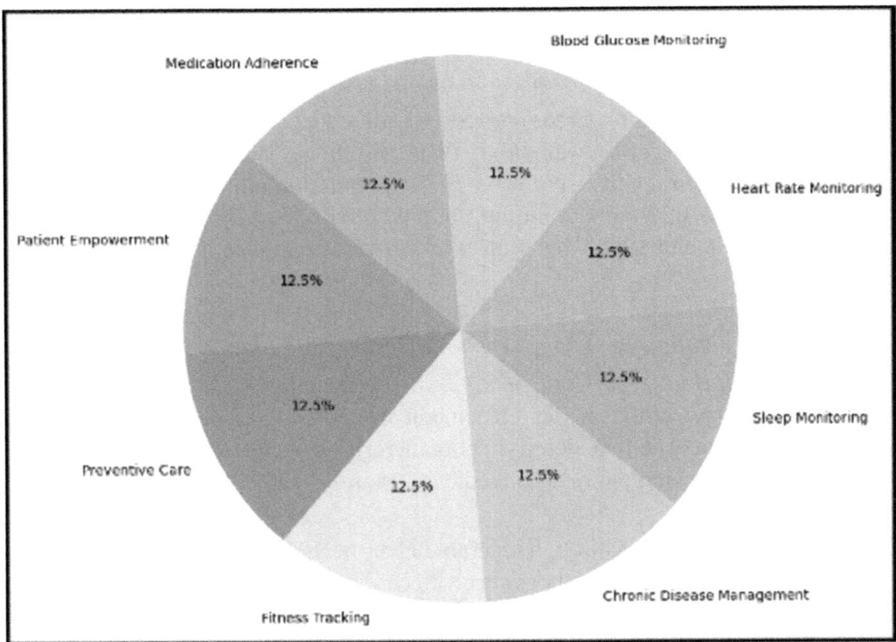

FIGURE 7.1 Applications of Wearable Health Technology.

7.2.2 Key Studies and Findings

7.2.2.1 Patient Empowerment through Wearable HealthTech

This paper, written in 2024, examined how wearable HealthTech enhances patients' autonomy in self-managing chronic illnesses. The research suggests that wearables enhance patient compliance, treatment schedules, and health results [8].

One study to be discussed is the psychological impact of wearable health technology on patients examined in 2024. The study showed that utilization of such devices has a positive continued impact on mental health through enhancing independence and self-esteem while dealing with health [9].

7.2.2.2 Preventive Care and Early Detection

We went further in the October 2024 study to show how wearable devices can help reduce the risk of sickness by detecting signs of risk beforehand. The devices have proven useful in faster identification of abnormal heart rhythms, signs of diabetic conditions, and other diseases [10].

An analysis of several studies on fitness trackers showed that continuous use of the Lose It! wearables promoted positive changes in the user's eating habits and physical activity that could substantially reduce the risks of diseases related to particular lifestyles [11].

7.2.2.3 Methodologies Used in Wearable HealthTech Research

7.2.2.3.1 Randomized Controlled Trials

7.2.2.3.1.1 Meaning and Significance Randomized controlled trials (RCTs) are best recognized as a tool to evaluate medication efficacy and safety within clinical trials. Randomization involves partitioning the population into two different groups, including members of the intervention group who will be using the wearable gadget in this case, and members of the control group who are given a placebo or regular treatment [12].

7.2.2.3.2 Application in Wearable HealthTech

7.2.2.3.2.1 Randomized Controlled Trials Systematic RCTs provide essential information on how utilizing wearable medical technologies performs in different contexts. These papers help in identifying not merely whether a tool is effective but also how it performs in relation to regular medical operations and other forms of remedy.

Example: Self-monitoring through wearable electrocardiogram (ECG) monitors was examined in a study that involved patients with cardiac disease. In this trial, participants were divided into two groups: In one, the researchers employed a wearable ECG monitor, while the other was based on standard monitoring techniques. It was evident from the outcomes that through wearing the device, individuals with heart problems received enhanced treatment by detecting vital issues on time adding to therapeutic value [13].

7.2.2.3.3 Observational Studies and Surveys

7.2.2.3.3.1 Definition and Importance Exploratory research often involves observing subjects or processes without interfering, which helps in gaining insights into realistic usage and outcomes.. Surveys and physical and online tools capture information regarding users' experiences and perceptions through questionnaires/interviews.

7.2.2.3.3.2 Application in Wearable HealthTech These methods are especially useful to gain insights into the integration of wearables into daily life, the compliance of the user, and the behavioral effects of these technologies. The results offer a good understanding concerning customer satisfaction, possible obstacles to the use of the devices, and the efficiency of the devices from the users' perspective.

7.2.2.3.3.3 Observational Studies These studies look at how wearables become integrated into the user's life and how these affect the user's health.

Example: In using a fitness tracker, a specific research project might monitor the level of usage before and after as well as the factors that may influence users to continue using the device.

7.2.2.3.3.4 Surveys Self-administered questionnaires provide qualitative information about user impressions, perceived benefits, or difficulties associated with the devices.

Example: Surveys would provide insight into the level of compliance that users demonstrate toward the technology, the various behavioral aspects associated with it, and how people integrate wearables into their lives. From the perspective of the user, these surveys provide information on the general effectiveness of a device and possible hindrances to its use as well as user satisfaction.

7.2.2.3.4 Combined Approach

Despite the richness of the data, one might combine two approaches to observational studies and surveys for a further comprehensive view of wearable health devices. While surveys give the author client/user opinions of their experiences with the product, observational data gives the author factual usage information.

Example: A meta-synthesis on wearable sleep trackers may combine survey results on people's subjective experience of using the device and their amount of sleep and quality as measured by the trackers.

Thus, promising methodological approaches to the study of wearable health technologies are RCTs, observational research, and internet-based surveys. RCTs provide a clear indication of efficiency in a controlled environment, while surveys are important for depicting usage patterns, satisfaction levels, and behavioral consequences in real life. In using these approaches, the scholars are equipped with details regarding the efficiency and usability of wearable medical devices to increase the efficiency of health interventions.

The methodologies utilized in wearable health technology research are depicted in Figure 7.2. They demonstrate how data gathering, sorting, and evaluation procedures are used throughout RCTs, observational studies, and surveys, offering an extensive review of wearable health devices.

7.2.2.4 Data Privacy and Security Concerns

The study addressed the privacy risks associated with wearable health technologies and underscored the need for robust data protection measures. It was found that widespread adoption of these technologies requires ensuring both the security and confidentiality of users' health information [14].

This report examined the legal frameworks for wearable health devices and provided recommendations for ensuring data security and privacy, highlighting the role of lawmakers in protecting user data [15].

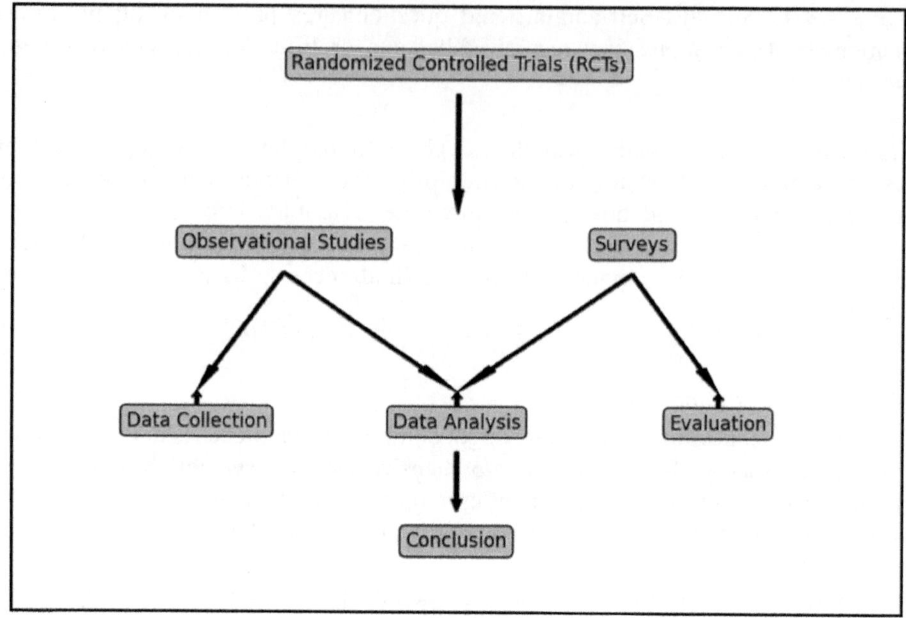

FIGURE 7.2 Methodologies Used in Wearable HealthTech Research.

7.2.3 Identified Gaps and Areas for Further Exploration

7.2.3.1 Long-term Impact Studies

Longitudinal studies are essential to ascertain how wearables will influence patient behavior and health outcomes in the future, even if a lot of research focuses on the immediate benefits of these devices.

7.2.3.2 Diverse Population Studies

Most research has been done on specific populations, usually in industrialized nations. It is necessary to conduct research on the applicability of wearable health technologies in disadvantaged and diverse populations [16].

7.2.3.3 Integration with Healthcare Systems

Further research is needed to ascertain how wearable health technology may be simply integrated into the present healthcare systems to enhance care delivery and coordination.

7.2.3.4 Cost-effectiveness Analysis

More investigation is warranted to evaluate the wearable device's cost-effectiveness, accounting for both the original investment and the long-term savings on healthcare due to early detection and preventive therapy.

7.2.3.5 User Experience and Engagement

This study can be significant to those who are interested in what motivates long-term usage of wearable devices and sustained user interest in them. Sometimes it is helpful to think about what users value, what drives them, and what they may find difficult; in turn, this will help designers create objects that can be used effectively and efficiently while accomplishing the latter's goals. This is evidenced by numerous studies and how wearable health technology has the capability to enhance patient care and even preventive care. Past literature has established a strong foundation on which to understand the advantages and the problems associated with these gadgets. Nevertheless, there are still numerous questions that require further research. To this end, wearable health technology gets to be fine-tuned in the way it tackles these gaps in the journey toward the improvement of patient successes and, consequently, the efficiency of services provided in the healthcare sector.

7.3 EVOLUTION OF WEARABLE HEALTHTECH

7.3.1 Early Beginnings

The journey of wearable health technology started modestly with the development of basic devices like pedometers and early heart rate monitors in the early 20th century. These innovations laid the groundwork for what would later become a revolution in healthcare technology.

7.3.2 The Holter Monitor: A Pioneer in Continuous Heart Monitoring

In the 1960s, Dr. Norman J. Holter made one of the most significant advancements in wearable medical technology with the invention of the "Holter monitor". This portable ECG recorder allowed for continuous monitoring of heart activity over a prolonged period, usually 24-48 hours. The Holter monitor transformed cardiology, enabling doctors to detect heart rhythm disorders and other cardiac irregularities that might not appear during a brief clinical ECG.

7.3.2.1 The Rise of Activity Trackers

Wearable activity trackers for consumers were available in the 1990s. Initially, the aerobic specimen incorporated equipment such as the Polar heart rate monitor and the Fitbit Classic. These devices, designed to measure heart rate, physical activity, and fitness, encouraged a healthier lifestyle by showing how much progress has been made by users.

7.3.2.2 Smartwatches: A New Era in Wearable HealthTech

Smartwatches are therefore considered a real revolution within the area of wearable health technologies. These devices were fitted with the best-developed sensors and connectivity and indeed propelled wearable devices to another level. The surge began in 2015 with the Apple Watch, which enabled users to monitor their pulse, track their exercise, and receive notifications about potential health issues, such as arrhythmia.

7.3.2.3 The Impact of the Apple Watch

In this sense, it is relevant to note that such a device as the Apple Watch not only secured the largest share of the smartwatch segment but also initiated the level of wearables focusing on health. Because of its link with smartphones and other devices, it was the main health control dashboard. Recording ECG, alerting emergency services, and detecting falls are the features that came out as very useful to save lives, making this invention one of the lifesavers.

7.3.2.4 Advancements in Sensor Technology

Wearable devices have continued to develop and incorporate more sensors, with their functions also being broadened. The health monitoring and management system has been expanded by these advancements to provide an enhanced understanding of the users' health status.

7.3.2.5 Continuous Glucose Monitoring

For individuals living with diabetes, for instance, technology such as continuous glucose monitoring (CGM) has been developed. Current models like Abbott FreeStyle Libre and Dexcom G6 provide CGM and hence the chances of complications are minimized.

7.3.2.6 Advanced Cardiac Monitoring

From the Holter monitor' experience, today's wearables – Apple Watch Series 4 and onward can take an ECG, detect atrial fibrillation (AFib), and much more, putting heart health at your fingertips. The presented data allows for timely identification of potentially problematic situations and can improve the value of the assistance offered to the users.

7.3.2.7 Sleep and Mental Health Monitoring

Wearable health technology also gradually moved to the next level where it started including sleep tracking and mental health tracking. Some of the wearables include the Fitbit Charge series and Oura Ring which monitor sleep, its duration, and stage/quality. Additionally, the Apple Watch and Fitbit Sense keep track of stress levels to provide information about the mental state of a user.

7.3.2.8 Integration with Healthcare Systems

One of the major advancement specifics in wearable health technology is connectivity with the patient's electronic health records (EHRs). This enables the healthcare provider to remotely monitor their patients, which makes it easy for patients to be checked on a regular basis, especially those with constant illnesses. This integration has the possibility of decreasing the high in-person visits rate and at the same time continuing uninterrupted care.

7.3.3 Future Directions

Wearable health technology is still developing. Future developments will likely focus mostly on improving communication, creating more sophisticated sensors, and extending the life of batteries. With ML and AI integrated, wearables will be able to provide more personalized health insights and recommendations.

7.3.3.1 Innovations on the Horizon

7.3.3.1.1 Flexible and Wearable Electronics

Advances in materials research may lead to the development of even more discrete and flexible wearable electronics, which might be applied momentarily, akin to temporary tattoos, or integrated into clothing.

7.3.3.1.2 Implantable Devices

These devices might also offer streaming data on a number of physiological parameters for enhanced and objective surveillance that does not need external wearables.

7.3.3.1.3 Better Artificial Intelligence and Data Analytics

AI can make health patterns recognizable by researchers, help to predict some problems, and advise on preventive actions based on wearable data analysis.

Wearable health technology is one of the best examples of the growth rate of technology, which could be a dramatic shift in healthcare. From just the basic step counters, it has evolved to smartwatches, if not more. As wearable technology continues to develop, it will keep playing an important role in patient engagement and disease prevention, opening new possibilities for improving health like never before.

The future directions and their relations in the context of wearable health technology are depicted in Figure 7.3. This refers to possible fields such as flexible and wearable electronics, implantable applications, and improved data analysis and AI.

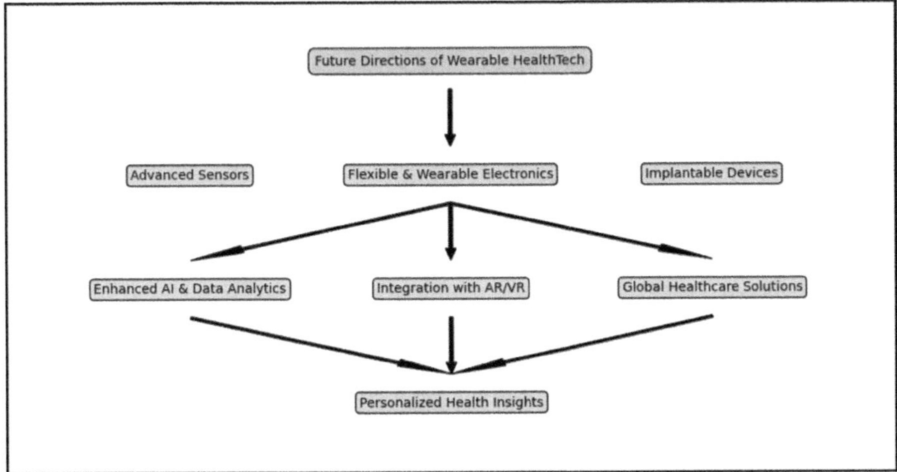

FIGURE 7.3 Future Directions of Wearable HealthTech.

Furthermore, it reveals how technological innovations are extending their integration with AR and VR to enable new healthcare progress. Figure 7.3 depicts the future direction of wearable HealthTech in the integration of both AR and VR and how these technologies will improve the treatment, education/training, and diagnosis of patients.

7.4 TYPES OF HEALTHTECH WEARABLES

Wearable health technology encompasses a vast category of devices, each designed to serve diverse health requirements and convenience. These devices can be categorized into various types, which are discussed below.

7.4.1 Fitness Trackers and Smartwatches

Two of the oldest and most well-known categories of wearable medical devices are smartwatches and fitness trackers. They are still popular nowadays because of their full features and functions that can be useful.

Examples:

- **Apple Watch:** Renowned for its wide range of health-tracking features, including fall detection, heart rate monitoring, and ECG capabilities.
- **Samsung Galaxy Watch:** Offers similar health and fitness tracking features as the Apple Watch, with a strong focus on user health.
- **Fitbit:** A leader in the fitness tracker market, providing detailed insights into heart rate, sleep patterns, and physical activity.
- **Garmin:** Popular among athletes for its precise activity tracking and advanced Global Positioning System (GPS) features.

Functionalities:

- **Heart Rate Monitoring:** Continuous heart rate tracking to detect irregularities and provide cardiovascular insights.
- **Activity Tracking:** Tracks steps, distance, and calories burned to help users achieve their fitness goals.
- **Sleep Tracking:** Monitors sleep patterns to improve sleep quality and habits.
- **GPS Tracking:** Accurately tracks outdoor activities such as running, cycling, and hiking.
- **Calorie Counting:** Estimates calories burned based on physical activity and metabolic rate.

7.4.2 Biosensors

Biosensors are electrical and biological components used to measure biological parameters in real time. They are these devices are used in controlling long-term illnesses and in identifying illnesses in their preliminary stages.

Examples:

1. **Continuous Glucose Monitors (CGMs):** New-generation devices like Abbott's FreeStyle Libre and Dexcom G6 give out real-time blood glucose levels making diabetes management easier.
2. **ECG Monitors**: Portable equipment used for the detection of cardiac disorders by recording the electrical activity in the heart.
3. **Blood Pressure Monitors**: Smart clothing that keeps monitoring pressure to help manage high blood pressure.
4. **Temperature Sensor**: Another type of device and equipment is one that records and always checks body temperature which is important in assessing fever and conditions that affect temperature regulation.

Functionalities:

- **Real-Time Vital Signs Monitoring:** Constantly monitors parameters such as glucose levels, blood pressure, pulse rate, Mach number, etc.
- **Chronic Disease Management:** Provides time-based and event-based information and notifications for diseases such as diabetes and hypertension.
- **Early Health Issue Detection:** Facilitates early recognition of potential health risks so that necessary action may be taken.

7.4.3 Remote Monitoring Systems

Supervisory care technologies or telemedical systems are aimed at offering constant health checks, especially for patients who are being discharged from hospitals, who have undergone surgery, or who have certain chronic illnesses. These devices can be worn, enabling healthcare practitioners to remotely monitor their patients and take timely action when necessary..

Examples:

- **Smart Clothing:** Wearable devices in apparel report the state of health by recording blood pressure, heart rate, and other physiological parameters [17].
- **Wearable Patches:** These adhesive patches track many health parameters, such as blood glucose level, ECG, and fluid balance.
- **Implantable Devices:** These are appliances that are inserted under the skin and monitor some specific physical characteristic consistently, for instance, heart rate or blood sugar.

Functionalities:

- **Continuous Monitoring:** Provides healthcare professionals with continuous access to patient data, allowing them to track the patient's health in real time.
- **Remote Care:** Enables medical professionals to deliver care and support without needing to be physically present with patients.
- **Early Intervention:** Helps identify changes in health that may require medical attention, potentially preventing complications and hospitalizations.

7.4.4 Augmented Reality and Virtual Reality Wearables

Overview: The notion of health wearables in the form of AR and VR devices now lies in the next phase of human innovation. These devices offer virtual experiences that can be loosely applied in therapeutic intervention, patient sensitization, and medical skill development, thus solving some of the most challenging problems in healthcare delivery.

Examples:

- **Microsoft HoloLens:** An AR headset that overlays digital data on the physical world, widely used in surgical training and planning.
- **Oculus Rift:** A VR device designed to create immersive environments for patient therapy and rehabilitation.
- **HTC Vive:** Another VR headset, similar to Oculus Rift, used for patient education and virtual therapy sessions.

Functionalities:

- **Immersive Health Experiences:** Offers patients engaging, dynamic environments that can aid in their rehabilitation and healing.
- **Surgical Training:** Provides a virtual platform for medical professionals to practice surgical techniques before operating on actual patients.
- **Patient Education:** Enhances the way doctors inform patients about their conditions and treatments through interactive and visual experiences.
- **Virtual Therapy Sessions:** Facilitates therapy for conditions like Post-Traumatic Stress Disorder (PTSD), anxiety, and phobias through safe, controlled virtual environments.

Wearable health technology makes health records, analysis, and management a part of life without interruption. The abovementioned technologies will play an ever-greater role in the future of healthcare as patients become their bosses, preventive care increases, and targeted treatment outcomes become better and quicker.

7.5 FUNCTIONS AND USES

Wearable health technology thus offers the user an interface for managing his/her health and well-being in one way or the other. Key functionalities and applications include the following.

7.5.1 Real-Time Health Monitoring

Real-time monitoring is central to wearable health technology as users can track their physiological and other parameters in real time. It offers the users prompt health information and responses.

Key Features:

- **Continuous Vital Signs Monitoring:** Smart Trackers and smartwatches track the blood pressure rate, heart rate, and respiratory rate. First of all, the Apple Watch is able to detect AFib – an irregular heartbeat – due to the ECG feature readily available on the device.
- **Activity Tracking:** Wearables are designed to track physical activity that ranges from the number of steps taken, distance covered, and calories consumed. Apparel such as Fitbit and Garmin provide data on the general activity of the user for the current day, week, or month.
- **Sleep Tracking:** Wearables track the amount of time and type of sleep, including light, quality, and rapid eye movement sleep. They can also recognize concerns like sleep apnea from the other metrics and sleep pattern algorithms introduced.

Applications:

- **Wellness and Fitness:** It allows users to restrict the number of points for activity, track their fitness goals, and receive feedback in the form of rewards and offline gifts.
- **Chronic Condition Monitoring:** Supervision of important physical characteristics is useful in identifying diseases such as arrhythmias and hypertension in their early stages.

7.5.2 Chronic Disease Management

Overview: Because wearable health technology provides guided information on the symptoms, it helps in the avoidance of repercussions in the management of chronic diseases [18].

Key Features:

- **Diabetes Management:** Due to CGMs such as the Abbott FreeStyle Libre and Dexcom G6, users can now manage their blood sugar level more accurately if they get real-time glucose level readings.
- **Cardiovascular Disease Monitoring:** For some wearables with ECG functionality, including AliveCor's KardiaMobile, or with tracking heartbeat, the possibility of distinguishing between pathological and deviations from the norm is possible.
- **Respiratory Disease Management:** Wearables that track oxygen saturation levels and breathing patterns are crucial for the proper treatment of conditions like asthma and chronic obstructive pulmonary disease (COPD).

Applications:

- **Improved Sickness Control:** Real-time data enhances the management of sickness as it involves timely response because feedback is quickly obtained.

- **Telehealth Integration:** Telemonitoring and teleconsultation can improve the quality of the patient's outcomes and decrease hospitalization time through sharing of wearable data to the healthcare gurus.

7.5.3 Rehabilitation and Physical Therapy

Wearable technology enhances physical therapy and rehabilitation with accurate motion tracking and fast feedback, improving patient outcomes and engagement.

Key Characteristics:

- **Wearable Motion Sensors:** Devices such as the MyoPro orthotic and the ReWalk exoskeleton track movements and assist with rehabilitation exercises.
- **VR Systems:** MindMaze provides VR systems that enhance the effectiveness and engagement of therapy by using immersive environments to get patients moving again through exercises.
- **Enhances Rehabilitation:** The devices help therapists and patients assess progress and adjust the strategy with the use of input from wearables [19].
- **Patient Engagement**: Incentives such as those used in VR systems show how patients are more motivated and enforce the completion of treatment regimens.

7.5.4 Stress and Mental Health

Smartwatches can also track the physiological signs that may be related to mental health and provide users the information and techniques for better mental health and coping with stress.

Important Elements:

- **Monitoring Physiological Signals:** Currently, gadgets like the Fitbit Sense and the Garmin Venu use skin conductance as well as heart rate variability (HRV) to measure stress.
- **Mindfulness and Stress-Reduction Techniques:** There are numerous wearables for stress management, such as biofeedback devices, and guided breathing exercises.

Uses:

- **Stress Detection:** By tracking the data daily, the wearables enable users to learn what factors cause stress and how to deal with it in more efficient ways.
- **Support for Mental Health:** Wearable devices also offer opportunities for accessing neurological assistance – mental health support through the practice of calming breathing and other stress-relief techniques, for instance.

7.5.5 Medication Adherence and Reminders

Some of the most useful reminders that the wearable provides to the users include reminders of when to take prescribed medications.

Key Features:

- **Reminders and Notifications:** Applications like MediSafe can sync with smartwatches to alert users when it is time to take their medication.
- **Tracking Medication Intake:** Advanced wearables can monitor medicine consumption and provide adherence data.
- **Improves Adherence:** Regular reminders help prevent missed doses, leading to better health outcomes.
- **Chronic Disease Management:** Proper medication management is crucial for controlling chronic diseases and avoiding complications.

7.5.6 Personalized Health Insights and Recommendations

Wearable health technology combined with AI and ML generates personalized health recommendations based on user data.

Important Characteristics:

- **AI and ML Algorithms:** These advanced algorithms analyze wearable data to offer tailored health advice, such as personalized exercise and diet plans.
- **Predictive Analytics:** Wearables can detect early health risks and disease progression, allowing for proactive intervention.

Applications:

- **Customized Health Plans:** Personalized advice helps users make informed health decisions.
- **Preventive Care:** Predictive analytics enable the early identification of potential health issues, preventing serious complications and facilitating timely intervention.

Wearable health devices help individuals take charge of their health, encourage preventive measures, and facilitate quick action. These technologies offer the possibility to move the healthcare domain from a more generic to a more patient-tailored approach.

7.6 ARTIFICIAL INTELLIGENCE, MACHINE LEARNING, AND BIG DATA ANALYTICS INTEGRATION

Wearable health devices offer health solutions that interconnect with AI, ML, and big data analytics, transforming raw data into big data intelligence and personalized health guidance. All these further enhance surveillance, early diagnosis, and differential therapy.

7.6.1 Screening and Preemptive Medicine

It uses ML and statistical algorithms to produce knowledge concerning possible future diseases and health risks to allow early intervention.

Important Characteristics:

- **Pattern Recognition:** Wearable technologies generate a great volume of health data; AI and ML then search for such patterns that may suggest a disease such as AFib, diabetes, or sleep apnea.
- **Risk Prediction:** Lasting predictive models inform of the risk of contracting specific diseases, and then the user can adopt preventive measures. For instance, wearables may help in forecasting future ways of developing risky cardiac events via HRV.
- **Uses of Early Intervention:** This allows physicians to address the conditions as early as possible before they aggravate to dangerous diseases like stroke and irregular heartbeat.
- **Preventive Measures:** Risk factors are identified well in advance, making it easier for the users to change some of the behaviors leading to chronic diseases.

7.6.2 Personalized Health Recommendations

Wearable data is then combined with AI to give personalized health recommendations based on an individual's health data.

Key Elements:

- **Customized Health Plans:** AI-generated recommendations that correspond to a person's aims and health issues.
- **Dynamic Adjustments:** AI systems receive new information on diseases or on how people live, and they alter the subsequent recommendations they provide.

Uses:

- **Lifestyle Modifications:** Tailormade suggestions guide users in making the right decisions when consuming food, exercising, and handling stress.
- **Improved Health Outcomes:** Personalized information increases the number of individuals committed to their goals and regular exercise and enhances their health.

There needs to be constant tracking and evaluation of the said arrangements. Given below is the explanation regarding why this is necessary in the following segments and discussion.

This way, there is the ability to monitor health deviations, giving constant real-time feedback and alerts.

Key Elements:

- **Real-Time Data Analysis:** AI is permanently engaged in the assessment of the data received from wearable to identify trends of health or a marked shift.
- **Timely Alerts:** It alerts users and healthcare providers about health risks and appropriate measures are taken.

Uses:

- **Early Anomaly Detection:** Continuous monitoring can spot early signs of health issues like abnormal heart rates or high blood sugar levels.
- **Progress Tracking:** Users can monitor their improvement over time and make necessary adjustments to their health routines.

7.6.3 Collaborative Decision-Making

Digital health data of wearable devices can link to EHRs to help clinicians and patients make a single, comprehensive patient-centered decision.

Key Elements:

- **Data Integration:** Wearable technology becomes integrated with EHRs, thereby enhancing a multisystem view of the patient data.
- **Better Clinical Insights:** Such information is then integrated with the other data, analyzed using AI algorithms, and, most importantly, helps in diagnosing and developing treatment plans.

Uses:

- **Extensive Health Assessments:** The availability of full health information gives physicians the opportunity to develop more adequate diagnostic and therapeutic management strategies.
- **Improved Patient Outcomes:** Integration of collaborative decision-making with AI helps enhance treatments, thus ameliorating patient outcomes.

7.6.3.1 Case Study: Cardiovascular Disease Risk Assessment

The Cleveland Clinic was led by the initiative of using data from wearables and EHRs to provide patients an estimated risk of cardiovascular disease.

Key Components:

- **Data Collection:** Wearable devices and EHRs have information related to HRV, physical activity, and other aspects of the patient's life.

- **Predictive Modeling:** Data regarding lifestyle patterns is further processed using sophisticated computer algorithms to arrive at a prognosis of probable incidence of cardiovascular disease.
- **Customized Recommendations:** They provide preventive suggestions for patients using a Personal Exercise and Nutrition recommendation list.

Results:

- **Risk Assessment:** Existing members complete a riskometer test to determine their risk of developing cardiovascular disease.
- **Preventive Action:** Patients can also reduce their risk through some stringent activities such as proper and balanced diet and regular exercise.

7.7 PREVENTIVE CARE AND PATIENT EMPOWERMENT

Wearable health technology allows patients to take charge of their health by making them diagnose their diseases early, provide them with proper and timely treatment, and even prevent diseases from occurring through such actions.

7.7.1 Managing Diabetes

Real-time CGM tools like the Dexcom G6 and Abbott's FreeStyle Libre have really turned the tables in the diabetes management stakes by supplying dynamic glucose data. These tools help patients know the necessary actions for making the right choice of food, proper exercise, and the correct medication, thereby improving blood sugar control and reducing complications.

- **Dexcom G6:** The product works continually every 5 minutes to record the blood glucose and connects with smartphones to display the data clearly. Users get notifications on high or low blood glucose levels, and they can discuss with their providers to get a personalized, more precise, and tailored treatment plan.
- **Abbott's FreeStyle Libre:** This flash glucose monitoring device reduces the fingertip-blood-drawing frequency, as the sensor on the arm of the patient provides instant readings. This tool portrays the glucose data, and it shows specific colors that are to be interpreted by the user so that they may make the best decisions in the management of their diabetes.

7.7.2 Cardiovascular Health

Wearable ECG monitors, such as the KardiaMobile, can identify AFib, a primary cause of stroke, allowing for early intervention and preventive measures. Devices that monitor heart rate and physical activity can motivate users to adopt more active lifestyles, thereby reducing their risk of developing cardiovascular problems.

KardiaMobile: This portable ECG device that connects to cellphones allows users to take a 30-second ECG anytime, anywhere. It accurately identifies tachycardia, AFib, and bradycardia. Users can provide their doctors access to the data for further analysis.

Fitness Trackers: Fitbit and Apple Watch are two examples of gadgets that measure physical activity, tally steps taken on a regular basis, and monitor heart rate. They encourage consistent exercise, provide insights, and help users define and meet fitness objectives.

7.7.3 Physical Therapy and Rehabilitation

Rehabilitation programs are increasingly using VR technology and wearable motion sensors to assess patients' progress, provide immediate feedback, and enhance the therapeutic experience. This strategy promotes patient involvement and therapeutical adherence, leading to better results, shorter recovery time, and a lower probability of complications.

- **Motion Sensors:** BioStampRC and MyoWare Muscle Sensors are the devices that monitor muscle activity and movement providing exact data on the status of physical performance and recovery.
- **VR Systems:** The MindMotion and VHealth systems have introduced VR to form and establish immersive therapy sessions. The patients perform exercises in a virtual environment and gain feedback and motivation; through the process, they are also interacting with real-world elements.

7.7.4 Stress Management and Mental Health

Wearable devices are capable of monitoring physiological indicators like skin conductance and HRV, which, in turn, are used for measuring stress levels. The proper practice of stress-reducing activities, such as mindfulness and guided breathing, will not only allow individuals to manage their own mental health but also act as a sign of their mental well-being to themselves and others.

- **HRV Monitors:** Wearables like the WHOOP Strap and Oura Ring measure HRV. This, again, is very useful for monitoring stress and health. One of the major features of these devices is the personalized advice they provide, helping users engage in activities which make their mental state healthier and cope with stress.
- **Mindfulness Tools:** Devices like the Muse headband are among the gadgets that facilitate meditation and mindfulness.

This will significantly enhance users' ability to manage stress and contribute to building their mental toughness.

7.7.4.1 Case Study: Diabetes Management with Continuous Glucose Monitoring

According to a clinical study, the University of Virginia looked at type one diabetes in young people and how CGM affected it. The study showed that CGM users had a substantial decrease in HbA1c levels – a critical marker of long-term blood sugar control – compared to those using the traditional finger-stick test. Additionally, CGM users claimed better glycemic regulation, enhanced quality of life, and an increased level of self-assurance with diabetes self-care.

The studies showed that over a period of more than six months, CGM users achieved an average reduction of 0.5% in HbA1c. In addition, CGM users rated their diabetes management better and experienced fewer instances of severe hypoglycemia that required hospitalization.

The quality of life: CGM users were less anxious and more confident in controlling their diabetes, which led to blood sugar drops and better well-being.

7.7.5 Future of Wearable Health Technology

The wearable health technology in the health tech industry is constantly evolving, with new innovations emerging daily.

Advances in flexible electronics can be regarded as enabling wearables that are more flexible, durable, and comfortable. For instance, sensors may be integrated into clothing or applied directly to the skin to provide continuous, non-invasive health monitoring. Examples include e-skin patches tracking vital signs, smart clothing checking posture, and flexible sensors that adapt to the human body shape.

Implantable Technology: Implantable devices provide accurate, real-time continuous scan of all health parameters the body needs to monitor from within. They offer real-time information and can even deliver automated treatments. Examples include implanted glucose sensors for continuous monitoring of blood sugar levels, heart monitors for detecting arrhythmias, neurostimulators, and devices for managing chronic pain or neurological conditions

Health and Well-being Gamification: Wearable technology uses gamified features such as challenges, rewards, and social interactions to involve the users increasingly. This process boosts users' motivation and helps them stay focused on their health goals. To train the users to live healthier lives, this integration of social sharing, rewards, and challenges into fitness groups helps. VR-based gamification of rehabilitation programs makes therapy more amusing and enjoyable.

Wearable health technology is revolutionizing healthcare through a culture of preventive care and proactive health management. As the field continues to evolve, one will expect more innovations that will enhance health outcomes and quality of life in the entire world.

7.8 ROLE OF INTEGRATING REMOTE PATIENT MONITORING IN TELEMEDICINE

7.8.1 Wearable Technology Integrated into Telemedicine

Wearable technology and telemedicine are working hand-in-hand to offer virtual consultations, monitor patients remotely, as well as provide and share data between the patient population and healthcare professionals without complications. This integration has enabled continuous and timely interventions, appropriate for improved delivery of healthcare.

Remote Patient Monitoring (RPM): Wearables capture information related to real-time data on health metrics, such as vital signs and activity levels. This information is then dispatched to healthcare providers through telemedicine platforms for continuous monitoring, especially in the case of chronic patients.

Virtual Consultations: Data from wearables could be used by the patient during his or her virtual consultation with healthcare providers. More informed decision-making and more personalized care plans can be considered.

These factors not only enhance access to healthcare for people but also provide timely advice on medical issues, especially in rural or underserved areas where access can sometimes be difficult.

7.8.2 Case Study: Use of Telehealth Monitoring for Chronic Illnesses

The Veterans Health Administration researched how veterans with chronic illnesses, including diabetes and heart failure, could benefit from remote monitoring. With wearable devices and data transmissions, vital signs could be monitored remotely. Management of chronic conditions improved with reduced hospitalization rates.

Study Results: Hospital admissions were 25% lower, while patients were better at controlling their illnesses. Feedback from patients indicated that they preferred remote monitoring due to its convenience, and this led to greater overall satisfaction with their care.

7.8.3 Augmented Reality/Virtual Reality Integration

7.8.3.1 Immersive Health Experience

Wearable health technology is now coming together with AR/VR to open up new avenues in providing immersive health experiences, both in the form of therapeutic practice, teaching, and training.

Virtual Therapy Sessions: For example, in "SnowWorld," virtual therapy sessions provide an immersive environment to assist people in dealing with pain and anxiety by engaging patients in virtual activities that reduce the need to take pain medications so that patients do not focus much on their discomfort.

Surgical Training Simulations: AR and VR systems offer highly lifelike simulations that train the medical professionals. Surgeons can be trained to hone their more complex procedures in a virtual setting, avoiding, at least in a significant way, the risk of going wrong during such procedures.

Patients can be educated using interactive materials that are accompanied by AR and VR. For example, a model of a human body can help patients understand their conditions or the treatment process.

7.8.3.2 Case Study: Virtual Reality in Pain Management

Researchers at Cedars-Sinai Medical Center developed the VR system known as "SnowWorld," designed to help surgical patients or patients recovering from injuries control their pain. When combined with wearable biosensors that monitor the patient's pain, this immersive VR experience has reduced the feeling of pain and, thus, the demand for painkillers.

Findings: Patients who were on "SnowWorld" experienced 50% reduced pain during interventions and overall required lesser pain medications.

Patient Experience: The VR environment immersed these patients in such a way that it dramatically reduced their anxiety and discomfort levels during their medical procedures.

7.8.4 Cutting-Edge Sensor Technology

7.8.4.1 Developments in Sensory and Nanotechnology

Advancements in sensor and nanotechnology research are making it possible to monitor many biomarkers and vital signs continuously, non-invasively, and with higher precision.

Flexible and Stretchable Sensors: With advancements in sensor design, it is now feasible to use sensors as temporary tattoos or to incorporate them into clothing. These sensors provide continuous monitoring of vital signs like heart rate, respiration, and blood pressure.

Non-Invasive Monitoring: Because of developments in nanotechnology, sensors that can detect biomarkers in sweat, saliva, or interstitial fluid have been created, providing non-invasive alternatives to blood testing.

Wearable Health Patches: Small, flexible devices called "wearable health patches" adhere to the skin and monitor a range of health metrics. Companies that have developed wearable health patches include VitalConnect and MC10. These patches can track respiration and pulse rates as well as detect signs of dehydration.

The BioStamp from MC10: When worn on different body parts, this flexible sensor measures heart rate, muscle activity, and other characteristics. It is used in sports science, clinical research, and rehabilitation.

VitalConnect's HealthPatch is a fantastic tool for telemedicine and RPM because it can detect arrhythmias and continuously assess vital signs.

7.8.5 Accessories for Particular Groups

7.8.5.1 Particular Wearables and Their Applications

The development of wearable health technology aims to meet the specific health needs of various populations, such as young people, athletes, and the elderly.

Elderly: Seniors require fall detection sensors and emergency response systems. When a fall is detected, fall detection technologies on gadgets like the Medical Guardian and Apple Watch alert carers or emergency services.

Athletes: Performance monitoring gadgets such as the WHOOP Strap and the Polar Vantage series assist athletes maximize their performance by providing detailed insights into training load, recovery, and sleep habits.

Children: Parents can rest easy knowing that wearables, such as the Owlet Smart Sock, monitor critical signs like heart rate and oxygen saturation levels.

7.8.5.2 Fall Detection for the Elderly

The Apple Watch's fall detection feature uses gyroscopes and accelerometers to detect severe falls. If the watch detects a fall, it notifies the user that they may need to contact emergency services. If the wearer does not respond within a preset period of time, the watch will automatically notify emergency services and pre-designated contacts.

User Feedback: Many elderly users and their families report feeling more secure and at ease knowing that help is nearby in the event of a fall.

7.8.6 Handling Global Health Issues

7.8.6.1 Improving Healthcare Equity and Access

Wearable health technology promises to improve healthcare access and equity in remote and impoverished areas by offering remote monitoring, timely interventions, and better illness management.

Remote Monitoring: By using wearable technology to continuously monitor patients in remote places, medical personnel can limit the need for in-person visits and provide timely interventions.

Timely Interventions: Wearable technology can enhance patient outcomes and ease the burden on healthcare systems by assisting in the early detection of health problems and the rapid treatment of patients.

Disease Management: Wearable technology can help control chronic illnesses like diabetes and hypertension by reducing complications and improving quality of life.

7.8.6.2 Wearables in Child and Maternal Health

In a setting of scarce resources, wearable technology is applied to monitor the health status of mothers and their babies. Devices, for example, are wearable fetal monitors as well as portable ultrasound systems such as Philips Lumify, which monitor vital signs such as heart rate for both mothers and fetuses, helping to detect possible problems early on and intervene in treatment promptly.

Impact: Early intervention devices may help reduce maternal and neonatal mortality rates by avoiding late medical intervention and ensuring better access to care before delivery.

In summary, the immense potential of wearable health technology, when integrated with telemedicine, AR/VR, advanced sensors, personalized wearables, and global health initiatives, is transforming healthcare in its most effective form. Together, these innovations address major global health challenges, empower individuals, and build up prevention itself.

7.8.7 Data Visualizations and Experimental Outcomes

In this section, the results from the experiments and data visualizations of experiments and real-world applications of selected studies are presented, explaining how wearables can empower and assist patients with regard to preventive care.

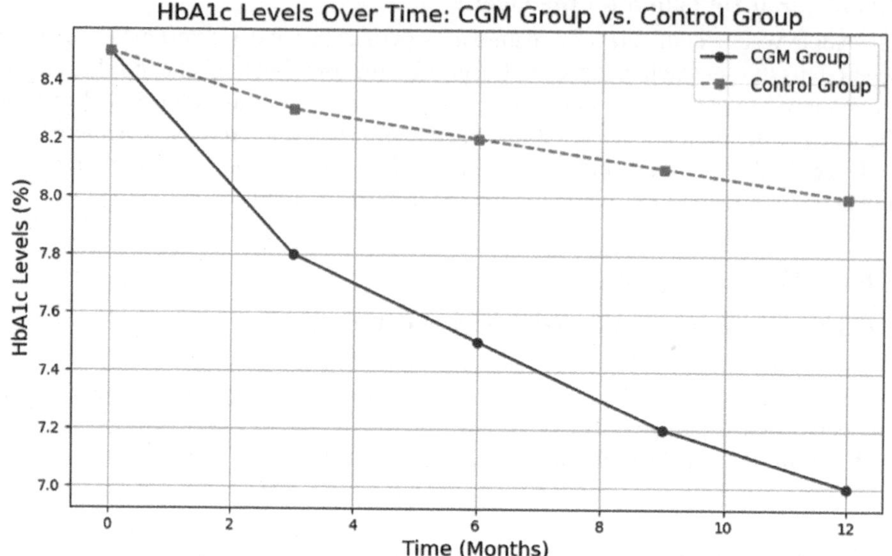

FIGURE 7.4 Line Graph Showing HbA1c Levels Over Time for CGM Group vs. Control Group.

7.8.7.1 Glucose Monitoring for Diabetes through Continuous Observations

The University of Virginia conducted a clinical study that determined how CGM affects diabetes management in young adults and adolescents. A good report was shown of a lower HbA1c level appearing in those who used a CGM device, rather than in those who used finger-stick monitoring. Those using CGMs appeared to experience better glucose control and increased confidence in managing their condition, resulting in an improved overall quality of life.

Figure 7.4 shows the difference in HbA1c level at six months to be markedly changed between the CGM group and the control group.

7.8.7.2 Heart Health and Wearable Electrocardiogram Devices

Cleveland Clinic conducted a research study to determine the feasibility and effectiveness of wearable ECG monitors in identifying AFib at an early stage. AFib is one type of common heart arrhythmia. Patients in whom an ECG monitor was placed for a more extended time were recorded based on the potential presence of any kind of arrhythmia developing in the patient. The data collected was then analyzed by the standardized procedure.

Figure 7.5 shows a histogram comparing the number of AFib events detected by wearable ECG devices with those detected by traditional ECG monitoring. The figure represents a histogram that shows a comparison in terms of count between the traditional ECG monitoring and the newly emerged wearable ECG devices capturing AFib events. The outcome indicates that there is a possibility of a better performance

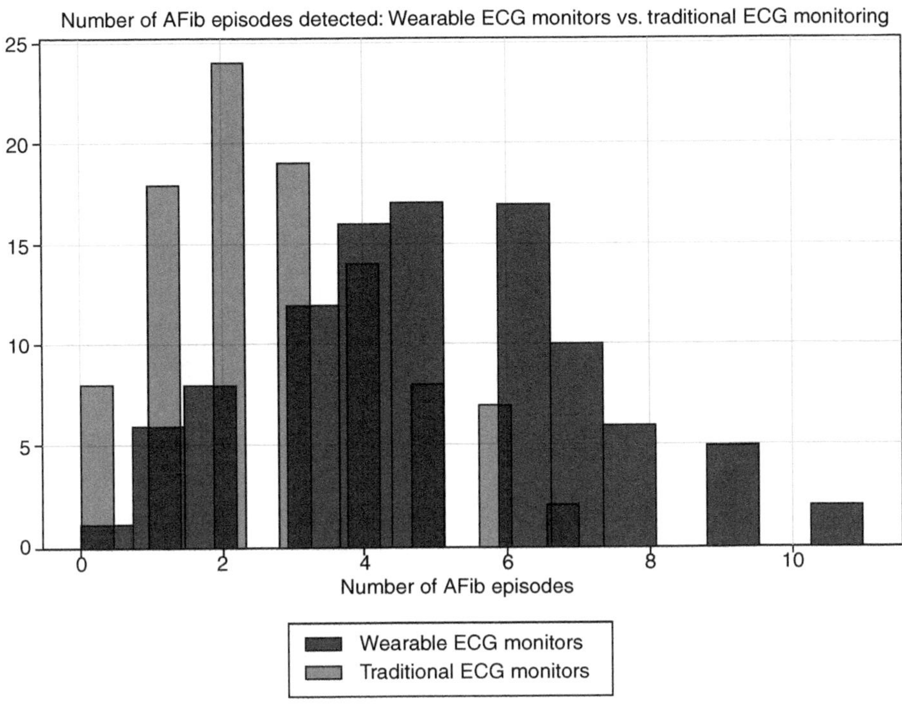

FIGURE 7.5 Histogram Comparing the Number of AFib Episodes Detected by Wearable ECG Monitors vs. Traditional ECG Monitoring.

by wearable technology to capture more significant numbers of AFib episodes so that they may be diagnosed early for proper treatments on time.

7.8.7.3 Monitoring Physical Activity and Fitness

According to an analysis in 2019 published in *PLOS ONE*, long-term fitness tracker wear affects the level of physical activity levels as well as sedentary behavior. In this study, within the followed period, activity tracking devices that enabled tracking day-to-day step counts and patterns recorded participant data for a year [2].

Figure 7.6 displays the mean daily step counts of participants by time in the study. The figure illustrates a tremendous increase over the first months of wearing fitness trackers, suggesting these devices might foster an active lifestyle.

7.8.7.4 Wearables in Child and Maternal Health

Wearable technology in resource-limited settings is being used to monitor the health of mothers and their babies. This may include wearable fetal monitors and even portable ultrasound systems, such as Philips Lumify, through which monitoring of vital signs, like maternal and fetal heart rate, becomes possible. Such data becomes significant for the early and timely onset of intervention, followed by treatment if necessary.

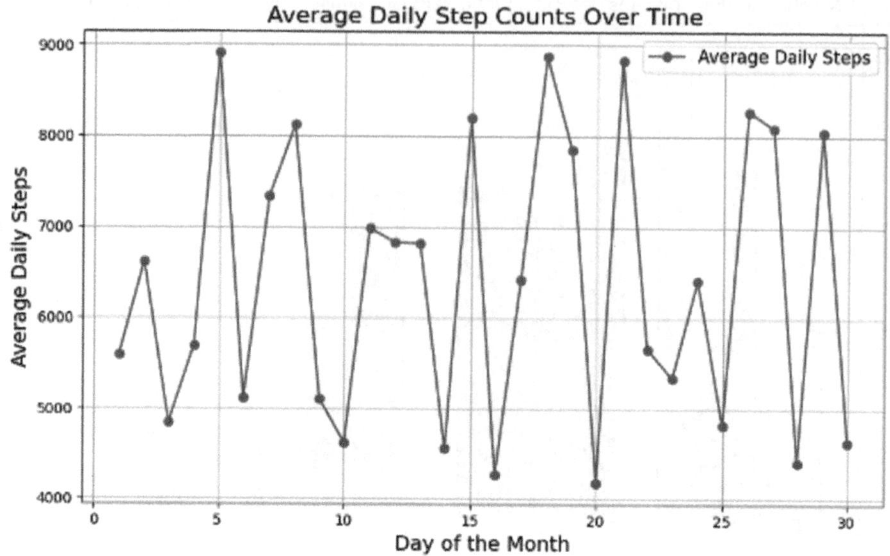

FIGURE 7.6 Line Graph Showing Average Daily Step Counts Over Time.

Impact: These devices are demonstrated with contributions to reduce the count of maternal and neonatal mortality rates, as these devices promote early medical interventions and availability of prenatal care.

In sum, wearable health technologies, combined with telemedicine, advanced sensors, and international health initiatives, hold great promise in mitigating many of the important health concerns. They empower and enhance preventive care and serve as a backbone for improving healthcare systems throughout the world.

7.8.8 Data Visualizations and Experimental Outcomes

This section presents data and visualizations from real-world studies and deployments, illustrating the impact of wearable health technology on patient empowerment and preventive care.

7.8.8.1 Continuous Glucose Monitoring in Diabetes Management

The University of Virginia conducted a clinical study in which CGM was assessed for its impact on the management of diabetes in adolescents and young adults. Outcomes from the research revealed that users of CGM had much lower levels of HbA1c, a long-term marker of blood sugar control, compared to those using traditional finger-stick monitors. Participants reported improved quality of glucose management, greater confidence in their diabetes self-management, and enhanced quality of life.

Figure 7.4 shows a comparison of HbA1c levels at up to six months for the CGM group and the control group. The figure illustrates the role that CGM devices play in glycemic control.

7.8.8.2 Wearable Electrocardiogram-Based Devices in Atrial Fibrillation Diagnosis

Cleveland Clinic studied the utility of a wearable ECG in the early detection of AFib, which is a relatively common irregular heart rhythm. The participants in the study used the ECG devices for several days to be monitored with respect to the start of arrhythmia; this data was thoroughly analyzed.

Figure 7.5 presents a histogram comparing AFib events recorded by wearable ECG monitors and traditional ECG methods. The results show that higher numbers of AFib episodes were picked up by wearables, with faster diagnosis and treatment.

7.9 CHALLENGES AND CONSIDERATIONS

Although wearable health technology holds a lot of promise, various challenges must be addressed before it achieves successful adoption in healthcare systems. This section discusses the core issues and advises on how to overcome them.

7.9.1 Data Protection and Security

The challenges that lie with wearables: Every second they gather and transmit sensitive personal health information, for instance, heart rate, glucose levels, and activity. This is sensitive data, and unless properly secured, it may be prone to breaches. Fears of who may access this and use it could lead to unwillingness of consumers to utilize the technologies.

Solutions:

- **Encryption:** Data is safely received and stored with the help of strong protocols, due to which it is encrypted in the correct endpoint, avoiding the improper channels for access.
- **Users' Consent:** Construct transparent means of consent from users so that they may fully understand precisely what data will be collected and how that data will be used. Explicit consent creates trust.
- **Data Security Procedures:** Regularly evaluate and enhance security protocols, ensure compliance with regulations such as General Data Protection Regulation (GDPR) and Health Insurance Portability and Accountability Act (HIPAA), and provide secure cloud storage solutions.

7.9.2 Regulatory and Ethical Considerations

Challenges: Wearable health technologies are evolving at breakneck speeds, while regulatory frameworks struggle to keep pace. Devices may enter the market with minimal oversight, raising significant ethical concerns about data ownership and usage.

Solutions:

- There is clear regulatory guidance. There should be well-defined guidelines developed by the regulatory bodies such that guidelines on the design, development, and utilization of wearable health technologies exist with safety and efficacy as well as data handling practices.
- **Ethical Standards:** Introduce relevant ethical requirements that would ensure to provide accountable guidance with respect to transparency over data, privacy, and consent from a patient while dealing with this technology.

7.9.3 Standardization and Interoperability

Challenges: Most wearables are produced by diversified companies, which puts them at a very serious disadvantage when it comes to integration into current healthcare systems. Wearables that lack standardization may not share data properly, possibly leading to fragmented care.

Solutions:

- **Industry Standards:** Industry standards are developed to enforce standards on formats of data, protocols for communication, and interoperability. Some examples of organizations leading these efforts include Institute of Electrical and Electronics Engineers (IEEE) and Health Level Seven International (HL7).
- **Collaboration:** Instruct the device developers, healthcare providers, and regulatory bodies to collaborate with each other, thus ensuring that the manufactured devices are interoperable, thereby not compromising patient care.
- **Use open Application Programming Interfaces (APIs):** This would mean that wearable devices could interface with EHRs and further efforts toward holistic care for patients.

7.9.4 User Adoption and Adherence

Challenges: The success of wearable health technologies depends primarily on user adoption and continued adherence. Devices that are uncomfortable, intrusive, or lack sufficient functionality may see a low uptake. In addition, users may discontinue usage if they do not perceive some form of immediate benefit.

Solutions:

- **Wearing Experience:** The product design should ensure comfort and functionality with the aesthetics. Involving users will also help refine and enhance the usability of a product.

- **Engagement Strategies:** Motivation strategy and other tactics, such as gamification, must be embedded in a design that will engage the user in achieving his/her health goals. This can further be supported by feedback and coaching to further increase long-term adherence.
- **Education and Support:** Educational materials that equip the consumer with extended after-sales support to assist the consumer in learning the benefits developed from wearable health technology and how to use it properly.

7.9.5 Cost and Accessibility

Challenges: The price tag for wearable devices, along with accompanying services, maybe a considerable barrier to low-income populations. The high cost will increase health disparity by limiting it to those who really need these technologies.

Solutions:

- **Innovative Financing Models:** Explore financing options such as leasing, subscription-based services, or installment payment plans to make devices more affordable.
- **Cover in Insurance:** Cover wearable health devices in insurance companies as cost-effective and, in the long run, benefits the health.
- **Subsidies and Grants:** The government through subsidies or non-profit organizations can fund poor people to use wearables. Public health programs can concentrate on providing services in underserved communities for these devices.

7.9.6 Addressing the Challenges

These challenges must be addressed through collaborative policies among policymakers, technology companies, healthcare providers, and researchers.

The key strategies

- **Privacy and Security Strengthening:** Use encryption, anonymization, and authenticated secure methods, and strengthen the security protocols regarding emerging threats.
- **Regulatory Involvement:** Involve regulatory authorities at an early stage of development of the device to deliver compliance with national and international standards.
- **Promote Standardization:** Promote common data standards and protocols to enhance interoperability.
- **Involving the User in the Design:** Involve patients and healthcare providers in designing devices so that they meet the needs of both and lead to adherence by the users [20].

In this regard, by addressing some of these challenges, wearable health technology can be further integrated into the healthcare system for purposes of patient empowerment and improvement of preventive care.

7.10 CONCLUSION

Wearable health technology is rapidly changing the delivery model of healthcare so that people are empowered to take charge of their health through real-time monitoring, which gives insight and provides actionable recommendations. This makes early detection of diseases and proactive management possible, resulting in timely intervention with ensured better health outcomes and reduced healthcare expenses.

Beyond this, the available case studies reveal the positive role that wearables play in the management of chronic diseases, such as diabetes and cardiovascular disease, rehabilitation, and mental health. Therefore, all these and more emerging trends – such as the rising integration of telemedicine and advancement of sensor technologies – will further strengthen the influence of wearables in solving global health issues, especially in underserved regions.

Despite well-known challenges related to data privacy, regulation, and user adoption, further collaborative efforts can ensure the responsible integration of wearable health technology. In the end, these innovations are changing the focus from reactive treatment toward proactive prevention and helping people live healthier lives.

REFERENCES

[1] Abaidoo, S. (2021). Technology-mediated transformation of health care and consumer empowerment: An examination of confluence of health-related sociotechnical movements. *International Journal of Technology, Knowledge and Society*, 17(2), 11.

[2] Bauer, U. E., Briss, P. A., Goodman, R. A., Bowman, B. A. (2014). Prevention of chronic disease in the 21st century: Elimination of the leading preventable causes of premature death and disability in the USA. *The Lancet*, 384(9937), 45–52. https://doi.org/10.1016/S0140-6736(14)60648-6

[3] Aggarwal, P. K., Jain, P., Mehta, J., Garg, R., Makar, K., Chaudhary, P. (2021). Machine learning, data mining, and big data analytics for 5G-enabled IoT. In: Tanwar, S. (eds) *Blockchain for 5G-Enabled IoT*. Springer, Cham. https://doi.org/10.1007/978-3-030-67490-8_14

[4] Haldorai, A., Ramu, A., Murugan, S. (2019). Machine learning and big data for smart generation. In: *Computing and Communication Systems in Urban Development. Urban Computing*. Springer, Cham. https://doi.org/10.1007/978-3-030-26013-2_9

[5] Plester, B., Sayers, J., Keen, C. (2022). Health and wellness but at what cost? Technology media justifications for wearable technology use in organizations. *Organization*, 31(2), 358–380. https://doi.org/10.1177/13505084221115841

[6] Aminabee, S. (2024). The future of healthcare and patient-centric care: Digital innovations, trends, and predictions. In *Emerging Technologies for Health Literacy and Medical Practice* (pp. 23). IGI Global. https://doi.org/10.4018/979-8-3693-1214-8.ch012

[7] Tariq, Muhammad Usman. (2024). Advanced wearable medical devices and their role in transformative remote health monitoring. In: *Transformative Approaches to Patient Literacy and Healthcare Innovation*. IGI Global, 308–326.

[8] Wendrich, Karine, Krabbenborg, Lotte. (2024). Negotiating with digital self-monitoring: A qualitative study on how patients with multiple sclerosis use and experience digital self-monitoring within a scientific study. *Health* 28(3), 333–351.

[9] Semeraro, Federico, et al. (2024). Cardiac arrest and cardiopulmonary resuscitation in the next decade: Predicting and shaping the impact of technological innovations. *Resuscitation* 200, 110250.

[10] Husnain, Ali, et al. (2024). A precision health initiative for chronic conditions: Design and cohort study utilizing wearable technology, machine learning, and deep learning. *International Journal of Advanced Engineering Technologies and Innovations* 1(2), 118–139.

[11] Sammy, Yousef. (2024). Impact of wearable health technologies on physical activity levels in sedentary individuals in Egypt. *American Journal of Computing and Engineering* 7(2), 27–38.

[12] Sivakumar, C. L. V., Mone, V., Abdumukhtor, R. (2024). Addressing privacy concerns with wearable health monitoring technology. *WIREs Data Mining and Knowledge Discovery* 14(3), e1353. https://doi.org/10.1002/widm.1535

[13] Yao, Xiaoxi, et al. (2024). Realtime Diagnosis from Electrocardiogram Artificial Intelligence-Guided Screening for Atrial Fibrillation with Long Follow-Up (REGAL): Rationale and design of a pragmatic, decentralized, randomized controlled trial. *American Heart Journal* 267, 62–69.

[14] Khatiwada, Pankaj, et al. (2024). Patient-Generated Health Data (PGHD): Understanding, requirements, challenges, and existing techniques for data security and privacy. *Journal of Personalized Medicine* 14(3), 282.

[15] Salehzadeh Niksirat, Kavous, et al. (2024). Wearable activity trackers: A survey on utility, privacy, and security. *ACM Computing Surveys* 56(7), 1–40.

[16] Ushaa, S. M., Madhavilatha, M., & Rao, G. M. (2011). Design and analysis of nanowire sensor array for prostate cancer detection. *International Journal of Nano and Biomaterials*, *3*(3), 239–255. https://doi.org/10.1504/IJNBM.2011.042132

[17] Zhao, Jinwei, et al. (2024). Wearable sensors for monitoring vital signals in sports and health: progress and perspective. Sensor Review 44(3), 301–330.

[18] Eswaran, U., Eswaran, V., & Sudharshan, V.B. (2013). Human like biosensor disease simulator, disease analyzer and drug delivery system. In: 2013 IEEE Conference on Information and Communication Technologies, Thuckalay, India. ICT (pp. 1033–1038). doi: 10.1109/CICT.2013.6558250.

[19] Megalingam, Rajesh Kannan, et al. (2023). Wearable hand orthotic device for rehabilitation: Hand therapy with multi-mode control and real-time feedback. Applied Sciences 13(6), 3976.

[20] Stiglbauer, B., Weber, S., Batinic, B. (2019). Does your health really benefit from using a self-tracking device? Evidence from a longitudinal randomized control trial. Computers in Human Behavior, 94, 131–139. https://doi.org/10.1016/j.chb.2019.01.018

8 Blockchain and Data Security

Safeguarding Patient's Information

Divyashree Duggegowda, Umadevi Ramamoorthy, and Hemanth K.S.

8.1 INTRODUCTION

In the contemporary era and the information age, privacy and security are the major concerns in the healthcare sector. Safeguarding medical information is vital, and blockchain technology emerged as a groundbreaking substitute to boost data security. Centralized databases are susceptible to unauthorized access, data modification, and hacking. Blockchain technology addresses these issues by providing immutable and transparent architecture. The health data consists of empathetic information, enclosed with personal, financial, and medical details [1]. Protecting the sensitive information of patients from data breaches and digital attacks is extremely essential. The safeguarding of medical data conforms to patient trust and the General Data Protection Regulation (GDPR), which will ensure the integrity of the healthcare sector.

The conventional centralized database methods of protecting data are inefficient and vulnerable to medical fraud, data breaches, and unauthorized access [2]. The immutable and decentralized properties of blockchain technology give a favorable solution for these issues. The evolution of blockchain technology after the bitcoin cryptocurrency, assimilate over different sectors, including healthcare. The increased research on the healthcare sector by leveraging blockchain technology is proving to provide enhanced access control, interoperability, and data security. An electronic health record (EHR) is a digital form of maintaining test reports, scanned reports, and doctor prescriptions of patient medical history [3]. The creation of EHR over the internet enables patient data to be instantly available for real-time access. Digital data sharing ensures that medical officers, hospitals, and stakeholders can access data globally through EHRs. At present, there are many EHR systems around the world with their own definition created by hospitals. Mutual correspondence is required to communicate between these EHR systems for global digital access.

The major challenges in EHR are interoperability, system security, data sharing, and mobility [4]. The healthcare sector has problems with system security, authentication, and access control of patient records. The patient data stored on a decentralized

DOI: 10.1201/9781003516163-8

database requires privileged security to safeguard patient information. Data sharing is another concern; many healthcare records end up fragmented. As individual patients' information can be stored in different centralized databases, accessing this data globally is a challenging task. Interoperability in accessing and sharing patient records among various sources is another main limitation of the healthcare sector. Huge medical data are generated every day and stored in a centralized database, which is the main cause of medical data fragmentation and lack of data access for medical research.

In this chapter, we will delve into the capability of blockchain technology and transform the healthcare sector against data breaches and unauthorized access. We will embark on an evolving landscape of EHRs, addressing data breaches and unauthorized access. We will understand the storage of healthcare data in a decentralized, transparent data storage. We will then continue with blockchain-based data security and building a secure and efficient healthcare ecosystem. Throughout the case studies, we will exemplify the advantages of blockchain technology in magnifying healthcare data security. We will also discuss ongoing development and innovation in blockchain technology and the potential of blockchain for integrating other emerging technologies with blockchain technology. Finally, the reader will obtain a conceptual understanding of how the implementation of blockchain technology is beneficial to the healthcare sector in safeguarding patient information against data breaches and unauthorized access.

8.2 THE EVOLVING LANDSCAPE OF HEALTHCARE DATA SECURITY

8.2.1 Growing Reliance on Electronic Health Records

The implementation of blockchain has made an evolutionary benefit in the healthcare sector. The blockchain offers an advantage in solving interoperability issues like recording, accessing, and storing patient data [5]. The healthcare data in EHRs as modern healthcare offers innumerable benefits in accessing patient data globally by safeguarding against data breaches and unauthorized access. The digitalization of medical data intensifies efficiency and leads to cost savings. Automated EHRs rationalize operational efficiencies such as scheduling appointments, billing, and prescription refills. The advancement of EHRs enhances the interoperability of the healthcare sector and is also valuable for data analytics and medical research.

8.2.2 Heightened Vulnerability to Data Breaches and Unauthorized Access

Blockchain integration in the healthcare sector indicates a comprehensive step toward intensifying the integrity, privacy, and security of healthcare records. Despite its potential, blockchain systems are prone to vulnerabilities and data breaches. Blockchain is a decentralized ledger where data is distributed across various nodes of the blockchain network. The consensus mechanism of blockchain technology ensures security from data tampering; the compromising of a single node will lead to unauthorized access [6]. In healthcare, data integrity is a prominent preference; any breach can have various consequences that violate accuracy and patient privacy. In addition, the self-executing smart contracts are directly written into code in many blockchain applications as an agreement. The poorly written smart contracts could allow hackers to bypass the security protocols, which lead to data breaches.

8.2.3 Consequences of Data Breaches: Patient Privacy, Financial Losses, and Reputational Damage

The health sector has sensitive data, which can have notable multifarious effects on data breaches. The primary consequence of a data breach is the violation of patient privacy. Blockchain, while implicitly securing healthcare data due to its decentralized nature, is not impermeable to data breaches. The unauthorized access leads to the exposure of patients' confidential information, including treatment plans, health histories, and individual identities. Another consequence of a data breach is financial loss, such as forensic investigations, breach response, legal fees, and regulatory fines. Europe's GDPR imposes massive penalties for data protection failures. In the context of blockchain technology, reputational damage is also one of the significant outcomes of data breaches. When organizations are affected by data breaches, it can not only tarnish their reputation but also affect the technology [7]. Issues of such incidents generally spread quickly through media and social networks. Trust is paramount; erosion of trust may result in clients switching to competitors.

8.2.4 Limitations of Traditional Data Security Measures

The traditional data security quantified in healthcare has various limitations, especially reliance on centralized databases, which are vulnerable to single points of failure. If an intruder attacks the central database, they gain access to all the stored data, leading to massive data breaches [8]. Centralized data storage also leads to insider threats, where people in the organization might misuse their access. Another vital limitation is the difficulty in ensuring data integrity. Traditional security measures focus on safeguarding data from unauthorized access and data breaches but fail to maintain the authenticity and immutability of data.

Additionally, traditional systems for data security frequently struggle with data sharing and interoperability issues. According to Health Insurance Portability and Accountability Act (HIPAA), ensuring secure data sharing is challenging among different stakeholders in the healthcare industry.

8.3 THE PROMISE OF BLOCKCHAIN TECHNOLOGY IN HEALTHCARE

8.3.1 Blockchain Concepts: Decentralization, Immutability, and Transparency

Blockchain technology was designed for bitcoin cryptocurrency initially and carries transformative capability for several domains, including healthcare. The key fundamentals of blockchain are immutability, decentralization, and transparency [9]. Blockchain technology provides a powerful framework for enhancing integrity, efficiency, and security. Figure 8.1 describes the architecture of healthcare EHRs by leveraging blockchain technology. The patient records remain secure in a healthcare database and cloud storage. The decentralized network spread across the networks verifies the blockchain and ensures data redundancy. The consensus mechanism ensures that all the nodes agree on the same state to safeguard integrity. The smart contracts run on blockchain platforms automatically enforce an agreement among users.

- **Decentralization** is a core principle of blockchain technology. In this system, there is considerable enhancement in the security of data as decentralization renders it challenging for an individual or team to intrude on the system. Patient records kept on blockchain can be maintained as off-chain data that are encrypted, and decryption is done using the coins for which each patient holds the cryptographic key. This strong security posture is an effective safeguard against the security threats associated with breaches and unauthorized access common in centralized systems.
- **Enhanced Data Sharing and System Interoperability:** The patient data is encrypted before storing it on blockchain and is accessible only through cryptographic keys, ensuring private information remains safe and tamper-proof.
- **Immutability** means that the data records under a blockchain cannot be altered or changed once initiated. When using blockchain technology, it is virtually impossible to change or erase the information stored on the blockchain [10]. Integrity and reliability of records in the healthcare sector are of supreme importance; hence, features of blockchain that ensure that the patient ledger,

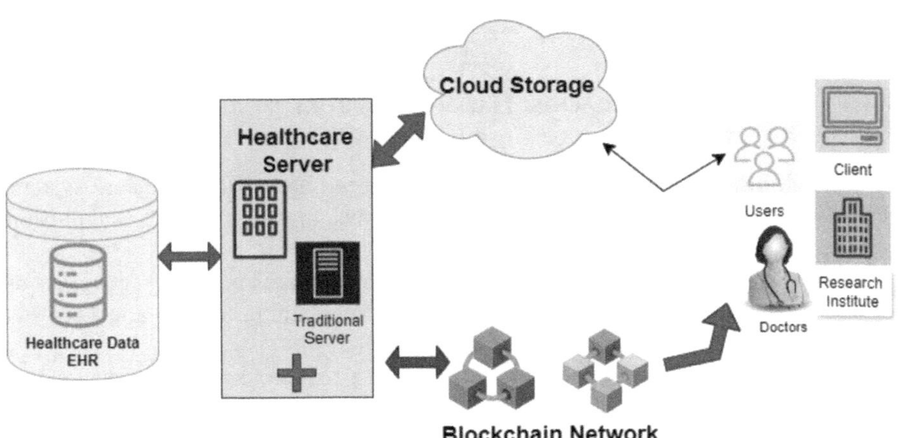

FIGURE 8.1 Blockchain Technology in Healthcare System.

clinical trial, and treatment records remain independent and are immune to alteration can greatly help in reducing the probability of inconsistent records.
- **Transparency** in blockchain is attained through its open ledger system, where all the transactions are recorded and transparent to authorized ones. In the context of the healthcare sector, transparency can increase the engagement of patients by empowering them with protected access to their own health records.

8.3.2 Potential Benefits of Blockchain for Data Security: Enhanced Privacy, Improved Auditability, and Stronger Access Control

Blockchain technology has brought transformation in healthcare by providing enhanced privacy, improved auditability, and strong access control, thereby safeguarding healthcare records. Blockchain uses advanced encryption techniques to encrypt patient data and store it across a decentralized network [11]. Cryptographic keys are used to access patient data, which gives control over the data breaches. All the transactions in the health sector are stored permanently in the blockchain, and the immutable nature of the blockchain will not allow for modification of transactions stored in the blockchain, which ensures improved auditability. The blockchain provides an extra layer of access control through smart contracts and decentralized authentication mechanisms. The access policies are automated by smart contracts that certify the authorized access.

8.4 ADDRESSING UNAUTHORIZED ACCESS AND DATA BREACHES WITH BLOCKCHAIN

Healthcare data breaches put patient integrity and privacy at the forefront, resulting in hospitals facing failures ranging from financial loss and identity theft to reputation damage [12]. All these data breaches can be avoided, and this requires effective mitigation strategies to stop them.

8.4.1 Types of Data Breaches: Hacking, Insider Threats, and Accidental Disclosures

- **Hacking:** External attackers gain unauthorized access to healthcare systems. Such type of a data breach is done through ransomware, malware, and phishing techniques.
  - **Phishing:** To obtain the credentials of healthcare employees, attackers use illusive emails or ambiguous links. After gaining access, attackers steal patient records and sensitive information.
  - **Malware and Ransomware:** They are malicious software designed to harm computer systems. They encrypt information and demand a ransom for its release. These types of data breaches disrupt healthcare operations by endangering patients' lives.

- **Insider Threats** are intentional or unintentional threats arising from individuals within the healthcare institution, such as contractors, employees, or business partners, and are difficult to identify and prevent.
    - **Malicious Intent:** The abuse of advantages by workers or contractors for monetary gain or selfish purposes. An employee could, for instance, take patient information to reveal institutional flaws or to resell on the illegal market.
    - **Negligence:** Staff may unwittingly cause data breaches through their negligence. They can also be a threat to security by handling sensitive data inappropriately, providing weak passwords, or breaching safety standards.
- **Unintentional Disclosures:** These occur when confidential medical information has been obtained by unregistered people [13]. The primary causes for these data breaches are either modern technology failures or human error.
    - **Human Mistake:** Inadvertent disclosures like leaving the computer screen unattended or sending an inaccurate message about patient information are instances of human mistakes.
    - **System Failures:** Data leaks may stem from technical mistakes such as software errors, poorly intended databases, or inadequate access controls. For instance, improperly established databases disclose patient data to the general public domain, making it readily accessible to anyone.

8.4.2 Strategies for Mitigation

To avoid such types of impacts on medical data, extreme safety precautions must be taken. Robust encryption techniques provide protection from unauthorized access. Regular audits and access restrictions to edge data access, in addition to staff training on phishing and cybersecurity threats, can aid in monitoring to avoid vulnerabilities and prevent data breaches. By implementing these tactics, healthcare organizations can lower the risks related to data breaches and enhance the protection of sensitive patient data.

8.4.3 Real-World Examples of Healthcare Data Breaches (Specific Incidents Mentioned Without Confidential Details)

Data breaches in healthcare have reflective impacts on patients' sensitive information. Vigorous cybersecurity procedures are required in regulating data breaches. This chapter determines the impact of data breaches and discovers numerous substantial data breaches in healthcare. Numerous medical organizations have suffered from data breaches; the UnityPoint Medical organization suffered from a data breach twice in 2018 exposing patient sensitive information from phishing attacks. The testing company Quest Diagnostics underwent a data breach in 2019 through unauthorized access by a billing retailer that caused more than 12 million health records to be breached [14]. The vast reputational and monetary damage produced by the American Medical Collection Agency (AMCA) in 2019 affected around 25 million patient data by third-party retailers linked to the Quest Diagnostics medical data breach.

The U.S. Department of Veterans Affairs disclosed a data breach affecting 46,000 veterans in September 2020. Payment data for community healthcare providers was stolen when unauthorized users obtained access to a web program. Increased monitoring of the affected accounts and a review of safety measures were caused by the data breaches. In 2019, the testing company, a Canadian laboratory, was affected

TABLE 8.1
Identification of Massive Breach of Healthcare Data

Year	Event	Type of Data Conceded	Data Breach	Entities Affected
2022	Advocate Aurora Health	Patient-sensitive data	Use of third-party tracking	3 million people
2022	Shields Healthcare group	Medical records and insurance information	Cyber-attacks	2 million individuals
2022	Morley Companies	Sensitive information and medical data	Unauthorized access	5,21,000 individuals affected
2021	Broward Health	Social security numbers and employee information	Unauthorized access	1.3 million individuals
2021	Nephrology Associates of Northern Illinois	Medical information	Cyber-attack leading to data theft	89,000 individuals
2021	Eskenazi Health	Online data theft of patient data	Ransomware attack	1.5 million individuals
2021	UF Health Central Florida	Encryption of patient data	Ransomware attack	70,00,000 patients
2021	American Anesthesiology	Unauthorized access to email patient data	Unauthorized access	1.2 million individuals affected
2021	Florida Healthy Kids' Corporation	Patient personal data and social security numbers	Website vulnerability	3.5 million people
2020	U S Department of Veterans Affairs	Financial and Personal Information	Unauthorized access	46,000 individuals
2019	American Medical Collection Agency	Patient data	Third-party retailers	25 million individuals
2019	Quest Diagnostics	Medical-sensitive data	Unauthorized access	12 million individuals

by a data breach by intruders who hacked sensitive data, including the lab test results. Table 8.1 presents massive healthcare data breaches that occurred in the past 5 years, providing details like the year the data breach occurred, details of the organization affected by the data breach, the type of data conceded, the number of affected entities, and the type of data breach.

8.4.4 Impact of Data Breaches on Patients, Providers, and Healthcare Systems

- **Patients:** The data breaches impact patients by violating their personal information and privacy. The patients do not have trust in healthcare sectors due to the impact of unauthorized vulnerabilities, which leads to confidential patient data disclosure [15]. The immediate loss of sensitive information damages the trust and reputation of the health sector. Generally, the data breaches comprise the patient's private information, like insurance particulars, medical private data, financial and personal details, and social security. Other than the evident adverse impacts, breaches decrease patient confidence in the capacity of healthcare professionals to safeguard their private data. This might result in people being less likely to provide private medical data in the future, which might decrease the quality of care they receive.
- **Health Providers:** Data breaches can have major consequences for healthcare providers in terms of significant monetary expenses related to breach mitigation efforts. These costs include forensic investigations, legal fees, as well as offering credit monitoring services to patients who might have been affected. There are additional regulatory penalties to take into account. For example, breaches of HIPAA could end up with substantial fines from agencies like the Office for Civil Rights (OCR) of the Department of Health and Human Services (HHS). Negative publicity for health providers may impact both current and new patients. The ransomware attacks may interrupt medical systems and the patient treatment may get delayed and threaten patient lives.
- **Healthcare Systems:** The data breaches in healthcare systems disrupt regular operations by causing a financial load. The healthcare system has to take preventive measures to control data breaches: investing in cybersecurity may cost more. Furthermore, the public's trust in the healthcare system as a whole may be undermined by frequent or severe breaches, which may result in a decrease in patient engagement and involvement [16]. This can hamper the creation of healthcare services further by generating cascading effects like reduced involvement in health attempts and resistance to embracing new technologies.

8.5 HOW BLOCKCHAIN MITIGATES DATA BREACHES

The core principle of the blockchain is storing data in a decentralized system and its immutable nature mitigates the data breaches. Here are some ways in which blockchain minimizes the threat of data breaches.

8.5.1 Decentralized Storage: Eliminating Single Points of Failure and Reducing Attack Vectors

Centralized databases, which store all of the data in a single repository, are the basis of traditional data storage systems. Due to the single point of failure that this centralization generates, the system is open to breaches, technological problems, and insider threats. The data stored on a centralized server is easily breached by the intruder, where all the data is compromised at a single point. The blockchain networks store data in a decentralized way, where each node in a blockchain keeps a copy of data by eliminating the single-point failure [17]. The data stored in a blockchain is accessible to all the other nodes on a network, even the other nodes are conceded. The attacks on decentralized data storage are not an easy task for intruders, as, in a centralized system, intruders need to breach the mainstream of all the nodes to gain access to decentralized storage.

8.5.2 Cryptographic Hashing: Ensuring Data Integrity and Preventing Unauthorized Modifications

The major challenge of the healthcare sector is safeguarding data integrity and avoiding unauthorized access. To safeguard data from tamper-proof and data breaches, cryptographic hashing with blockchain is a robust solution. The cryptographic hashing as a digital fingerprint takes an input to produce a fixed-size hash output, which is unique to each input. The hashing cryptographic algorithms like SHA512, SHA256, MD5, and MD4 are used to ensure data integrity, as they produce fixed distinctive output for the given input. The advanced cryptographic hashing techniques assist in maintaining transparency, safeguarding data, and supporting the enhancement of medical outcomes. Conquering the current obstacles will result in an effective and secure healthcare system.

8.5.3 Permissioned Access Control: Granular Control Over Who Can Access Patient Data

Permissioned access control systems are essential to achieve integrity and confidentiality and ensure that only authorized persons access or modify confidential medical data. Permissioned access control is a regulatory security mechanism to control access to healthcare data. It controls the access to who can have a provision to modify or view the data. These controls are serious in medical settings, where the confidentiality of patient data is officially mandated. The various key mechanisms used in permissioned access control systems, like mandatory access control (MAC), role-based access control (RBAC), and attribute-based access control (ABAC), when strict monitoring of data access is required, are used to provide data security by a central authority, depending on the classification of security [18]. RBAC mechanisms are used when only specific access needs to be given to an individual in an organization. An ABAC mechanism is considered based on the user location, time access, and data requested; it is generally based on multiple attributes.

8.5.4 Immutable Audit Trail: Complete Transparency in Data Access and Modifications

Immutable audit trail is the concept, where once the transactions are recorded in a block, they cannot be altered or modified, ensuring the integrity of medical records. An immutable audit trail is achieved by implementing blockchain and cryptographic techniques. The blocks in a blockchain store data and have a cryptographic hash value. Each block contains the hash of the previous block's hash value; modifications to the block are practically not possible, ensuring it remains tamper-proof. The key benefits of an immutable audit trail in healthcare are improved data integrity, transparency, enhanced security, and regulatory compliance. Maintaining the complete log history without modification in data fosters accountability and transparency. The decentralized nature of data storage in blockchain technology avoids tampering with data. The immutable audit trail supports meeting the requirements of regulatory compliance. The medical organizations mandatorily adhere to GDPR and HIPAA regulations in data access. The Immutable Audit Trails meet the regulations of GDPR and HIPAA.

8.6 CASE STUDY: IMPLEMENTATION OF A BLOCKCHAIN-BASED ELECTRONIC HEALTH RECORD SYSTEM

The recent 2024 case study of a healthcare provider in New York, Medblock Health, launched a project to set up an EHR system constructed on blockchain.

Figure 8.2 illustrates Medblock Health's blockchain-based EHR system. The flowchart describes a comprehensive assessment to identify key requirements in implementing blockchain-based EHR over traditional methods. It also describes the multiple tests conducted during the project to deploy blockchain-based EHR.

The initiative is to overcome the interoperability issues and security data breaches. This case study inspects the challenges and benefits met during the implementation process. Medblock Health has treated over a million patients in a range of preferences [19]. The core objectives of implementing blockchain-based EHR are to improve data security, interoperability, ensuring data integrity, and simplifying regulatory compliance. The challenges faced by Medblock were inefficient sharing of data among sources, making sure that patients' confidential data was inaccessible, and security was required due to the rise in data breaches. A comprehensive assessment and planning were done by healthcare professionals, legal advisors, and IT experts to identify the key requirements to implement the EHR in Medblock. A detailed project plan was developed by evaluating the various blockchain platforms. A private blockchain, Hyperledger Fabric, was chosen to avail a permissioned network for controlled access. Blockchain technology was used to store the data confidentially, and smart contracts were used to automate the process of access control. In the development of blockchain-based EHR, all the requirements were met, and testing processes were carried out to test the reliability and performance. Extensive training was provided for healthcare staff and practitioners to handle the problems in maintenance and assistance. The challenges faced by Medblock during the implementation of

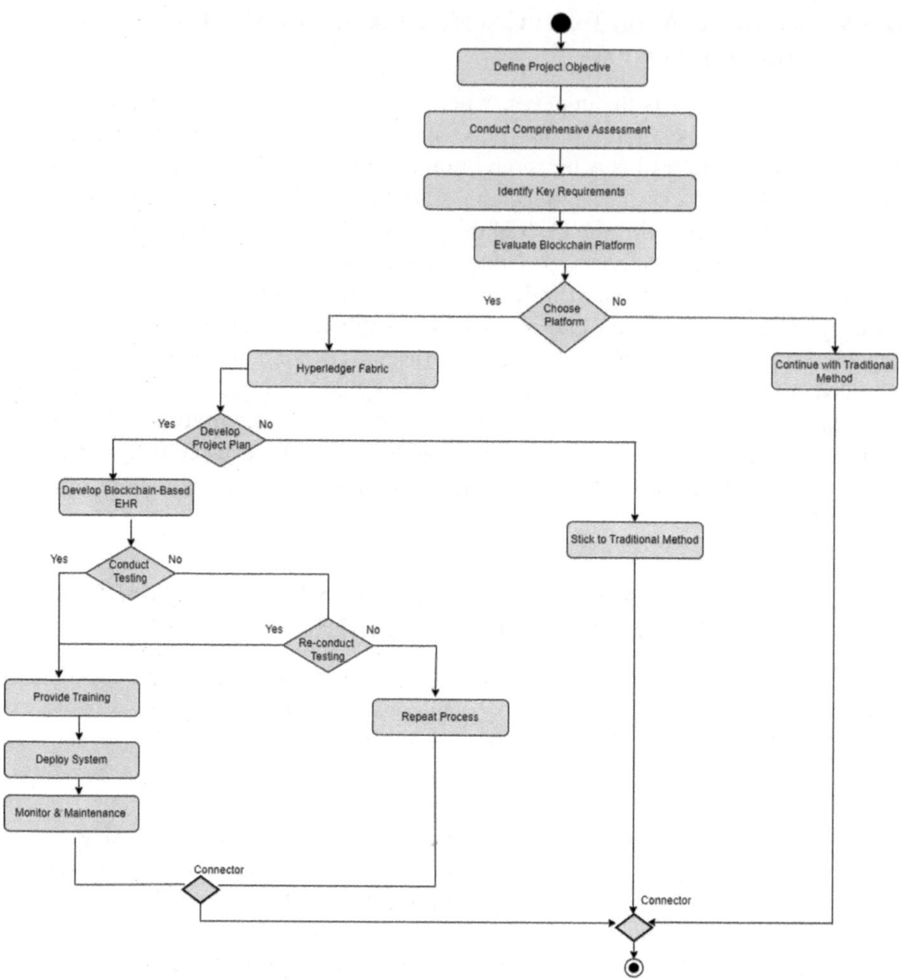

FIGURE 8.2 Flowchart Description of Medblock Health Organization Based EHR System.

blockchain-based EHR are complexity in technical setup, scalability to handle large volumes of data, buy-in stakeholders, and ensuring compliance with regulations.

8.7 DECENTRALIZED AND TRANSPARENT MEDICAL RECORD STORAGE

The blockchain and cryptography techniques are used to attain decentralization and transparency in the storage of medical records. The integration of cryptographic encryption techniques assures resistance to modification of each record and also boosts the integrity, accessibility, and security of medical data. This approach obviates the need for a single point of archive and decreases the risk of data breaches from attackers. The key benefits of decentralized and transparent medical record storage are transparency, interoperability, data integrity, and improved security. The immutable characteristics of blockchain guarantee that once data is stored, it cannot be deleted or altered. The vulnerability minimizes cyberattacks, and an immutable audit trail ensures feasible data access.

8.7.1 Challenges with Traditional Electronic Health Record Systems

Traditional EHR systems have a number of major shortcomings, while digitizing patient records is essential. Data silos: traditional EHR system have interoperability issue and could prove challenging in sharing patient data among various medical organizations [20]. Traditional healthcare is substantial in maintenance, installation, upgrading of the system, employee education, and technical support expenses. The security risks with traditional EHR systems are sensitive; centralized EHR systems are easily prone to cyberattacks. Ensuring the accuracy of EHR systems is a kind of battle that never ends. The sensitive information in patient records can be exposed by inadvertent deletions, illegal modifications, and data entry errors. Another major challenge is usability issues with EHR, which may intensify healthcare providers, while complex interfaces may hinder productivity. Regulatory compliance is another challenge in traditional EHR, as remaining on the forefront of all the regulations of healthcare can be difficult.

8.7.1.1 Lack of Interoperability Between Different Healthcare Providers

The most critical challenge in EHR systems is lack of interoperability; efficient communication of patient data is hampered, causing several issues. The fragmented patient care issue results in repeated tests of patients and a lack of comprehensive patient histories. The increased errors are another challenge; inconsistent exchange of data may raise medical errors. The administrative burden is another issue; healthcare professionals share a large quantity of information throughout the system manually for a period of time; expenses and load of administration are increased by this inefficiency. Patients frequently become frustrated when asked to share their information with multiple healthcare centers, which influences patient dissatisfaction. The potential solutions to these issues are adopting standards in protocols and maintaining structured data formats to enhance interoperability. Integrating blockchain technology offers the safety, accuracy, and availability of medical records. Cloud-based solutions are also the optimal solution for making data integration and data exchange easier.

8.7.1.2 Data Silos Hinder Patient Care Coordination

The data silos are fragmentations of patient data among various departments. Data silos hinder the coordination of patient care and seamless access. The healthcare information may not be available to medical practitioners if patient data is dispersed among separate systems. Providers may request redundant procedures or tests unintentionally despite a unified view of the patient record, which may result in unnecessary costs and annoyance for patients [21]. The medical mistakes and adverse effects increase if essential patient data is not easily available. Implementing integrated EHR systems to facilitate seamless data sharing among different departments can mitigate data silos. Secure and efficient exchange of data can be achieved via the implementation of Health Information Exchange (HIE), while adopting interoperability standards enhances data compatibility.

8.8 BENEFITS OF BLOCKCHAIN-ENABLED ELECTRONIC HEALTH RECORDS

The implementation of blockchain in EHRs ensures various advantages, such as improved security, integrity, privacy, auditability, interoperability, cost efficiency, immutability, and access control.

8.8.1 Secure and Permanent Storage: Data Immutability Prevents Tampering and Ensures Long-Term Recordkeeping

Blockchain technology provides a safe environment by ensuring that once data is recorded, it cannot be altered or deleted. Each block stores a hash of the previous block, encrypted cryptographically, that forms a chain of blocks. It ensures that once data is recorded on a block it is permanent and immutable. The intrusion of a single node on blockchain is safe and will not affect the other nodes on the blockchain network. The long-term recordkeeping in blockchain has tremendous benefits from blockchain immutability. This secure, long-term preservation concept assures maintaining the integrity of medical data and other confidential information.

8.8.2 Improved Interoperability: Seamless Data Sharing Across Healthcare Networks

Implementation of blockchain technology overcomes interoperability issues in healthcare, as it stores data on decentralized platform, making data accessible globally and sharing secure. This also helps to eliminate incompatible technologies among various vendors [22].

Figure 8.3 describes the architecture of the Fast Healthcare Interoperability Resource (FHIR) protocol, as shown the image. The framework of FHIR in an EHR system typically comprises several fundamental components: data sources such as hospitals; clinical labs are the primary sources of patient's information, FHIR servers are the resource repository that stores standardized healthcare data; and the application programming interface (API) layer facilitates secure exchange of data through RESTful APIs. EHR systems act as an interface with the FHIR server to retrieve patient data. The security layer will ensure the authorization and authentication of patient access through the OAuth2 protocol or similar protocols.

Blockchain allows smooth sharing of healthcare data through blockchain communication protocols like Health Level (HL7) and FHIR, assuring data is accessible globally without compromising security. To facilitate the digital transfer of healthcare data between various medical organizations, the HL7 standards introduced the advanced FHIR interoperability standard protocol. The FHIR is the recent

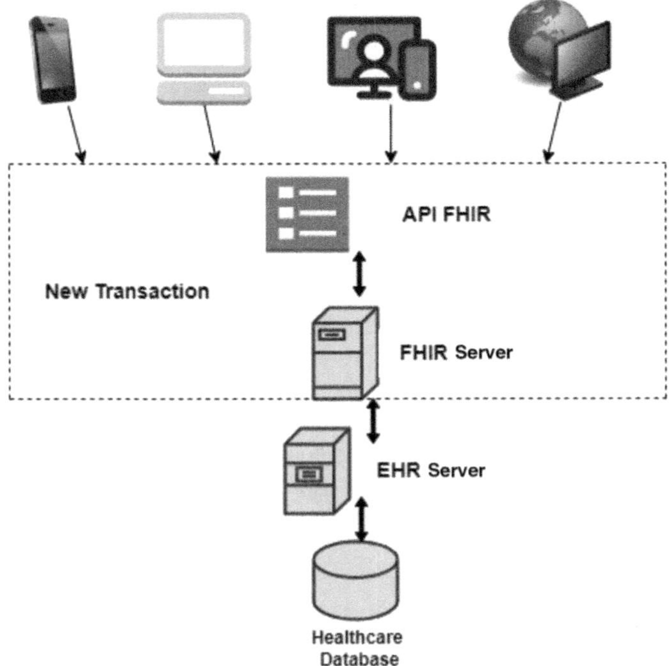

FIGURE 8.3 Architecture of FHIR Interoperability Protocol in EHR.

interoperability protocol that understands the existing theoretical and logical models. HL7 is a simpler interoperability protocol that maintains data integrity and transfers data among medical applications.

The FHIR protocol utilizes APIs to allow various applications to plug in to an operating system and provides workflow with all the pertinent data to the providers. The FHIR standard protocol supports various forms of data, including documents, services, and messages for resource sharing. FHIR is designed to meet the expectations of the user in the increasing complexity of medical standards, providing an internet-based method for interacting between several distinct parts [23]. Data sharing requires comprehensive mechanisms between various healthcare applications. FHIR improves the potential for data communication and expedites the implementation process for application developers of healthcare.

8.8.3 Patient-Centric Data Ownership: Empowering Patients to Control Access to Their Medical Records

The EHRs are made discoverable and easily accessible to stakeholders; FHIR protocol ensures this functionality as patients move around the healthcare ecosystem. The primary goal of the FHIR protocol standard is to achieve digitization to meet healthcare industry growth while maintaining the integrity of confidential patient data. The FHIR interoperability protocol is designed to support machine learning or artificial intelligence (AI). Automated clinical decision support systems make flexible interfaces for patients to gain control access of their own.

8.8.4 Enhanced Care Coordination: Facilitates Collaboration between Healthcare Providers by Providing a Single Source of Truth

In contemporary healthcare, improving care coordination is a crucial tactic that significantly improves patient results. The method of single source of truth guarantees that all team members have access to current patient data. The main advantage of care coordination via a single source of truth is the decrease in clinical errors. A patient seeing different doctors might have their healthcare history and current treatments to avoid unnecessary testing and drug interactions, as the healthcare practitioners have access to the same data through a decentralized database. The treatment plans, medical history, and test results are all stored in a single location that maintains all patient data in a single source refers to a single source of truth. In addition, health providers spend less time looking for patient information and spend more time to provide patient care, which improves the efficiency of medical services.

8.9 IMPLEMENTING BLOCKCHAIN-BASED DATA SECURITY IN HEALTHCARE

The primary advantage of the healthcare industry is to secure patient data, as ordinary healthcare databases are susceptible to data breaches and cyber-attacks. As blockchain keeps data on a network of computers rather than a single server, it minimizes the risks of cyber-attacks and data breaches. The hackers find it very difficult to alter or modify data because of its decentralization storage.

- **Simplifying Management Process:** Blockchain maximizes efficiency and substantially reduces costs in the healthcare sector by simplifying management processes. The concept of smart contracts is embedded into code, which are self-executing agreements with certain constraints that can automate the management processes, including billing, insurance processing, and chain management. To reduce the fraudulent act, the smart contracts process information automatically, saving time and effort.
- **Encouraging Innovation and Research:** Blockchain is an ideal solution for research and innovation; the transparent and immutable design of blockchain safeguards the integrity of clinical research.
- **Enhancing Data Accessibility and Interoperability:** Patient data is frequently scattered among several providers and systems. Blockchain ensures that healthcare providers can communicate patient data securely on an easily accessible single platform by making sure that all parties have a thorough understanding of a patient's healthcare history. This soft data exchange improves effective treatment and the accuracy of diagnoses.

8.10 PRACTICAL CONSIDERATIONS FOR ADOPTION

8.10.1 Interoperability with Existing Systems: Integrating Blockchain with Current Electronic Health Record Infrastructure

The integration of blockchain with the existing EHR system assures seamless integration and interoperability. The objective of this integration is to enhance privacy, data security, and interoperability without compromising the workflows of the current EHR [24]. Assessing the current state of EHR systems is essential, unlike traditional EHR systems, which pose problems like fragmentation, interoperability, and security. EHRs are digital copies of patients' paper documents and are are vital for keeping track of patient health data.

8.10.2 Robust Identity Management: Securely Verifying Participants and Preventing Unauthorized Access

The digitization of medical data and the invention of cutting-edge technologies like blockchain demand the safeguarding of medical data. Robust management is essential to handle and safeguard health information through authenticated access. This entails planning the technological tools to stop unauthorized access and boost the confidence of patients.

8.10.3 Essential Elements of Robust Identity Management

- **Verification and Authorization:** The RBAC and multi-factor authentication (MFA) techniques ensure the identity of users. Several verification techniques like biometrics, passwords, and one-time codes enhance security through RBAC and MFA techniques.
- **Biometric Verification:** Biometric verification is difficult to fake and is the only trustworthy way to validate a user's identification.
- **Managing Identities and Access (IAM):** To verify the proper identity and authorization of users, IAM systems are automated in user provisioning and deprovisioning to ensure the authorized access.

8.10.4 Regulatory Landscape: Addressing Legal and Compliance Concerns with Patient Data

Healthcare organizations must abide by the ethical handling of medical data and the management of patient data to safeguard patient privacy and security. The HIPAA regulates that patients' rights to privacy are respected; it restricts the use or sharing of patient's sensitive information without the consent of the patient. The Health Information Technology for Economic and Clinical Health (HITECH) mandates to report data breaches by healthcare providers to the HHS. The United States has data protection legislation that may set extra data protection obligations on medical professionals [25]. Taking care of compliance and legal issues can be achieved through regular audits and control access to guarantee regulatory compliance. Unwanted access attempts are traced by frequent audits and log monitoring.

8.11 THE ROLE OF SMART CONTRACTS IN DATA MANAGEMENT

Smart contracts are agreements embedded within code, which executes automatically when certain criteria are met between anonymous, identified parties. Smart contracts offer strong security safeguards on a blockchain network; it uses cryptography for protection. Smart contracts provide access control, immutability, and enhanced security. Smart contract handles automated permissions, ensuring that only required information is exchanged. It also guarantees real-time data exchange, giving faster access to vital information. A large amount of administrative work is automated by smart contracts to increase accuracy and reduce administrative burden. Smart contracts automate insurance claim procedures after a patient receives care, enabling automatic claim processing with insurance policies without human involvement. Billing can also be automated to generate invoices on their own.

- **Automating Data Access Controls: Defining Conditions for Granting and Revoking Access to Patient Data**
  Advanced technologies like smart contracts with blockchain automate access controls and enforce guidelines for denying or approving access to patients. To guarantee regulatory compliance and maintain data integrity, control access is essential in the medical sector. Automated data access is necessary to attain security by preventing unwanted access and lessening the workload to improve efficiency and transparent audit trails. Blockchain-based smart contracts facilitate open access management by granting access to patient data according to pre-established criteria, supported by automated data access controls. The essential prerequisites consist of contextual factors such as time of day, particular needs, location, and RBAC. An automated data access restricts the access to withdraw in certain circumstances; key prerequisites for removing access include a change in role, employment status, or end of treatment.
- **Ensuring Regulatory Compliance: Automating Workflows to Meet Data Privacy Regulations**
  The GDPR in the European Union and the HIPAA in the United States established data protection guidelines. These protection guidelines can be automated to comply with these requirements.
- **Streamlining Processes for Access Control and Data Encryption in Compliance**
  Automating encryption features, in encrypting data, that complies with GDPR and HIPAA's security rules. The RBAC system is also automated to ensure that sensitive information is accessed only by authorized persons.
- **Improved Accountability and Governance: Tracking Data Access and Usage for Audit Purposes**

Tracking and auditing data access in healthcare organizations may improve transparency, compliance, and security. To guarantee patient trust and data security, sustaining accountability and strong governance are essential [26]. The improved accountability and improved governance are enhanced security, by lowering the risk of data breaches; limited access to authorized persons; increased patient trust, ensuring their data is handled appropriately; regulatory compliance, which helps avoid expensive fines and legal issues; and operational efficiency, with automated tracking and auditing tools that reduce the administrative load.

8.12 BUILDING A SECURE AND EFFICIENT HEALTHCARE ECOSYSTEM

The healthcare institutes are digitally connected; development of an effective and safe healthcare environment is necessary, and strong systems are needed to manage and tackle escalating problems with data security, patient privacy, and operational effectiveness. The necessary elements of a safe and effective healthcare environment are information security, confidentiality, and encryption techniques. Smart contracts on a blockchain help to automate multiple administrative processes, such as billing, claim processing, and consent management. Healthcare procedures can be improved by combining machine learning and AI, like treatment planning, patient triage, and diagnosis, thereby also enhancing patient outcomes and resource allocation. EHRs assure well-informed coordination and combine data from clinics, hospitals, and labs. Enabling remote consultations for rural location patients can be expanded.

8.12.1 Benefits of Blockchain for Stakeholders

8.12.1.1 Patients: Increased Privacy Control, Improved Access to Their Medical Data, Enhanced Trust in Healthcare Providers

Patients can have tremendous benefits from blockchain technology; the way the healthcare industry manages and exchanges data has been influenced by its transparent, decentralized, and immutable nature. The primary advantages for patients are control over privacy; the data stored in decentralized systems renders it vulnerable to intruders; and approved access. On the other hand, enhanced cryptography methods are used in blockchain to assure that patient information stays secure. Likewise, enhanced healthcare data access is another advantage; the regular fragmentation of health records among various healthcare organizations is problematic for patients in obtaining a complete health history. Patients are empowered to access their health records from any location, any time, by integrating blockchain into healthcare. In addition, the ability of blockchain to encourage interoperability ensures easy data communication in healthcare. Another incredible advantage is increased confidence in health professionals; the relationship between patients and health providers relies on trust; the immutable property of blockchain may provide patients with a sense of comfort.

8.12.2 Healthcare Providers: Streamlined Data Sharing, Improved Care Coordination, and Reduced Administrative Burden

Blockchain technology presents numerous aids to healthcare providers by increasing the efficiency and efficacy of their services, such as minimized administrative burden, enhanced coordination, and faster data exchange. Streamlined data transfer is the imperative benefit for healthcare providers, data silos and jeopardize issues due to fragmentation of healthcare data are the common issues in healthcare. Blockchain overcomes these issues by generating immutable, decentralized records to assure security and data integrity for patients. Each piece of data uploaded to the blocks is encrypted and linked to each other through its hash value. Health providers can have real-time access to patient records, which decreases the possibility of oversights and mistakes. The health professionals can gain another benefit of better care coordination; chronic diseases need seamless collaboration among multiple providers for chronic diseases [27]. Blockchain assists with improved care coordination by providing a single source of authority for patient data. The transparency attribute of blockchain minimizes redundant tests and medical errors.

8.12.3 Healthcare Organizations: Enhanced Data Security, Improved Compliance with Regulations, and Potential Cost Savings

Healthcare organizations can be revolutionized by incorporating to enhance integrity, efficiency, security, and regulatory compliance. Blockchain technology also helps in possible financial savings; claims processing, verification, and data entry tasks are automated to reduce labor costs. Increased data security is one of the key benefits for healthcare organizations. Medical institutes are frequently targeted by cyber-attacks. Blockchain data is stored in a distributed ledger, where each node is connected to a previous node from a chain of nodes that provides data security. Protecting privacy and ensuring the accuracy of healthcare data are under strict regulatory guidelines. Compliance procedures can be simplified through blockchain by maintaining audit trails of all the data transfers; every entry in the blockchain is time-stamped, which makes it easy to prove compliance during audits. Due to the immutability and transparency of blockchain, it becomes easier to detect and prevent fraudulent activity, such as billing for services that were not provided or forging health records.

8.13 THE FUTURE OF BLOCKCHAIN IN HEALTHCARE

As technology advances further, blockchain technology claims to offer innovations that enhance organization efficiency, interoperability, patient care, and data security.

8.13.1 Ongoing Development and Innovation in Blockchain Technology

- **Improved Protocol Security:** The researchers gain advancements in upgrading the cryptographic security models to safeguard data from breaches. The primary focus of research is on security protocols and novel approaches, such as quantum computing and quantum-resistant algorithms, to safeguard blockchain networks from potential hazards. These advancements will offer data protection, preserving privacy and confidence in healthcare as utmost security.

- **Solutions for Interoperability:** As healthcare data is frequently fragmented among various systems, the interoperability issue is a key concern. Blockchain provides a promising solution to interoperability issues; the architecture of blockchain enabled effective and secure access to data sharing among healthcare institutions.
- **Combining Traditional and New Technologies:** When new technologies like AI and the Internet of Things (IoT) are integrated with blockchain, AI systems can be used to analyze huge data stored on blockchain to identify the trends to improve patient care. IoT devices can be used for real-time health monitoring, as they capture data and send to the blockchain securely.
- **Automation and Smart Contracts:** Self-executing agreement smart contracts are embedded into the code to automate supply chain management and insurance claims among other medical organizations. Smart contracts have the potential to execute insurance claims automatically, which saves time and reduces the risk of fraud compared to manual processing.
- **Prospects and Difficulties for the Future:** A lot of transactions cannot be handled by current blockchain networks; scalability issue remains an ongoing focus of research and development. The healthcare organizations may also be vulnerable to legal and regulatory barriers; blockchain must comply with current laws and norms of healthcare.

8.13.2 Potential for Integrating Other Emerging Technologies with Blockchain

The integration of blockchain with AI and IoT might boost data security and improve patient results. The blockchain ledgers augment capabilities of AI by offering authorized audit trail for the AI decision-making process and allowing interested parties to track the route and source of algorithmic judgments and data inputs, which resolve the black box issue of AI [28]. AI systems, for instance, can forecast the trends of healthcare by analyzing the patient data, which is private and immutable. The unauthorized access and data breaches can be avoided by encoding the IoT to the blockchain technology; it also provides secure data collection and safe transmission of data from IoT devices. For example, the automatic upload of data to a blockchain from a patient's device is accessed by an authenticated healthcare provider who can view it instantly. These real-time data can be extremely important for the early diagnosis of medical disorders and chronic diseases [29, 30]. Telemedicine and remote patient monitoring is another advancement in the healthcare industry. Data collected through telemedicine platforms and IoT devices is securely sent to blockchain and evaluated by AI to produce beneficial insights [31]. Quantum computing is another technology that can be integrated with blockchain, which gives a powerful solution to solve optimization issues. The quantum algorithms have the ability to tackle complex issues, which can be used to increase the transaction processing time in blockchain networks.

8.13.3 The Path Toward a More Secure and Patient-Centric Healthcare Ecosystem

To resolve the current issues faced by the healthcare sector, blockchain technology is the promising healthcare solution going forward in multiple ways [32]. The empowerment of patients to access their medical data as needed makes them feel more confident that their confidential data is handled safely, because of the transparency nature of blockchain. Furthermore, patients have the option to track who, when, and why their data is accessed; these help in building trust among healthcare professionals and patients. Blockchain gives access to anonymized huge data, which will speed up the treatments [33]. Blockchain has revolutionized the pharmaceutical supply chain by enabling the recording of every step from production to distribution, leading to improvement in tamper-proofing of records. This will also address the problem of counterfeit drugs. Remote care and telemedicine have rapidly advanced after the COVID-19 epidemic. Through blockchain, patients can access telemedicine services remotely, independently and securely. The real-time access to healthcare providers of patients from IoT devices are safeguarded through blockchain.

8.14 CONCLUSION

Blockchains enhance security protocols and ensure transparency, security, and integrity of data in EHRs. Blockchain with improved cryptographic techniques assures protection against data breaches and unauthorized access. Permission access control in the healthcare industry is essential as an evolution in healthcare digitization.

The immutable audit trail in healthcare sectors guarantees complete transparency in data access and is essential for preserving public confidence. In conclusion, the immutable, decentralized, and transparent nature of blockchain for health data storage is a viable way to upgrade the healthcare industry. EHRs enabled with blockchain are an incredible improvement in the healthcare sector by allowing interoperability, empowering patients, guaranteeing transparency, and providing quicker access. The integration of blockchain with the current EHR system safeguards confidential data of patients by verifying participants and avoiding unauthorized access. The strong security measures in the healthcare sector navigate the regulatory environment and build trust among patients. Smart contracts automate administrative processes and guarantee compliance. They tackle the data management issues in the healthcare sector and strengthen optimized data exchange. The integration of smart contracts in the healthcare sector is to achieve patient-centric healthcare networks, enhance patient outcomes, and resolve interoperability problems. Automation in administrative processes is the need of the hour in the healthcare sector to ensure integrity, privacy, and security of patient data. The robust compliance with laws according to HIPAA and GDPR that must be followed by healthcare will guarantee patient trust and safeguard patient data. Blockchain has the potential to shape the healthcare sector and enhance notable benefits by improving interoperability and privacy control. To sum up, the implementation of blockchain in healthcare sector is an important advancement that solves a lot of problems and can strengthen accuracy, efficiency, and security of healthcare data. It offers multiple advantages, such as improved regulatory compliance, superior data security, and possible cost savings, which will ultimately result in reliable, efficient healthcare. In conclusion, integrating blockchain with other advanced technologies can solve current issues. With the aid of blockchain-based technologies and the synergy of AI, IoT, and quantum computing, operations could be improved and optimal results should be achieved. . The abundance of hope in the future that AI and IoT technologies can completely revolutionize the healthcare sector. The convergence of these advanced technologies with blockchain is likely to result in groundbreaking advancement and tremendous benefits.

REFERENCES

[1] Sonkamble, R. G., Bongale, A. M., Phansalkar, S., Sharma, A., & Rajput, S. (2023). Secure data transmission of electronic health records using blockchain technology. *Electronics*, *12*(4), 1015.

[2] Butt, G. Q., Sayed, T. A., Riaz, R., Rizvi, S. S., & Paul, A. (2022). Secure healthcare record sharing mechanism with blockchain. *Applied Sciences*, *12*(5), 2307.

[3] McGhin, T., Choo, K. K. R., Liu, C. Z., & He, D. (2019). Blockchain in healthcare applications: Research challenges and opportunities. *Journal of Network and Computer Applications*, *135*, 62–75.

[4] Wenhua, Z., Qamar, F., Abdali, T. A. N., Hassan, R., Jafri, S. T. A., & Nguyen, Q. N. (2023). Blockchain technology: Security issues, healthcare applications, challenges and future trends. *Electronics*, *12*(3), 546.

[5] Kim, M., Yu, S., Lee, J., Park, Y., & Park, Y. (2020). Design of secure protocol for cloud-assisted electronic health record system using blockchain. *Sensors*, *20*(10), 2913.

[6] Sharma, Y., & Balamurugan, B. (2020). Preserving the privacy of electronic health records using blockchain. *Procedia Computer Science*, *173*, 171–180.

[7] Shi, J., Li, R., & Hou, W. (2020). A mechanism to resolve the unauthorized access vulnerability caused by permission delegation in blockchain-based access control. *IEEE Access*, *8*, 156027–156042.

[8] Liu, H., Crespo, R. G., & Martínez, O. S. (2020, July). Enhancing privacy and data security across healthcare applications using blockchain and distributed ledger concepts. In *Healthcare* (Vol. 8, No. 3, p. 243). MDPI.

[9] Nemec Zlatolas, L., Welzer, T., & Lhotska, L. (2024). Data breaches in healthcare: Security mechanisms for attack mitigation. *Cluster Computing*, *27*, 8639–8654.

[10] Jayabalan, J., & Jeyanthi, N. (2022). Scalable blockchain model using off-chain IPFS storage for healthcare data security and privacy. *Journal of Parallel and Distributed Computing*, *164*, 152–167.

[11] Hussien, H. M., Yasin, S. M., Udzir, N. I., Ninggal, M. I. H., & Salman, S. (2021). Blockchain technology in the healthcare industry: Trends and opportunities. *Journal of Industrial Information Integration*, *22*, 100217.

[12] Singh, S., Pankaj, B., Nagarajan, K., Singh, N. P., & Bala, V. (2022). Blockchain with cloud for handling healthcare data: A privacy-friendly platform. *Materials Today: Proceedings*, *62*, 5021–5026.

[13] Zaabar, B., Cheikhrouhou, O., Jamil, F., Ammi, M., & Abid, M. (2021). HealthBlock: A secure blockchain-based healthcare data management system. *Computer Networks*, *200*, 108500.

[14] Attaran, M. (2022). Blockchain technology in healthcare: Challenges and opportunities. *International Journal of Healthcare Management*, *15*(1), 70–83.

[15] Pandey, P., & Litoriya, R. (2020). Securing and authenticating healthcare records through blockchain technology. *Cryptologia*, *44*(4), 341–356.

[16] Pandey, A. K., Khan, A. I., Abushark, Y. B., Alam, M. M., Agrawal, A., Kumar, R., & Khan, R. A. (2020). Key issues in healthcare data integrity: Analysis and recommendations. *IEEE Access*, *8*, 40612–40628.

[17] Alzahrani, A. G., Alhomoud, A., & Wills, G. (2022). A framework of the critical factors for healthcare providers to share data securely using blockchain. *IEEE Access*, *10*, 41064–41077.

[18] Yadav, D., Shinde, A., Nair, A., Patil, Y., & Kanchan, S. (2020, May). Enhancing data security in cloud using blockchain. In 2020 4th International Conference on Intelligent Computing and Control Systems (ICICCS) (pp. 753–757). IEEE.

[19] Sharma, Y., & Balamurugan, B. (2020). Preserving the privacy of electronic health records using blockchain. *Procedia Computer Science*, *173*, 171–180.

[20] Kim, M., Yu, S., Lee, J., Park, Y., & Park, Y. (2020). Design of secure protocol for cloud-assisted electronic health record system using blockchain. *Sensors*, *20*(10), 2913.

[21] Jabbar, R., Fetais, N., Krichen, M., & Barkaoui, K. (2020, February). Blockchain technology for healthcare: Enhancing shared electronic health record interoperability and integrity. In 2020 IEEE International Conference on Informatics, IoT, and Enabling Technologies (ICIoT) (pp. 310–317). IEEE.

[22] Shi, J., Li, R., & Hou, W. (2020). A mechanism to resolve the unauthorized access vulnerability caused by permission delegation in blockchain-based access control. *IEEE Access*, *8*, 156027–156042.

[23] Liu, H., Crespo, R. G., & Martínez, O. S. (2020, July). Enhancing privacy and data security across healthcare applications using blockchain and distributed ledger concepts. In *Healthcare* (Vol. 8, No. 3, p. 243). MDPI.

[24] Alketbi, A., Nasir, Q., & Talib, M. A. (2018, February). Blockchain for government services—Use cases, security benefits and challenges. In 2018 15th Learning and Technology Conference (L&T*)* (pp. 112–119). IEEE.

[25] Baygin, N., Baygin, M., & Karakose, M. (2019, November). Blockchain technology: applications, benefits and challenges. In 2019 1st International Informatics and Software Engineering Conference (UBMYK) (pp. 1–5). IEEE.

[26] Politou, E., Casino, F., Alepis, E., & Patsakis, C. (2019). Blockchain mutability: Challenges and proposed solutions. *IEEE Transactions on Emerging Topics in Computing*, *9*(4), 1972–1986.

[27] McGhin, T., Choo, K. K. R., Liu, C. Z., & He, D. (2019). Blockchain in healthcare applications: Research challenges and opportunities. *Journal of Network and Computer Applications*, *135*, 62–75.

[28] Teymourlouei, H., & Jackson, L. (2019). Blockchain: Enhance the authentication and verification of the identity of a user to prevent data breaches and security intrusions. In Proceedings of the *I*nternational *C*onference on *S*cientific *C*omputing (CSC) (pp. 40–46). The Steering Committee of The World Congress in Computer Science, Computer Engineering and Applied Computing (WorldComp).

[29] Pereira, J., Tavalaei, M. M., & Ozalp, H. (2019). Blockchain-based platforms: Decentralized infrastructures and its boundary conditions. *Technological Forecasting and Social Change*, *146*, 94–102.

[30] David, S., Duraipandian, K., Chandrasekaran, D., Pandey, D., Sindhwani, N., & Pandey, B. K. (2023). Impact of blockchain in healthcare system. In *Unleashing the Potentials of Blockchain Technology for Healthcare Industries* (pp. 37–57). Academic Press.

[31] Ekblaw, A., Azaria, A., Halamka, J. D., & Lippman, A. (2016, August). A Case Study for Blockchain in Healthcare:"MedRec" prototype for electronic health records and medical research data. In Proceedings of IEEE *O*pen & *B*ig *D*ata *C*onference (Vol. 13, p. 13).

[32] Tanwar, S., Parekh, K., & Evans, R. (2020). Blockchain-based electronic healthcare record system for healthcare 4.0 applications. *Journal of Information Security and Applications*, *50*, 102407.

[33] Settipalli, L., & Gangadharan, G. R. (2024). QFBN: Quorum based federated blockchain network for healthcare system to avoid multiple benefits and data breaches. *IEEE Consumer Electronics Magazine*, *13*(2), 24–35.

9 Ethical Considerations in HealthTech

Balancing Innovation and Privacy

Anjuli Goel and Chander Prabha

9.1 INTRODUCTION

For many years, research and development on artificial intelligence (AI) have been ongoing [1]. AI is the capacity of a computer to perform tasks by mimicking human cognitive processes, including inference, judgement, generalisation, and experience-based learning, without explicit instructions [2]. AI is fast gaining recognition as a disruptive force in the healthcare sector with the ability to improve clinical trials, drug discovery, patient care, sickness detection, and operational efficiency. However, there are a number of ethical and legal issues that come with incorporating AI into healthcare; therefore, they should be carefully considered.

Eugenio [3] acknowledged that the United States spent $2,487.7 billion on AI in the healthcare sector in 2019. According to a recent report by Reports and Data, investments in AI in the healthcare sector are expected to expand at a significant rate over the next several years [4]. By 2027, their estimates place the market value at $61.59 billion. According to Zakaryan's projections [5], the healthcare industry's computer-generated growth rate (CAGR) for AI investments would rise by 41.8% and reach a total of $120.2 billion by 2028.

The growing demand for better healthcare services and the proliferation of digital health technologies have generated a wealth of data across healthcare settings. AI, particularly machine learning, has the potential to harness this data for the benefit of patients and healthcare practitioners. Unlike traditional computational algorithms, AI systems can adapt, learn, and reason, opening new avenues for insights into healthcare delivery. AI in healthcare typically comprises both software and hardware components. Artificial neural networks, resembling the human brain's interconnected neurons, are central to AI algorithms. These algorithms analyse vast datasets, learning and improving over time [6].

While AI–clinician collaboration holds promise in diagnosis, drug discovery, personalised care, and operational efficiency, a robust governance framework is imperative to mitigate potential ethical and legal pitfalls. AI has found applications in diverse healthcare areas, including electronic health records (EHRs) analysis, drug

DOI: 10.1201/9781003516163-9

development, and clinical care optimisation. AI's ability to uncover clinical best practices, analyse clinical trends, and improve healthcare delivery models presents several opportunities for better patient outcomes [6].

Numerous advancements in the use of AI have given rise to several ethical concerns. Among these concerns are data security for patients [7, 8], and the doctor–patient relationship is in jeopardy [9].

It seems that HealthTech is a synonym for Digital Health, the intersection of health and technology. Integrating technology into healthcare, commonly referred to as HealthTech, has brought about revolutionary changes in patient care and medical research. However, this rapid innovation raises significant ethical concerns, particularly regarding data privacy [10]. The use of organised knowledge and abilities in the form of tools, medications, vaccinations, processes, and systems created to address health issues and enhance people's quality of life is known as health technology. Therefore, "health technology" can refer to a wide range of actions inside a healthcare system. Among the instances are [11]:

- Interventions related to prevention and rehabilitation (such as immunisation campaigns).
- Systems within which health is safeguarded and maintained.
- Methods (like surgery).
- Pharmaceuticals.
- Health-related gadgets.
- The industry known as "health tech," or "health technology," includes digital goods and services intended to advance healthcare delivery and/or promote health.

The chapter's main purpose is to present a thorough summary of the ethical considerations to be followed in practice related to HealthTech. It explores various technologies to be explored in HealthTech. It presents an ethical AI framework demonstrating the various phases involved.

The chapter is structured as follows: Section 9.2 presents the AI perspective in HealthTech along with their benefits. Section 9.3 presents ethical considerations and their relationship with human values. Section 9.4 briefly describes the ethical AI framework, followed by data privacy concepts and challenges in Sections 9.5 and 9.5.1, respectively. Section 9.6 presents the regulatory framework in HealthTech. The concept of patient consent in HealthTech has an important role and is described in Section 9.7. Further, Section 9.8 explores stakeholders' role in HealthTech for shaping ethical practices. Later, Section 9.9 describes the challenges and future direction. Finally, Section 9.10, concludes the chapter.

9.2 ARTIFICIAL INTELLIGENCE IN HEALTHTECH

AI in healthcare is one of the most important technology developments of the past several years, with enormous potential advantages for patient care, research, and healthcare administration. AI systems may use machine learning and deep learning

TABLE 9.1
Various Benefits of AI in HealthTech

Benefits	Explanation
Capacity to process vast volumes of data reliably and swiftly	• AI systems can spot patterns and trends in patient data that human practitioners might overlook by examining data from tests, imaging scans, medical histories, and other sources. • Tailored treatment regimens and quicker, more accurate diagnoses might ultimately result in improved patient outcomes.
Enhance patient management in healthcare	• AI systems can monitor patients' vital signs continually, so they can alert doctors to issues before they become critical. This improves patient outcomes by allowing healthcare providers to take prompt action to avert adverse events. • AI can analyse patient data to identify those who are more likely to contract illnesses, enabling more specialised care and preventative measures.
Boost the effectiveness of the healthcare system	• AI can potentially improve the effectiveness of medical services by handling tasks automatically like medication refills and appointment scheduling. AI can free up doctors' time so they can devote more of their attention to patient care. • Furthermore, AI-powered chatbots can triage patient inquiries, providing timely information to patients while freeing up healthcare providers to handle more complex cases.

approaches to evaluate vast volumes of data to spot patterns, forecast results, and provide treatments. This is often something that these technologies can accomplish faster and more precisely than people.

AI has enormous advantages in the healthcare sector, revolutionising it in several ways. AI algorithms play a key role in increasing diagnostic accuracy by facilitating the faster and more accurate diagnosis of diseases like cancer, which can have a substantial influence on treatment results. AI also aids in the optimisation of hospital operations through cost reduction, process simplification, and efficient resource allocation—all of which raise the standard of patient care overall. Additionally, AI rapidly identifies potential remedies, which shortens research timeframes compared to traditional methods and accelerates the creation of new medications [12].

9.2.1 Benefits of Artificial Intelligence in HealthTech

In the field of healthcare, AI holds significant promise for improving patient outcomes. Table 9.1 lists the several advantages along with an explanation [11].

9.3 ETHICAL CONSIDERATIONS IN HEALTHTECH

Health technology ethics encompasses various topics, including consent, data privacy, openness, and equity. Patient data protection and responsible use are essential for establishing and preserving public confidence. In addition to protecting patient rights, ethical behaviour enhances the legitimacy and standing of health technology businesses [10]. Even while AI can potentially improve healthcare, integrating it also poses significant ethical issues that need to be resolved first. Table 9.2 explains different ethical issues, concerns, and solutions.

9.3.1 Key Human Values and Ethical Issues in Artificial Intelligence for Healthcare

Many AI applications use software engineering, which typically disregards human values. It is untrue, despite popular belief, that deliberately matching AI with human values may lead to several advantages, including better patient engagement and cancer care. In contrast, a host of ethical issues surface when human ideals are transgressed. Four values were found to be the most often referenced in a review of recently released publications by software engineers: autarchy, universalism, security, and compassion. Figure 9.1 presents these human values as well as the ethical standards linked with them [13].

- **Non-Maleficence:** In terms of discrimination, invasion of privacy, physical injury, and contributions to well-being, non-maleficence entails a duty to reduce foreseen harm. Because it is so prevalent in the current AI standards, one may argue that preventing damage is a more vital purpose of AI than causing good. Owing to AI's quick advancement in healthcare, there is concern that negative effects will not be recognised until after they happen and then dealt with.

  Safety is a main concern in AI for healthcare now because only a few of the tested methods are evidence-based. Nonetheless, technical malfunctions, such as AI chatbots that cease functioning correctly or AI programs that stop working when there is a network outage, can lead to unpredicted results. In addition, AI may not possess enough interpersonal skills or cultural knowledge, which may be barriers between the client and the therapist, and consequently, the client may suffer from additional mental health problems.
- **Self-Direction:** Self-direction is a term used to describe a certain degree of individual autonomy, which is a combination of the moral precepts of autonomy, privacy, and dignity. To be considered free and autonomous, one must provide informed permission, disclose pertinent facts, demonstrate comprehension, and engage voluntarily. Obtaining permission for the use of opaque methods and big datasets is quite challenging. Respecting human dignity involves preserving human rights and decency as well as addressing any emotional harm that AI may cause to clients in therapeutic settings. Although privacy is a human right, the use of AI in healthcare raises questions regarding data management, collection, and utilisation of social media. Bad security procedures, inaccurate portrayals of mental states, a lack of anonymisation, and the retention of data even after a user's withdrawal are among the issues in this respect.
- **Benevolence:** Benevolence is the application of moral precepts like charitableness, authority, faith, translucency, and unity to "good" behaviour on a personal and social level.

TABLE 9.2
Different Ethical Issues, Concerns, and Solutions

Ethical Issue	Concerns	Solutions
Autonomy	The increasing prevalence of AI technologies in the healthcare sector may lead patients to feel sidelined in making their healthcare decisions, potentially resulting in heightened mistrust and decreased patient satisfaction.	Healthcare professionals should make sure that patients understand exactly how AI is being applied to their treatment and should give them the chance to weigh in on decisions.
Bias	Biased data will unavoidably appear in AI systems as they can only be as objective as the training set. This might result in disparities across the patient individuals' standards of care, particularly for disadvantaged backgrounds.	Healthcare workers should constantly monitor AI systems to ensure that any biases are promptly detected and corrected and that the systems function as intended. This necessitates a commitment to ongoing AI system development and review to lower the risk of patient harm.
Privacy	For healthcare organisations, protecting patient privacy and safely storing all collected data should come first. Building trust and giving patients the best treatment possible depend on protecting sensitive information.	Assuring that patients have authority over their health information and establishing clear policies and processes for gathering, keeping, and using patient data are crucial.
Trust and Communication	As AI becomes increasingly prevalent in the medical field, people run the risk of thinking of AI as their primary healthcare provider rather than a medical professional. This might lead to a breakdown in the communication and confidence needed to provide patients with high-quality care.	To improve clinical decision-making, healthcare practitioners must make sure AI is applied in a way that complements rather than undermines human interaction. AI is just one tool in the healthcare provider's toolkit, and patients should be aware that they still have the last word in all matters of decision-making.

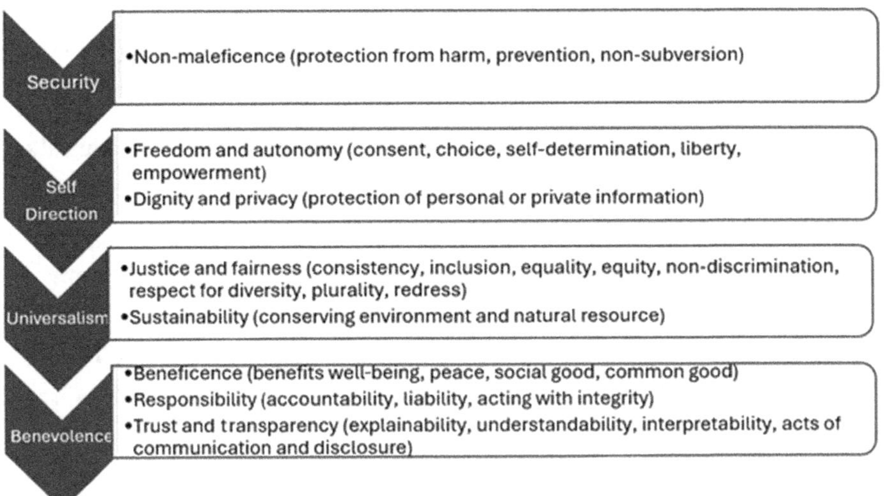

FIGURE 9.1 Ethical Standards Linked with Human Values.

- **Beneficence:** There are ethical quandaries related to the use of AI for the health of individuals and society, especially the metaphor in which AI takes over the doctor's decision-making, where AI cannot find out the dangerous cases and could turn into fulfilling a prophecy.
- **Responsibility and Trust:** Trust in AI systems can only be built on principles such as accountability, transparency, and security. However, new technologies often create ambiguities in the distribution of responsibility for the outcomes of their application. Trust can be forfeited because of wrong findings, incompetence, or the unauthorised use of public data.
- **Transparency:** Explainability and interpretability of AI decisions are key points in the discussion on transparency, yet "black box" algorithms are one of the reasons why it is difficult to achieve this. One of the pitfalls is also the revelation of AI's shortcomings such as false results, and bias as the "weak spots" of the technology to discuss.
- **Solidarity:** Disadvantaged populations and low-income groups are at risk of exclusion from the AI healthcare revolution and AI might also be the reason for harm or its application may be such that it will be used for manipulative forces, like insurance premium increases for risky entities.
- **Universalism:** Universalism encompasses respect for both people and the environment, including the moral precepts of justice, equity, and ecology.

Justice and Fairness: Representing a diverse community, addressing prejudice against marginalised groups, and permitting challenges to AI-based choices are all necessary for justice and fairness in AI. Restricting research and development of AI to specific social groups may be an example of misaligned goals confirming pre-existing inequalities, and applicability of biases that might already exist in training data. Implementers must analyse the validity of the dubious outputs, and in the case of perilous cases similar to algorithms that predict suicide, AI judgements need to be questioned because they are not always accurate. Source and decision-making allocation to automated systems must be looked at with a critical eye.

Sustainability: Sustainability calls for minimising the ecological imprint of AI projects and taking the environment into account. All AI programs should take this seriously, as important healthcare-specific elements have not yet been determined.

9.4 ETHICAL ARTIFICIAL INTELLIGENCE FRAMEWORK FOR HEALTHTECH

Even though a lot of work has gone into mapping the ethical principles of AI for healthcare, it is difficult to turn this knowledge into useful applications on its own. Figure 9.2 presents an approach to applying ethics to AI in healthcare across the development lifecycle to close this gap. First, developers' and users' professional practices; their organisation's governance; and the law's regulation of individuals and groups are all factors that contribute to ethical AI. Second, the AI lifecycle consists of three main phases that must be gradually completed before the next phase is started, as explained in Table 9.3 [13, 14].

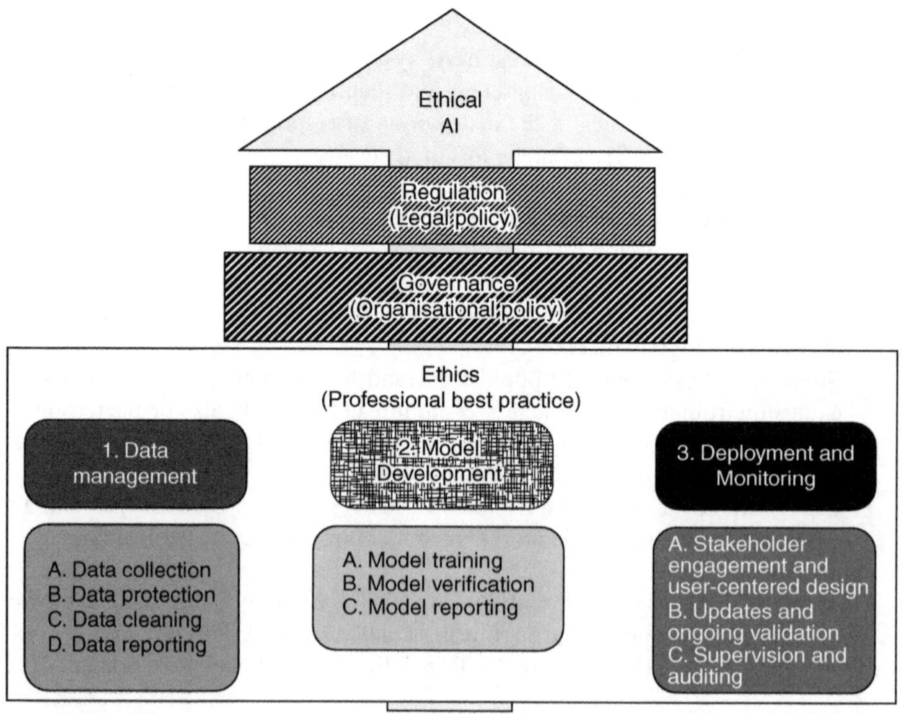

FIGURE 9.2 Ethical AI Framework.

TABLE 9.3
Explanation of Various Phases of Ethical AI Framework in HealthTech

Phase	Sub-Parts	Description
Data Management	A. Data Collection	Gather inclusive and varied data; stay away from biased datasets and superfluous data kinds. Honour personal space and think about de-identifying. Collect data from marginalised communities and preprocess it to enhance its quality.
	B. Data Protection	Using optimal security practices, such as de-identification and privatisation, and routinely upgrading data privacy and security safeguards are necessary to defend health data systems from assaults. Different settings of privacy can be employed, and procedures for sharing of data must be open and demand express agreement.
	C. Data Cleaning	Unbiased data for vulnerable populations is essential to ensuring justice in AI. It is best to steer clear of biased or incomplete datasets and utilise cleaning methods like MLClean, HoloClean, Activeclean, and Universal Cleanser.
	D. Data Reporting	Give datasets comprehensive documentation to promote openness and aid ML developers in identifying problems with training data. Motivation, composition, the gathering method, pre-processing, uses, dissemination, upkeep, impact, and ML problems should all be included in the documentation. The logic for curation, diversity in linguistics, speaker and interpreter groups, voice environment, features of content, and quality of recordings should all be covered in NLP documentation. By giving customers and regulators auditable information on purpose, performance, safety, and security, AI service FactSheets can help foster trust in AI systems. A template that outlines the situations in which AI systems are created and used is accessible.
Model Development	A. Model Training	A prior analysis approach should be adopted to develop responsible ML models that must specify objectives, technological strategies, research questions, desired results, and limitations based on values and ethics. For openness and confidence, interpretable models are favoured.
	B. Model Verification	Consider factors such as prioritising a small number of false positives or false negatives when selecting performance indicators for AI algorithms. Analyse how well the algorithm works for under-represented groups and use subset techniques to pinpoint underperformance.

(continued)

TABLE 9.3 (Continued)
Explanation of Various Phases of Ethical AI Framework in HealthTech

Phase	Sub-Parts	Description
	C. Model Reporting	Transparency and fostering faith in the technology depend heavily on the model's characteristics and verification environment, as well as on the source of data, contributors, predictors, and results being reported. For reuse, models across other phenotypic, ethnic, or demographic groups should be evaluated and recorded. Transparency and increased interpretability of models may be achieved using ad hoc and external post hoc strategies.
Deployment and Monitoring	A. Stakeholder Engagement and User-Centred Design	All phases of the AI lifecycle should engage stakeholders, including deployment. This involves users, decision-makers, and information specialists, with an emphasis on highlighting sociocultural diversity. Users should receive the necessary training, and there should be a clearly defined clinical condition that has to be treated. Patients should have access to download the final AI after notifying them of its use and limitations. It is important to consider patient preferences and ensure that the AI system's terminology does not perpetuate unjust preconceptions.
	B. Updates and Ongoing Validation	AI systems should be able to adapt to changes in the world and gain knowledge from user activity to remain relevant. It is a major concern to consider comments given by users and provide a way for unfair errors to be corrected.
	C. Supervision and Auditing	Because AI systems may function autonomously and at large scale, they provide both new and current hazards in the healthcare industry. The application of ethical concepts necessitates active governance, encompassing rules, processes, and standards. Ethics-based auditing may support governance through organised methods to check adherence to ethical norms, algorithmic-use risk assessments, and audits (inside and outside).

9.5 DATA PRIVACY CONCEPTS IN HEALTHTECH USING ARTIFICIAL INTELLIGENCE

In the context of healthcare IT, data privacy is a multi-faceted concept encompassing several critical aspects [15]:

- **Confidentiality:** This refers to the obligation to keep personal health information private, sharing it only with those who need to know how to provide healthcare and with the patient's informed consent. Confidentiality is fundamental in building trust between patients and healthcare providers.
- **Data Protection:** Data protection involves implementing technical and organisational measures to ensure that personal data is processed safely, securely, and by legal and ethical standards. In healthcare IT, this includes protecting data from unauthorised access, disclosure, alteration, and destruction.
- **Information Security:** Closely related to data protection, information security is specifically concerned with protecting information systems and databases from cyber threats. Various techniques like encryption, access controls, and secure data transmission and storage involve guaranteeing the availability, confidentiality, and patient data integrity.

9.5.1 Challenges of Data Privacy

The adoption of IT in the healthcare sector has ushered in a massive plethora of benefits such as better enhanced patient care, increased efficiency, and the promotion of medical research. However, these developments also pose a substantial threat to data privacy, which implies the following:

- **Technical Vulnerabilities:** Healthcare systems are intricate and combine with a lot of other systems, which leads to several potential points of weakness. These may entail flaws in the software, using old systems, and lacking proper encryption, which are the routes through which cybercriminals take advantage to corrupt the system and access the sensitive data the organisation did not intend to expose [16].
- **Data Breaches:** It is a major concern in the healthcare field. The healthcare sector has sensitive and priceless data, which is why criminals target this sector the most. Data breaches can be committed through different means such as hacking, phishing, insider threats, or even accidental disclosures. The effects of these breaches are serious and can include, among others, financial loss, loss of patient trust, and even possible injury to patients' health [17].
- **Unauthorised Access:** Unauthorised access to healthcare data can be a result of both external threats as well as internal organisation members. This may occur because of improper access controls, the non-existence of employee training on data privacy, or misuse of data by the staff. Guaranteeing that only authorised personnel have access to the sensitive information and are using it properly is a constant challenge [18].
- **Mobile and Cloud Technologies:** Mobile devices and cloud-based services have developed in the healthcare sector bringing in the required efficiency and flexibility. Yet, these advances in technology escalate the new risks for data privacy, including the loss or theft of devices and lack of control over where data is stored and how it is secured in the cloud [19].

- **Interoperability and Data Sharing:** The sharing of health data between researchers, providers, and third parties can benefit as well as facilitate medical progress. However, it is not without its complex privacy problems. The challenge of securely sharing data, ensuring compliance with patient consent, and meeting legal requirements is an immense task [20].

9.6 REGULATORY FRAMEWORKS

To tackle these issues and safeguard the privacy of persons, many legislative frameworks have been instituted worldwide:

- Europe's General Data Protection Regulation, or GDPR: The GDPR establishes strict guidelines for the processing of personal data, including health information, of people residing in the European Union (EU) and the European Economic Area (EEA). Consent, data minimisation, and people's rights to view and manage their data are among the values it highlights. Healthcare companies are required to comply with GDPR, which includes putting strong data protection measures in place, quickly reporting data breaches, and making sure that health data is processed lawfully [21, 22].
- The United States' Health Insurance Portability and Accountability Act (HIPPA): Patients who own personal health information are granted several rights under HIPAA, which also offers federal safeguards for such information. Included in it is the Privacy Rule, which establishes guidelines for safeguarding patient medical records and other private health information, and the Security Rule, which establishes guidelines for protecting digitally protected health information [23].
- Healthcare IT is impacted by data privacy legislation in several different nations and areas. For instance, the Privacy Act in Australia and the Personal Information Protection and Electronic Documents Act (PIPEDA) in Canada both contain the Australian Privacy Principles (APPs), which provide guidelines for the protection of personal information, including health data [15].

9.7 CONCEPT OF PATIENT CONSENT IN HEALTHTECH

Based on the moral duty to uphold patient autonomy and the right to self-determination, informed consent is a fundamental concept in both healthcare and research. To enable people to make an educated and free choice regarding their care or participation, they must be fully informed on the nature of the medical treatment or study, including its risks, advantages, and alternatives. Consent in Healthcare IT encompasses all aspects of patient data collection, usage, sharing, and storage. It ensures that technology improves patient care without sacrificing ethical norms by safeguarding patient privacy and fostering confidence between patients and healthcare professionals [24, 25].

Obtaining relevant permission from patients in the healthcare sector poses several challenges [15, 26].

- **Comprehension:** Patients may find it difficult to understand the technical aspects of data usage rules and digital health services. Complex terms of service, medical language, and the abstract nature of data processing can all operate as barriers that prevent patients from completely understanding what they are consenting to.
- **Consent Can Be Compromised:** When digital services are seamlessly integrated into healthcare, patients may feel that they have no option but to consent to the use of their data. Instead of agreeing, patients give their permission for consent as they are aware that it is mandatory for their treatment.
- **Digital Consent Complexity:** Filling the forms is difficult for users because the procedure is very long and is full of complications. Due to so much information, patients are more likely to mistakenly give permission. Also, it is a problem for them to interact with consent forms digitally due to their lack of touch and impersonal structure.
- **Difficulty in Obtaining Consent:** The use of patient data depends upon the time due to the evolving field of healthcare. It is very challenging to preserve the consent that considers the possible use of it in future.

Improving Consent Procedures in Healthcare IT needs methodical techniques that address its issues and leverage technology to encourage greater understanding and engagement [26].

- Documents about informed consent are simplified
- Evaluation of the patient's understanding
- Utilising information sheets and brochures in print
- Utilising audio–visual presentations and multimedia
- Lengthy conversations with patients
- Use of decisional aids to support patients in decision-making

9.8 THE ROLE OF STAKEHOLDERS IN SHAPING ETHICAL HEALTHTECH PRACTICES

Ethical issues play a very vital role in the fast-changing field of HealthTech as they ensure the proper development and application of technologies that affect human health. Diverse stakeholders such as academia, healthcare providers, industry, regulatory bodies, patients, and the public play an important role in generalising ethical standards in the healthcare sector. Here, contributions of subtleties and their intersection of point of view are explored [27]:

- **Industry Players: Balancing Profit and Responsibility**
  HealthTech companies are often in a difficult position to balance their profit motives with their ethical responsibilities. On the one hand, there is a drive to innovate to expand the market. On the other hand, the stakeholders at these companies must make an effort to think about the ethical implications of their decisions. For example, if a HealthTech startup develops a wearable device that

monitors vital signs, the company has to choose whether to give users data to third parties for research purposes. User privacy and informed consent are commercial interests that should be regarded as equal.

- **Regulatory Bodies: Setting Standards and Safeguards**
Regulatory agencies (such as the Food and Drug Administration (FDA), European Medicines Agency, or National Medical Products Administration) are a vital part of having ethical HealthTech practices. Safety standards are set, product submissions are examined, and compliance is enforced by them. Their choices affect patient's safety and technology acceptance. For instance, the FDA's approval process for medical devices guarantees that HealthTech products pass safety and efficacy tests. Stakeholders in clinical trials, data collection, and reporting must comply with these standards.
- **Healthcare Providers: Bridging Innovation and Patient Care**
Frontline stakeholders include doctors, medical practitioners, and nurses. Medical professionals always try to embed health technology within the patient's treatment. The viewpoint of healthcare providers influences the adoption rates, usability, and patient outcomes. For example, a telemedicine platform helps in linking physicians with patients who live far away. Healthcare professionals need to think about moral issues including informed consent, patient privacy, and fair access to technology. It is essential to maintain the balance between patient comfort and their well-being.
- **Patients: Empowering Informed Decision-Making**
HealthTech adoption is an activity that patients actively participate in. Their wants, requirements, and fears influence the ethical standards. Patient empowerment is one of the main pillars of informed consent, privacy rights, and data ownership. A patient using a health app to track fitness goals needs to keep in mind that the data is being used by the app. Transparency about data-sharing practices and the right to opt out are critical ethical considerations.
- **Academia and Research Institutions: Advancing Knowledge and Ethics**
Researchers, academics, and ethicists contribute to HealthTech ethics by studying emerging technologies, identifying risks, and proposing guidelines. Their work informs industry practices and regulatory decisions. An academic study reveals biases in an AI algorithm used for cancer diagnosis. Stakeholders across sectors must collaborate to address these biases and improve patient outcomes.
- **Public Perception and Advocacy Groups: Influencing Discourse**
Public perception shapes HealthTech adoption. Advocacy groups raise awareness, advocate for patient rights, and hold stakeholders accountable. A public outcry over a HealthTech company's data breach prompts regulatory action. Public discourse influences industry practices and drives ethical improvements [28].

9.9 CHALLENGES AND FUTURE DIRECTIONS

The integration of AI in the healthcare sector raises significant ethical questions. Four key ethical issues must be addressed to maximise AI's potential: informed consent for data usage, safety of data, transparency, algorithmic fairness, and data privacy. The classification of AI systems as legal entities is a contentious issue that requires careful consideration by policymakers [1, 3, 29, 30]. These legal entities can also be considered as future directions for practitioners and researchers.

- **Data Security:** Data security is crucial in HealthTech due to rising EHRs [31] and health information exchanges (HIEs), increasing data breach risks. Breaches can cause identity theft, insurance fraud, and compromised patient care. Cyberattacks in healthcare have grown.
- **Informed Consent:** Informed consent is vital in healthcare, ensuring patients understand the risks and benefits of medical procedures or research. In HealthTech, it includes informing patients about data collection, its purpose, and who accesses it [32].
- **Transparency in AI Algorithms:** AI in healthcare offers better diagnostics and treatments, but transparency in AI algorithms is essential for trust. Patients and providers need to grasp AI decision-making processes. The GDPR allows patients to request explanations for AI decisions [33].
- **Insufficient Information:** Data is a major component that AI systems use to provide precise forecasts and suggestions. Frequently, there is not enough high-quality data available to properly train AI systems. This constraint may hamper the effectiveness and precision of AI systems [34].
- **Interoperability Issues:** The smooth integration of AI into healthcare systems is significantly hampered by interoperability difficulties as AI integration frequently necessitates data exchange across several platforms and systems. It is therefore extremely difficult to ensure the safe transfer of this data while preserving its integrity and confidentiality [35].
- **Reluctance to Accept:** One of the biggest obstacles to integrating AI into healthcare is acceptance resistance. Healthcare workers may be reluctant to adopt AI-driven solutions due to a lack of familiarity with the technology, worries about how it will affect their job security, or changes in workflow.
- **Bias Mitigation:** Fair and representative algorithm development for a variety of demographics is crucial. Sustained endeavours will centre on detecting and reducing biases in training data, thereby guaranteeing fair healthcare results for diverse populations.

9.10 CONCLUSION

In a digital world, HealthTech is known as digital health, integrating the technology into a medical field which helps in taking care of patients and their treatment. It is a sector related to the products and services in the medical field digitally. AI is one of the most trending and implementable technologies in health, AI helps in collecting data, analysing results, and providing advice on the required treatment to patients. AI in HealthTech has its potential benefits such as processing data quickly and accurately, improving data management procedures, and increasing the efficiency of healthcare delivery. It was emphasised how crucial ethical theories and values are in directing healthcare activities by mapping ethical considerations with human values. Although the application of AI in healthcare has the potential to revolutionise patient care, there are important ethical issues that need to be resolved. To protect patient data privacy, maintain patient autonomy over healthcare decisions, and stop bias in AI systems, healthcare practitioners are essential. Healthcare professionals may use AI to improve medical outcomes while maintaining patient autonomy by addressing these ethical concerns. Here, the AI framework in HealthTech has been explained as the solution provided to avoid risks in using the application of AI healthcare. AI framework works in different layers to operate the ethics in an easy way for healthcare practitioners and developers. Challenges and future directions are also mentioned so that upcoming researchers can do their research on these with their full potential.

Upholding moral principles is crucial in the ever-changing field of healthcare information technology. Our ethical frameworks, rules, and practices need to change as technology advances to safeguard patient rights, maintain privacy, and promote confidence in the healthcare system. All parties involved technologists, patients, legislators, and healthcare providers must work together on this. We can fully use the enormous potential of healthcare IT to enhance patient care and public health while maintaining the core principles of justice, autonomy, and privacy by giving ethical concerns top priority in the development and application of this technology.

REFERENCES

[1] S. M. Saleem and S. M. Salim Khan, "The ethics of artificial intelligence in healthcare: balancing innovation and patient autonomy," *Journal of Integrative Medicine and Public Health*, vol. 2, no. 1, pp. 7–9, 2023.

[2] C. Kooli and H. Al Muftah, "Artificial intelligence in healthcare: a comprehensive review of its ethical concerns," *Technological Sustainability*, vol. 1, no. 2, pp. 121–131, 2022.

[3] E. J. Zuccarelli, "3 AI trends that will revolutionise healthcare," https://towardsdata science.com/3-ai-trendsthat-will-revolutionise-healthcare-da4198dbb31d (Accessed 15 Sept 2024).

[4] Reports and Data, "Artificial intelligence (AI) in healthcare market size worth $61.59 billion by 2027 | CAGR of 43.6% by Reports and Data," www.globenewswire.com/news-release/2021/01/19/2160281/0/en/Artificial-Intelligence-AI-in-Healthcare-Market-Size-Worth-61-59-Billion-By-2027-CAGR-of-43-6-By-Reports-and-Data.html (Accessed 15 Sept 2024).

[5] V. Zakaryan, "AI future in healthcare: improving the effectiveness of medical care," https://postindustria.com/ai-future-in-healthcare-improving-the-effectiveness-of-medical-care/ (Accessed 18 Sept 2024).

[6] B. Lenin, "The AI revolution in healthcare: balancing innovation with ethics and law," www.linkedin.com/pulse/ai-revolution-healthcare-balancing-innovation-ethics-law-biplab-lenin (Accessed 20 Sept 2024).

[7] R. Challen, J. Denny, M. Pitt, L. Gompels, T. Edwards, and K. Tsaneva-Atanasova, "Artificial intelligence, bias and clinical safety," *BMJ Qual. Saf.*, vol. 28, no. 3, pp. 231–237, 2019.

[8] A. Choudhury and O. Asan, "Role of artificial intelligence in patient safety outcomes: systematic literature review," *JMIR Med Inform*, vol. 8, issue 7, pp. 1–30, 2020.

[9] D. A. Hashimoto, G. Rosman, D. Rus, and O. R. Meireles, "Artificial intelligence in surgery: promises and perils," *Ann. Surg.*, vol. 268, no. 1, pp. 70–76, 2018.

[10] Mayank Patel, "Ethical considerations in health tech: balancing innovation with data privacy," www.linkedin.com/pulse/ethical-considerations-health-tech-balancing-innovation-mayank-patel-co0nf (Accessed 20 Sept 2024).
[11] Eupati, "What is a health technology?," https://learning.eupati.eu/mod/page/view.php?id=423 (Accessed 22 Sept 2024).
[12] K. N. Sarfaraz, "The coming of age of AI/ML in drug discovery, development, clinical testing and manufacturing: the FDA perspectives," *Dovepress*, pp. 2691–2725, 2023.
[13] B. Al Halmuni, "The ethics of AI in healthcare: balancing innovation with privacy and security," www.birzeit.edu/en/community-affairs/institutes-centers/center-continuing-education/blog/ethics-ai-healthcare-balancing (Accessed 23 Sept 2024).
[14] P. Solanki, J. Grundy, and W. Hussain, "Operationalising ethics in artificial intelligence for healthcare: a framework for AI developers," *AI Ethics*, vol. 3, no. 1, pp. 223–240, 2023.
[15] A. O. Adeniyi, J. O. Arowoogun, C. A. Okolo, R. Chidi, and O. Babawarun, "Ethical considerations in healthcare IT: a review of data privacy and patient consent issues," *World J. Adv. Res. Rev.*, vol. 21, no. 2, pp. 1660–1668, 2024.
[16] B. Farahani, F. Firouzi, and M. Luecking, "The convergence of IoT and distributed ledger technologies (DLT): opportunities, challenges, and solutions," *J. Netw. Comput. Appl.*, vol. 177, p. 102936, 2021.
[17] A. H. Almulihi, F. Alassery, A. Irshad Khan, S. Shukla, B. Kumar Gupta, and R. Kumar, "Analyzing the implications of healthcare data breaches through computational technique," *Intell. Autom. Soft Comput.*, vol. 32, no. 3, pp. 1763–1779, 2022.
[18] N. Patel, "Social engineering as an evolutionary threat to information security in healthcare organizations," *J. Adm. Kesehat. Indones.*, vol. 8, no. 1, p. 56, 2020.
[19] M. Javaid, A. Haleem, R. P. Singh, S. Rab, R. Suman, and I. H. Khan, "Evolutionary trends in progressive cloud computing based healthcare: ideas, enablers, and barriers," *Int. J. Cogn. Comput. Eng.*, vol. 3, pp. 124–135, 2022.
[20] G. I. Ahmad, J. Singla, and K. J. Giri, Security and Privacy of E-Health Data, In: *Multimedia Security*, Singapore: Springer Singapore, 2021, pp. 199–214.
[21] C. Kuner, L. A. Bygrave, C. Docksey, L. Drechsler, and L. Tosoni, "The EU general data protection regulation: a commentary/update of selected articles," *SSRN Electron. J.*, 2021, pp. 1–332. https://ssrn.com/abstract=3839645 or http://dx.doi.org/10.2139/ssrn.3839645
[22] C. Ryngeart and M. Taylor, "The GDPR as global data protection regulation?," *Symposium on the GDPR and International Law*, vol. 114, pp. 5–9, 2020.
[23] B. Krzyzanowski and S. M. Manson, "Twenty years of the health insurance portability and accountability act safe harbor provision: unsolved challenges and ways forward," *JMIR Med. Inform.*, vol. 10, no. 8, p. e37756, 2022.
[24] V. Jaiman and V. Urovi, "A consent model for blockchain-based distributed data sharing platforms," *IEEE Access*, vol. 8, pp. 143734–143745, 2020.
[25] C. Thapa and S. Camtepe, "Precision health data: requirements, challenges and existing techniques for data security and privacy," *Comput. Biol. Med.*, vol. 129, no. 104130, p. 104130, 2021.
[26] R. A. Kadam, "Informed consent process: a step further towards making it meaningful!," *Perspect. Clin. Res.*, vol. 8, no. 3, pp. 107–112, 2017.
[27] FasterCapital, "Healthtech ethical issues navigating the ethical landscape in healthtech innovation," https://fastercapital.com/content/Healthtech-ethical-issues-Navigating-the-Ethical-Landscape-in-Healthtech-Innovation.html (Accessed 26 Sept 2024).

[28] D. Sharma and C. Prabha, Security and Privacy Aspects of Electronic Health Records: A Review. In: *2023 International Conference on Advancement in Computation & Computer Technologies (InCACCT)*, pp. 815–820, 2023.

[29] K. Luong, "Challenges of AI integration in healthcare," www.ominext.com/en/blog/challenges-of-ai-integration-in-healthcare (Accessed 1 Oct 2024).

[30] K. Pradhan, P. John, and N. Sandhu, "Use of artificial intelligence in healthcare delivery in India," *J. Hosp. Manag. Health Policy*, vol. 5, pp. 28–28, 2021.

[31] Gupta, S., et al., 2021. Voting Regression Model for Covid-19 Time Series Data Analysis. In: *3rd International Conference on Advances in Computing, Communication Control and Networking (ICAC3N)*, pp. 2041–2046, doi: 10.1109/ICAC3N53548.2021.9725524

[32] Sharma, G., et al., 2022. A Systematic Review for Detecting Cancer using Machine Learning Techniques. In: *International Conference on Advancement in Computation & Computer Technologies (ICACCT-2021), AIP Conference Proceedings*, Vol. 2555, p. 040007. https://doi.org/10.1063/5.0108888

[33] Kaur, G., et al., 2022. A Systematic Approach to Machine Learning for Cancer Classification. In: *5th International Conference on Contemporary Computing and Informatics (IC3I), Uttar Pradesh, India*, pp. 134–138, doi: 10.1109/IC3I56241.2022.10072474

[34] Sharma, D., et al., 2023. Security and Privacy Aspects of Electronic Health Records: A Review. In: *International Conference on Advancement in Computation & Computer Technologies (InCACCT), Gharuan, India*, pp. 815–820, doi: 10.1109/InCACCT57535.2023.10141814

[35] Mittal, P., Gahlot, K., and Phul, V. (2023). Smart Healthcare System Based on AIoT Emerging Technologies: A Brief Review. In: Singh, Y., Verma, C., Zoltán, I., Chhabra, J.K., Singh, P.K. (eds) *Proceedings of International Conference on Recent Innovations in Computing*. ICRIC 2022. Lecture Notes in Electrical Engineering, vol 1011. Springer, Singapore.

10 The Future of Clinical Trials

Accelerating Drug Development

Ujjwal Srivastava and Gaurav Kumar Singh

10.1 INTRODUCTION TO TECHNOLOGICAL INNOVATIONS

10.1.1 Digital Health and Wearable Devices and the Use of Artificial Intelligence

In this growing digitalized world, the digitalized healthcare system is also blooming using various artificial intelligence (AI)-based algorithms. In this digitalized era, wearable devices such as smart watches, smart tattoos, smart glasses, and many more are in common use these days. These devices are intelligent mechatronic devices or mechanical devices which have in-built sensors which are able to collect and analyse the data received from the body, and transmit the signals received in the form of digital format, which can be easily read [1] . These machines are also being used to monitor the vital signs of the body such as measuring oxygen concentration in the body, heartbeat, body temperature, blood pressure, etc. (see Figure 10.1). According to a report, the global market value size of wearables was valued around USD 61.3 in 2022 and is expected to expand at a compound annual growth rate (CAGR) of 14.6% from 2023 to 2030 [2]. These smart mechanical devices are worn on the wearer's body or on items of clothing, etc.; these devices use an effective and suitable transmission medium such as Bluetooth low energy (BLE), Zigbee, or Wi-Fi for the intercommunication using the human body [3].

Wearables which have in-built sensors are capable of capturing or tracking any change shown by the patients during their treatment from the hospital or clinic environment until the patient gets completely treated and moves freely. Such tracking records help the doctor or clinician in providing accurate treatment. The data provided by these wearables in the form of digital values through these biosensors can be used in the detection of various diseases such as Lyme disease, respiratory infection, cardiovascular diseases, coronavirus infection, Parkinson's disease, and many more [4]. The use of AI in the field of diagnostics enhances the capability of wearables in terms of wearable data alongside imaging modalities, clinical laboratories, etc. The use of multimodal AI in wearables which is

DOI: 10.1201/9781003516163-10

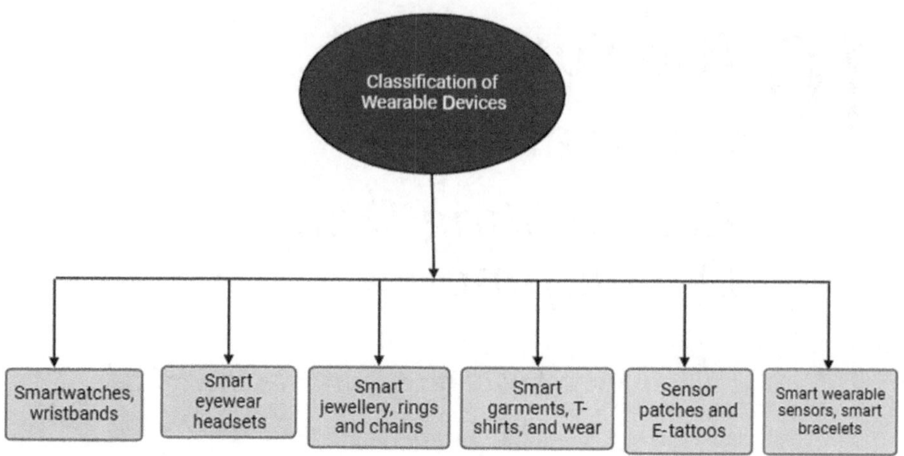

FIGURE 10.1 Classification of Various Wearable Devices.

based on the deep learning (DL) method shows transformative potential mainly for longitudinal layered data which can enhance the prognosis, diagnosis, and help improve treatment strategies [5]. Other commonly used AI-based tools rely on image-generated data such as computed tomography (CT) scans, magnetic resonance imaging (MRI), and endoscopy; other most commonly used AI tools in the medical field are electronic medical records (EMR) and textual data. These electronic data help the clinicians while performing any medical examination [6]. DL is a subset of machine learning (ML) which is a form of representation learning where these representations are produced in several layers, and each of these layers has a non-linear function, collectively called a neural network [6]. DL method networks are used for recognition of facial systems and are now also used in self-driving cars and to identify deep fakes as well. In 2011, International Business Machine (IBM) used Watson a computer-based system that was used for responding to natural language; later on, it was announced that Watson would be used for cancer management cases in New York hospitals. A similar machine named IDx-DR was approved by the Food and Drug Administration (FDA) in 2018; this device is useful as it can scan diabetic retinopathy by using the retinal scans uploaded to it [6].

10.1.2 Other Gadgets Used in Healthcare

The practice of using mobile health (mHealth), which means the use of mobile-based devices that are easy to carry such as mobile phones, patient monitoring devices, personal digital assistants (PDA), is now being commonly used as a healthcare monitoring device [7]. These devices are actively used in the monitoring of blood glucose levels, blood pressure, sleep tracking, heart rate, etc. Healthcare-based applications used on mobile phones are classified into general health and fitness-based applications, information on medicine-based applications, and applications for

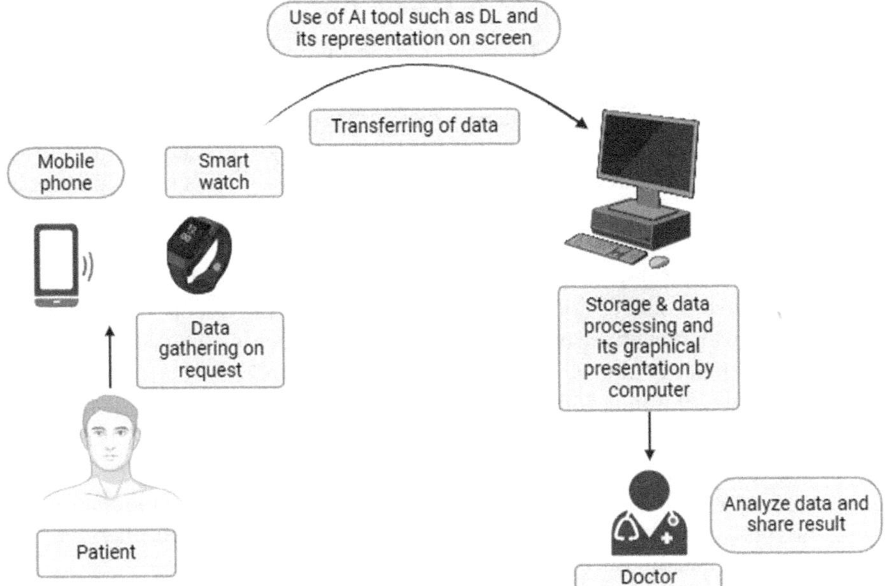

FIGURE 10.2 Processing of mHealth.

managing health care (see Figure 10.2) [7]. The ML algorithm used here in these mobile phones and other similar portables is an advanced AI that is used for Internet of Things (IoT), machine vision, driver assistance, and natural language processing which helps in the diagnosis of various diseases, including cancer research [7].

For the assessment of the potential and performance of the mHealth applications, several performance measurement indicators are used which are as follows:

1. **Usefulness:** This application allows the person to accomplish their daily goals, and also this application inspires people to use this application.
2. **Effectiveness:** This application also allows the user to achieve their goals but in the way the user expects it to.
3. **Veracity:** This application ensures trustworthiness, reliability with accuracy of data collected in healthcare. Like other indicators, this metric helps in the assessment of the data after achieving the goal.
4. **Interactivity:** This encourages the user to use mHealth, with a sense of engagement with the user.
5. **Customization:** This functions by allowing the user to use more than one healthcare domain as per the motto of mHealth, such as the detection of a disease, and its treatment, expert intervention, and recovery.
6. **User Satisfaction:** It can be understood by how well users perceive the quality, functionality, and effectiveness of mHealth applications in meeting their health-related needs.

10.1.3 Blockchain Technology in Data Integrity

It is a kind of distributed ledger technology that is promising in maintaining transparent, secure, and tamper-resistant record keeping. Blockchain technology was first introduced in the year 2008 which was capable of maintaining the security of data and was able to integrate with other information technology systems such as finance and admission systems [8]. Blockchain works by decentralization, blocks, cryptographic hashing, consensus mechanism, and immutability.

1. **Decentralization:** The data here is distributed across a number of systems (computers) called nodes. Every single node has a copy of the entire Blockchain, which ensures that no single entity controls the system.
2. **Block:** Each of the blocks contains a batch of records. Once the block is completed, it is then added to the chain, creating the chronological order of all transactions.
3. **Cryptographic Hashing:** Here each block is attached to another block by cryptograph hash which is a unique identifier generated by the data within the block. If any of the blocks gets tampered with or altered, then the hash changes, making the chain invalid.
4. **Consensus Mechanism:** Such kind of Blockchain network uses consensus mechanism, for example, use of Proof of Stake (POS) or Proof of Work (POW) to validate records and addition of new blocks.
5. **Immutability:** Such type of Blockchain uses tamper-proof mechanisms by interlocking the data stored in subsequent blocks. The data cannot be easily tampered without changing all the subsequent blocks, once the data is recorded in Blockchain. The change requires consensus from most of the network, which makes it a more secure and tamper-resistant Blockchain.
6. **Smart Contract:** These are the Blockchain self-executing contracts, where the terms and conditions are directly written into the lines of codes.

10.1.4 Role of Blockchain in Detecting Falsified Drugs

Drug counterfeiting is a challenge faced across the globe [9]. According to World Health Organization (WHO), one out of ten drugs in market circulation is a part of counterfeiting or a falsified drug. These falsified drugs which could contain inactive components or active components have inappropriate dosages of such components, which could cause potential threats to patients if consumed [9]. The same goes for the use of low-quality antimicrobials which cannot treat the patients but can rather increase antibiotic resistance, resulting in higher death rates and spreading the highly resistant strains across the world. This falsified drug not only increases the economic burden of the country but also reduces the belief of public on effective drugs [9]. The use of Blockchain, an electronic cryptographic ledger, adopts a decentralized networking model, which is a well-known, trustworthy, immutable tamper-resistant AI model. The decentralized networking model works by distributing and synchronizing the information across all nodes, unlike conventional cloud-based applications. These nodes gather true information in case of record duplication by using an algorithm which is synchronized within the network that reduces the chances of record duplication. After the information gets verified, it is then added to the hash value of the previous block, and the new sequence is hashed, which forms a new block by using the cryptographic hash function. This cryptographic hash is a string of unreadable letters and numbers of consistent lengths, making it immutable and tamper-free. These consistent letters and numbers contain information that can be used only by hash algorithm to retrieve information. This ability of Blockchain to send information via nodes makes it potent enough to track any falsified drug or chemicals through information verification of supply chain participants [9].

10.1.5 Types of Blockchains

Consortium (public permissioned), private, and public (permissionless) are the three types of Blockchains. Here, public (permissionless) Blockchain refers to anyone who can access the data that is made public and can join and contribute to both consensuses (theory) and changes to the software [8]. The permissionless Blockchain is widely used by people and is mainly used for cryptocurrencies, such as Bitcoin and Ethereum. In a consortium Blockchain, only a limited number of people have access, which means it is partially centralized. The other kind of Blockchain is the private one, in which only a certain number of nodes can participate in a network, but it is managed by one central authority [8].

10.1.6 Blockchain Used in Wearables

Wearables such as smartwatches and other human IoT help in gathering information from the body in the form of signals that can be read or seen on the screen.

TABLE 10.1
Type and Speciality of Block Chains: An Overview

Property	Public Blockchain	Consortium Blockchain	Private Blockchain
Agreement	All minors	Preferable set of nodes	One organization
Target audience	Open for all	Open for all or restricted	Open for all or restricted
Chances of tampering	Impossible	Chances of getting tampered	Chances of getting tampered
Capability	Less	High	High
Authoritative control	No	Partial	Yes
Grant of permission	No permission required	Permission required	Permission required

Source: Ref. [8].

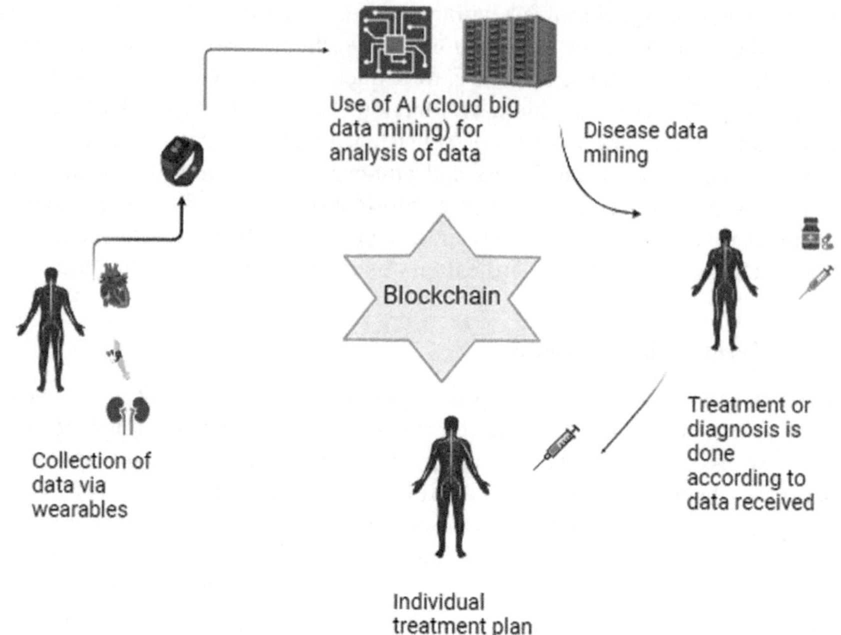

FIGURE 10.3 The integration between AI and Blockchain.

These wearables provide confined intelligence service by using field-programmable gate array capsulation for endpoint devices. The AI used in medical diagnosis, especially for chronic diseases, uses rule engines, big data mining, and DL, which process the health data within time limits and show effective results. The integration of Blockchain with AI in wearables has played a crucial role in data safety and management by providing patient privacy by realizing cross-chain patient interaction and by transferring the data of different Blockchain platforms via a unified consensus plugin. The amalgamation of AI and Blockchain in wearables helps in the automation of data and its security, which enhances the quality of management of chronic diseases (see Figure 10.3).

10.2 NOVEL CRITICAL TRIAL DESIGNS

10.2.1 Introduction to Clinical Trials

Clinical trials are the studies with respect to research that are conducted to check the safety, effectiveness, and potential side effects of medical devices, drugs, vaccines, or treatment. This requires a clearly articulated question and a proper answer which should be satisfactory [10]. The research question should include population, intervention, comparator, and outcomes to be measured. The population study should be based on gender, age, physical condition, and disease status. If we take a narrow population for our study, then the treatment precision will be better and homogeneity will be increased but because we have not targeted a large number of people in our study, treatment might not be effective for a larger population [10]. On the other hand, if we include a larger population for our study, which also includes youngsters, then homogeneity may be reduced, but the treatment effectiveness can be seen in a larger population. The choice of intervention should be clearly defined such as the amount of dose required, route of drug administration, and its time period [10].

10.2.2 Types of Clinical Trials

1. **Treatment Trials:** These trials are performed to study the efficacy of new drugs, new surgical procedures, or treatment methods.
2. **Prevention Trials:** Such trials are practised to prevent any disease or recurrence of any disease.
3. **Diagnostic Trials:** Such trials expose new methods for diagnosing diseases.
4. **Screening Trials:** These trials are performed to detect health or health conditions.
5. **Quality-of-Life Trials**: These trials support the quality of life of patients who are suffering from chronic diseases.
   - **Adaptive Trials:** Adaptive trials are a kind of clinical study that allows researchers to modify the research procedures based on a short period of data analysis without compromising the data integrity. There are various ways to achieve adaptive trials such as by increasing the number of subjects, narrowing the study focus or prior to treatment using various forms of randomization based on the responses of subjects, or by balancing treatment allocation [11]. Adaptive trials help the patients and healthcare providers both financially and ethically, and are considered to be an alternative to a fixed sample trial size in a given appropriate clinical circumstance [12]. Table 10.2 shows the types of adaptive trials.
   - **Platform Trials:** Platform trials can be defined as adaptive, randomized trials, without having an exact end date; as a result, it becomes possible in pathology to examine numerous interventions and make decisions by the addition or reduction of the treatment arms as per the previous (pre-established) rules [13]. It involves the initiation of key infrastructure which can be differentiated with various arms, one after the other to a common control group. The platform trials in comparison with other trials show some benefits such as establishing a model with master protocol, a fixed network of investigator sites with the trained team, possibility of shared control arms which helps in avoiding repeating creation of identical control groups, also by considering platform trial as a single trial which also reduces time limits (Roustit et al., 2023)

Examples of platform trial are as following:

1. **Stampede:** It stands for Systematic therapy in advancing or Metastatic prostate cancer: Evaluation of drug Efficacy (Stampede), which is a multiarm multistage adaptive clinical trial that is designed to assess different treatments for men with high risk, or locally advanced or metastatic cancer.

TABLE 10.2
Types of Adaptive Trials

Name	Description
Group sequential design (GSD)	This is a type of statistical methodology used in clinical trials that allows temporary analysis of data at various stages during the trial.
Sample size re-estimation	Used to reassess and potentially assess the sample size partway through the study based on data collected up to that point.
Adaptive randomization	In this clinical trial, the researchers are allowed to adjust the allocation of participants to different treatment groups depending upon the data received during the trial.
Internal pilot	This clinical trial is used to check the effectiveness of the trial and does not entertain any obstacles.
Multiarm multistage	This allows various treatments that are differentiated with a single control arm.
Expected value of perfect information (EVPI)	This is based on decision analysis concept used to quantify the maximum value that having perfect information would bring in a decision-making process under uncertainty.
Expected value of partially perfect information (EVPPI)	This quantifies the value of obtaining perfect information about the subset of uncertain variables rather than all uncertainties in a decision problem.
Expected value of sample information	This is used to assess the rate of particular research design according to which a decision can be made.
Economic evaluation	This clinical trial will assess both the cost and health outcomes associated with medical intervention.

2. **SPY 2:** It is basically used for women who are suffering from breast cancer. This clinical trial is used to detect triple-negative breast cancer, which is an aggressive stage of breast cancer that does not express the receptor for estrogen, progesterone, or human epidermal growth factor receptor 2 (HER 2).
3. **REMAP–CAP:** It stands for randomized, embedded multifactorial adaptive platform trial for community-acquired pneumonia (REMAP-CAP). This clinical trial is designed to assess treatment for community-acquired pneumonia (CAP).
4. **RECOVERY:** It stands for randomized evolution of COVID-19 therapy (RECOVERY), which is a multicentre clinical trial, used to evaluate potential treatment against COVID-19.
    - **Decentralized Trials (DCT):** A DCT is a clinical trial design that uses digital tools and technologies and other methods that open the gateway of patients for clinical research activities; it also enables the collection of remote data and to investigate and communicate between the investigators and participating subjects [14]. DCT makes a better option for patients who are of old age and cannot come to the research sites or due to any other clinical condition such as neuromuscular disease or even in some

cases logistics can be an issue. DCT studies are done for medium to lower complexities conditions, and not for long studies [14]. Due to its lower complexity, many pharmaceutical companies conducted DCT. For example, Pfizer in 2011 conducted DCT for the topic entitled 'Research on Electronic Monitoring of Overactive Bladder Treatment Experience (REMOTE)'. The results were published in 2014, and internet was used for subject enrolment; the investigational medicinal products were delivered to the patient's home [14]. The key point that makes DCT a good option as a clinical trial is that participants can engage in the trial from their homes, or local healthcare facilities, and remote participation can include virtual visits with healthcare providers, remote monitoring, and online data collection. Digital tools such as mobile phones, wearable devices, and telemedicine make it more feasible to fetch the data for study teams. DCT also reduces the burden on participants by minimizing travel and time commitments and cost efficiency [14].

10.3 REGULATORY INNOVATIONS

Regulatory Sandboxes: These are the controlled, experimental environments in which business especially those in emerging industries can test innovative products, services or business models under relaxed regulatory framework. The Regulatory Sandbox uses data driven innovation, including the use of financial driven technology [15]. Since Regulatory Sandbox provides safe atmosphere to work, the regulators require sandbox applicants to use appropriate safeguard to protect the market from risk of their innovative business [15]. A Regulatory Sandbox can also be considered as a framework within which the investors can test their ideas in a safe mode on a live market under a relevant regulator supervision. Here the regulators closely monitor the sandbox participants to understand the potential risk and benefits of new technologies or business models. Regulatory sandboxes boost the collaboration between the technology and investors ideas due to which regulators gets early insights of new technology and companies gets feedback on compliance and risk..

10.3.1 Accelerated Approval Pathways (Breakthrough Therapy Designation)

The USA FDA requires that pharma companies produce drugs which are not harmful to the patient in any condition. FDA supports the drugs which benefit the patients and outweigh the risk of consuming the drug [16]. One of the major challenges faced by the FDA is the timely launch of the drug in the market for those diseases that have limited medical treatment. Due to this urgent requirement for drugs and to enhance the process of the drug development process, the situation can become life-threatening during this expedition process. Therefore, FDA has developed enhanced approval pathways and designation by introducing the FDA Safety and Innovation Act of 2012 [16]. The newest designation is the breakthrough therapy designation (BTD). Drugs that treat life-threatening diseases are eligible for BTD. The BTD offers various advantages to the manufacturer like rolling review, response within 60 days, also frequent interaction with the FDA-approved team, so that sponsors can get guidance and assurance from the managers for the development and review of a drug (Herink et al., 2018). The other benefits of BTD are that patients with serious or life-threatening illnesses will receive the drugs more quickly as the streamlined approval process reduces time to market. Drugs can be approved earlier during their development process by the FDA if they show promising characteristics even if long-term outcomes are not fully understood.

10.4 PATIENT-CENTRIC APPROACH

10.4.1 Patient Recruitment and Retention Strategies

When a person suffers from a life-threatening disease such as cancer or stroke, then he/she might suffer from financial burden, which also includes worries about health insurance coverage for the clinical trials, logistics, and lack of resources, which makes it difficult for these people in enrolling themselves for clinical trials [17]. Moreover, restricted eligibility criteria set by the trial companies also play a role in the exclusion of certain patient populations because of which it can be observed that most people are left behind for this clinical trial and shows disparity between persons getting enrolled for trials and patients who are actually taking treatment for the disease who could be a part of trial [17]. One of the other reasons for the patients not enrolling themselves in these clinical trials is uncertainty about the success ratio of these trials, especially researchers and patients who are not sure of the outcome of such clinical trials. The strategies for recruitment and retention include the following:

1. Improving mutual understanding between the researchers and the patients.
2. Use of patient navigation and physician consideration of patient concerns, needs, and preferences to enable shared decision-making.
3. Use of questionnaires related to physical and psychosocial aspects that patient can ask their clinical teams during clinical visits.
4. Helping the patients in financial status, so that they can actively participate in the trials.
5. Addressing the patient's concerns.

10.5 DATA MANAGEMENT AND ANALYSIS

10.5.1 Role of Real-World Evidence

Real-world evidence (RWE) has an important role in clinical trials, by supporting regulatory decisions, guiding health policies, improving patient outcomes, etc. RWE is an analysis of real-world data (RWD). Here RWD helps in the collection of data from various sources that are beyond the reach of randomized control trials (RCTs) [18]. RWD includes the data collected from devices by many users such as sphygmomanometers, or self-checked glucometers, and such data cannot be read by conventional clinical trials. A large amount of data is obtained by EMR, especially the medical record, which is helpful for clinicians and researchers. These data gathered by EMR gives quality research [18]. The EMR uses a variety of data such as medical prescription, disease management, and treatment decision-making, which makes it as definitive data with the highest reliability among RWD. RCT is performed for a larger group of population, and it is such a reliable tool that it can include major affected population which makes it authentic and most of the clinical guidelines are based on the report of RCT's, but the disadvantage of RCT is that the patient might not visit the proposed clinical site due to illness or financial issues which could have contributed in representing the actual population size which includes the inclusion or exclusion data due to which there can be biasness among the actual population [18]. To overcome such biases, combining RWE with RCT should be used to make the data more reliable rather than competing with each other (Table 10.3). Here, for example, if RCT monitors the efficacy of the drug, then RWE should monitor the epidemiology, safety, and effectiveness of treatment or cost of treatment related to the drug [18].

The FDA has taken important steps to regularize the use of RWE in the decision-making process [19]. When the 21st Century Cures Act was passed in December 2016, the RWE gained momentum in its role. According to this act, FDA is required to formulate a programme that can access the use of RWE for the monitoring of already approved drugs and fulfil post-approval study requirements [19]. In 2018, the FDA made a framework for its RWA programme, and from then onward FDA has been making rules on its regulatory expectations regarding the use of RWE in medical use (approval of medical products), which is playing a critical role in the effectiveness of biopharmaceutical industries [19].

10.5.2 Data Sharing and Collaboration

Data sharing is the process of sharing raw or analysed data generated from clinical studies which are available to stakeholders, researchers, and clinicians. These data are mostly restricted to publicly funded research [20]. According to the selective reporting of a clinical trial, the comparison between the published drug trial with

TABLE 10.3
Differences between the Working of RWE and RCT

Variable	RCT	RWE
Motive	Overall potential	Productiveness
Role	Research	Real-world setting
Formation	Model	Commonly under trial
Therapy	Stable pattern	Irregular pattern
Population size	Same group of population	Different group of population
Clinicians/doctors involved	Principal investigators	Many clinicians
Control	Inactive drugs/interventions	Other alternative drugs
Patient focusing	Continuous/per protocol	Changeable

unpublished drug trial is the data which is procurable at the drug regulatory agencies that highlighted the benefit of published drug trials and they hide the potential threats of using these drugs which are underrated; consequently, people continue to use these drugs unknowingly [20]. Selective reporting has an adverse impact on clinical trials, for example, the use of class 1 anti-arrhythmic drugs caused the premature death of 50,000 Americans each year in the 1980s. This drug led to nine deaths earlier during a clinical trial, but it was never published. Recently, the rofecoxib (Vioxx) drug which is an anti-arthritis drug, and also a cyclooxigenase-2 (COX-2) inhibitor, caused around a lakh of unnecessary heart attacks in the US accompanied by 10,000 deaths, which could have been avoided earlier [20]. So data sharing is necessary for doctors as well as researchers for better and improved clinical trials. The benefits of data sharing are as follows:

1. The researchers or the doctors are made aware of ongoing clinical trials and the benefits and harm of a medicine.
2. The motive for cheating and immoral use can be reduced as the formulation or calculations are known to others.
3. Due to the effectiveness of the healthcare research, the questions can be answered from the previous trial.
4. Access to raw data can boost the meta-analysis in case of trials of similar interventions.
5. Sharing data from clinical trials can lead to faster discoveries of treatments, ultimately benefiting patients.

The demerit of record sharing is most obviously that anyone can tamper with the data for their own use like plaintiff's lawyers or anti-vaccination proponents. However, this could be possible to some extent because after the trials are made public the tampering or misuse of the data can be highly reduced as well.

10.6 IMPACT OF PERSONALIZED MEDICINE ON CLINICAL TRIAL

The use of personalized medicine has introduced greater precision in the clinical trial process, with the potential to improve treatment outcomes and reduce drug development times. As the technology is enhancing with the development of new emerging innovative technologies, the validation and identification of 'biomarkers' have now become the key element for personalized medicine [21]. Biomarkers are important biological markers that can be measured or evaluated. Based upon these evaluations, a doctor or clinicians can determine the normal pathological or biological process occurring in a patient [21]. These biomarkers help in the identification of diseases, and accordingly, personalized clinical trials for a particular drug are tested. For example, treatments in cancer patients are done by identifying the biomarkers taken from a tumour to help in the treatment, plan, diagnosis, and prognosis of the disease. The major role of personalized treatment is to provide personal treatment based on the personal characteristic or biomarker which can enhance or help further in the treatment [21]. Personalized medicine for patients refers to refined diagnosis of the disease free from trial-and-error period. Not every patient responds to personalized treatment; therefore, the researchers rely on biomarker-based patient stratification to target a larger population that is likely to show successful drug response. With the help of biomarkers, scientists or researchers are able to make personalized drugs, mostly for the diseases related to oncology and cardiology [21].

10.6.1 Application of Virtual Reality and Augmented Reality in Clinical Trials

Virtual reality (VR) and augmented reality (AR) are both technological breakthroughs that provide entertainment and communication worldwide [22]. Here, VR uses its three-dimensional virtual world for entertainment, whereas AR is linked with the real world and uses virtual elements with the real world. Both these applications are used for clinical trials in the field of healthcare. Recently, critical care published electronic choice of a system for intensive care relaxation (E-CHOISIR), which is the first cross-over randomized clinical trial that shows the beneficial effects of its virtual effect on patients suffering from stress, pain, and discomfort [22]. As per the patients' point of view, VR reduces stress and anxiety levels, and it also improves the communication level between the stakeholders, relatives, and others, thus aiding in maintaining coordination and understanding. The key role of VR, apart from reducing stress and anxiety, is that it can also reduce the pain level [22]. The concept of reducing pain by using VR technology emerged in the 1990s. Weakness acquired in intensive care units (ICUs) after prolonged stays or postoperative measures often leads to stress and anxiety. The VR rehabilitation programme has been found to reduce these stresses. Moreover the augmented reality (AR) can assist surgeons or clinicians in intubation or central line placement which shows the clear pictures while performing practical steps [22].

10.7 CONCLUSION

The amalgamation of AI with wearables is not only used to track health status but also to promote preventive healthcare. Most of the population, especially the young generation, is wearing smart wearables, which helps in tracking healthcare data using various AI tools. AI in these wearables can be used to provide reminders for water intake, measure hydration biomarkers, track intake of nutrients, etc. The use of wearables has become a game changer because of its ability to track health records and make you aware of these records. These records are now being extensively used in clinical trials to develop new technologies and overcome similar diseases. The role of DCTs and platform trials also contributes to the development of society. Overall, clinical trials are game changers if used for a larger population. As the population is growing, we are always surrounded by new challenges, so the production of newer drugs that should be promising and effective needs to undergo clinical trials, for which there is the requirement of equal participation of volunteers for the betterment of society. As the population is rising the data security of patients and even newer drugs is of utmost importance and due to which the researchers are commonly using various Blockchains to eradicate this problem. The use of Blockchains with AI can yield promising results in both data collection and record-keeping, while also ensuring security. The future of AI is demanding and AI should always be used for the betterment of society.

REFERENCES

1. D. Nahavandi, *Application of artificial intelligence in wearable devices: opportunities and challenges*, Elsevier, 2022.
2. Grand View Research, "Wearable technology market," [Online]. Available: www.grandviewresearch.com/industry-analysis/wearable-technology-market#. [Accessed: Oct. 7, 2024].
3. V. Vijayan, J. P. Connolly, J. Condell, N. McKelvey, and P. Gardiner, "Review of wearable devices and data collection considerations for connected health," *Sensors*, vol. 21, no. 5589, 2021.
4. S. Chakrabarti et al., "Smart consumer wearables as digital diagnostic tools: a review," *Diagnostics*, vol. 12, no. 9, p. 2110, 2022. doi:10.3390/diagnostics12092110.
5. T. B. Marvasti et al., "Unlocking tomorrow's health care: expanding the clinical scope of wearables by applying artificial intelligence," *Canadian Journal of Cardiology*, [Preprint], 2024. doi:10.1016/j.cjca.2024.07.009.
6. M. K. Sana et al., "Artificial intelligence in celiac disease," *Computers in Biology and Medicine*, vol. 125, p. 103996, 2020. doi:10.1016/j.compbiomed.2020.103996.
7. Z. F. Khan and S. R. Alotaibi, "Applications of artificial intelligence and big data analytics in M-health: a healthcare system perspective," *Journal of Healthcare Engineering*, vol. 2020, pp. 1–15, 2020. doi:10.1155/2020/8894694.
8. D. Elangovan et al., "The use of blockchain technology in the health care sector: systematic review," *JMIR Medical Informatics*, vol. 10, no. 1, 2022. doi:10.2196/17278.
9. P. Sylim et al., "Blockchain technology for detecting falsified and substandard drugs in distribution: pharmaceutical supply chain intervention," *JMIR Research Protocols*, vol. 7, no. 9, 2018. doi:10.2196/10163.
10. A. Schultz et al., "An introduction to clinical trial design," *Paediatric Respiratory Reviews*, vol. 32, pp. 30–35, 2019. doi:10.1016/j.prrv.2019.06.002.
11. F. P. Cerqueira, A. M. Jesus, and M. D. Cotrim, "Adaptive design: a review of the technical, statistical, and regulatory aspects of implementation in a clinical trial," *Therapeutic Innovation & Regulatory Science*, vol. 54, no. 1, pp. 246–258, 2020. doi:10.1007/s43441-019-00052-y.
12. L. Flight et al., "A review of clinical trials with an adaptive design and health economic analysis," *Value in Health*, vol. 22, no. 4, pp. 391–398, 2019. doi:10.1016/j.jval.2018.11.008.
13. M. Roustit et al., "Platform trials," *Therapies*, vol. 78, no. 1, pp. 29–38, 2023. doi:10.1016/j.therap.2022.12.003.
14. C. Petrini et al., "Decentralized clinical trials (DCTS): a few ethical considerations," *Frontiers in Public Health*, vol. 10, 2022. doi:10.3389/fpubh.2022.1081150.
15. A. Martin and G. Balestra, "Using regulatory sandboxes to support responsible innovation in the humanitarian sector," *Global Policy*, vol. 10, no. 4, pp. 733–736, 2019. doi:10.1111/1758-5899.12729.
16. M. C. Herink, A. N. Irwin, and G. M. Zumach, "FDA breakthrough therapy designation: evaluating the quality of the evidence behind the drug approvals,"

Pharmacotherapy: The Journal of Human Pharmacology and Drug Therapy, vol. 38, no. 9, pp. 967–980, 2018. doi:10.1002/phar.2167.

17. R. D. Nipp, K. Hong, and E. D. Paskett, "Overcoming barriers to clinical trial enrollment," in *American Society of Clinical Oncology Educational Book*, no. 39, pp. 105–114, 2019. doi:10.1200/edbk_243729.
18. H.-S. Kim, S. Lee, and J. H. Kim, "Real-world evidence versus randomized controlled trial: clinical research based on electronic medical records," *Journal of Korean Medical Science*, vol. 33, no. 34, 2018. doi:10.3346/jkms.2018.33.e213.
19. C. A. Purpura et al., "The role of real-world evidence in FDA-approved new drug and biologics license applications," *Clinical Pharmacology & Therapeutics*, vol. 111, no. 1, pp. 135–144, 2021. doi:10.1002/cpt.2474.
20. P. C. Gøtzsche, "Why we need easy access to all data from all clinical trials and how to accomplish it," *Trials*, vol. 12, no. 1, 2011. doi:10.1186/1745-6215-12-249.
21. P. Carrigan and T. Krahn, "Impact of biomarkers on personalized medicine," in *Handbook of Experimental Pharmacology*, pp. 285–311, 2015. doi:10.1007/164_2015_24.
22. R. R. Bruno et al., "Virtual and augmented reality in critical care medicine: the patient's, clinician's, and researcher's perspective," *Critical Care*, vol. 26, no. 1, 2022. doi:10.1186/s13054-022-04202-x.

11 Challenges and Roadblocks

Navigating the HealthTech Ecosystem

Shubham Gupta and Rajnish Kohli

11.1 INTRODUCTION TO THE HEALTHTECH ECOSYSTEM

HealthTech is a mature and evolving landscape that leverages bleeding-edge technology in health to bring a new nature and end points of healthcare as well as efficiency and personalization in healthcare delivery. This includes an electronic health record (EHR), telemedicine, mobile health (mHealth) apps, wearable devices, as well as newer technologies like artificial intelligence (AI), machine learning (ML), and blockchain. If executed well, it could revolutionize clinical care, administrative services, personal health tools, and public health management. We have AI algorithms that are better than human experts at interpreting medical images, wearables that constantly monitor our health, and telemedicine platforms, thus allowing us to consult the right doctors at any time, from anywhere in the world. The advantages include EHRs, making it easier to coordinate as well as reducing the chances of some manual errors in patient data management. While these advancements are welcomed, so too does the mainstreaming of AI and HealthTech integration come with its challenges. There has always been a challenge integrating systems and sharing data among disparate care systems, and, of course, data security comes to the top of mind when we talk about protecting patient health information from organizational breaches and cyber-threats. There are also regulatory and compliance considerations for startups in the space, as HealthTech solutions can fall under several global regulations that can be difficult to parse due to the national, fragmented nature of healthcare laws worldwide, not to mention very significant pieces of legislation like Health Insurance Portability and Accountability Act (HIPAA) in the United States and General Data Protection Regulation (GDPR) in Europe. Other widespread issues are financial constraints due to high upfront development and implementation costs, which require substantial investment and a clear return on investment (ROI) to stakeholders [1]. The adoption of new technology into practice is often met with organizational resistance and requires heavy re-training and up-skilling of the healthcare workforce. However, ethical and social concerns (e.g., patient privacy, the right to access, and the quality of HealthTech solutions being applied) need to be addressed to ensure that HealthTech

 DOI: 10.1201/9781003516163-11

solutions become more careful and equitable. Nonetheless, the HealthTech upside is compelling. Accurate diagnosis, personalized treatment, and continuous health monitoring promoted by HealthTech, in addition to increased operational efficiency and decreased costs, facilitate patient care and indicate a digital revolution occurring in healthcare. These technologies also engage patients, enable access to their health information, and support ways to manage proactive health. Advanced data analytics and real-time surveillance are helpful for public health initiatives, for timely detection, monitoring, and response in terms of health crises. The HealthTech ecosystem is enabling this future, with its challenges, complexity, and timeline for impact, making strides in curing diseases and keeping people healthy. Twenty-first-century technology companies will ensure health is no longer a matter of zip code, provide the power and resources to build the future of healthcare, and enable all humanity to be well. The progression of this ecosystem, as shown in Figure 11.1, will determine what the future of healthcare looks like, further reinforcing the need for greater interdisciplinary collaboration between healthcare providers, patients, developers, investors, and policymakers to build and deploy the next-generation healthcare innovations, long-anticipated by many.

HealthTech (Healthcare + Technology) is building technology solutions focused on improving the quality, access, and cost of healthcare services [2]. It encompasses the breadth of technological developments and applications, both physical and digital,

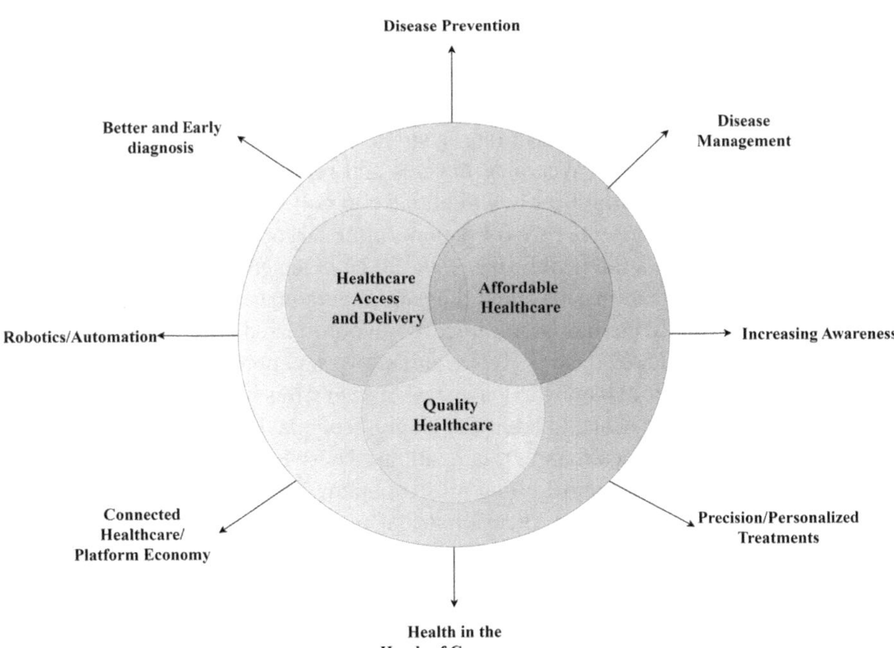

FIGURE 11.1 HealthTech Ecosystem.

as they all relate to bettering patient care, streamlining administrative services, and improving health and well-being. HealthTech covers the following areas:

- **Clinical Applications:** Any software tool or technology that supports the diagnosis, treatment, or monitoring of patients such as radiology and other imaging systems, digital pathology and medical imaging sharing services, surgical robots, Internet of Things (IoT) health wearables, and monitoring devices.
- **Administrative Applications:** These applications include EMRs, patient management tools, billing applications, etc.
- **Consumer Health Technologies:** Applications and wearables that empower consumers to track and manage their health and well-being, including activity trackers, food logs, remote health consultation applications, and more.
- **Public Health Technologies:** Technologies used by public health entities to monitor and manage public health issues (e.g., epidemiology tracking systems, health information exchanges [HIEs], and telehealth services for underserved populations).

11.1.1 Importance and Impact of HealthTech on Modern Healthcare

HealthTech has a profound significance and power to change the ways of medical services by improving patient care, operational efficiency, and healthcare delivery, regardless of the hierarchical structures. HealthTech is making a considerable difference on many levels, with one of the largest benefits of HealthTech advancement in healthcare being quantified precision and correct diagnostics because of the aid of advanced tools like AI and ML. For instance, AI algorithms are now increasingly capable of identifying medical images with a higher degree of accuracy than even human radiologists, providing earlier and more accurate diagnoses, especially in the fields of cardiology and oncology. Wearable devices and remote monitoring technologies not only make it easier to monitor health but also to collect real-time data to manage chronic conditions and provide care for patients after surgery. By monitoring continuously, in many instances the health issues would be detected before they can worsen and result in hospital readmissions, and the patient outcomes could be improved. The integration of telemedicine has even radically revolutionized healthcare reach to the distant and underprivileged locales. Telehealth allows a patient to consult and identify disease conditions without having to leave the house and this is very efficient because it can save time and health costs. In addition, HealthTech plays a huge part in enhancing operational efficiency in healthcare organizations. These EHRs are essentially patient data management tools and ensure that all the patient information is well-structured and accessible to the medical professionals, in turn, not losing or missing out on asylum vital pieces of information [3]. The improved access has eliminated the incentive for each interdisciplinary team to coordinate more widely with their administrative colleagues, needlessly burdensome, and reliant upon manual logging processes that could otherwise lead to errors. Additionally, HealthTech can provide economic savings by automating daily tasks, improving resource allocation, and enabling IoT-tech-driven predictive maintenance of medical devices. These efficiencies take on added importance in an era of price constraints on healthcare systems worldwide, along with an aging population and the demand for more efficient care delivery. It also enables patient empowerment with the tools they need to manage their health proactively. Just by learning about their health record and tracking health parameters, the engagement layer increases due to mHealth apps, and links to resources and communications for the patients with healthcare professionals on patient portals are upon your door step and finger tips (you can check my health any time) ergo good attitude and thoughts for self-care. Such empowerment is especially valuable in the care of chronic disease, in which patients cannot be passive dependents. This further enables population health trends to be identified using advanced data analytics and big data in HealthTech, helping public health initiatives and policymaking. By sensing changes in large data sources quickly, real-time data analytics enables us to effectively monitor disease outbreaks, follow vaccination coverage, assess the response to public health interventions, and therefore develop the capacity to respond better to public health. While HealthTech is advancing at a breakneck pace, existing challenges in HealthTech include cybersecurity and data protection, interoperability, and the necessity of regulatory landscapes that can properly protect the well-being and privacy of individual patients. Nevertheless, the impact that HealthTech can have on the transformation of healthcare delivery, as well as improving patient outcomes and system efficiency, is unquestionable. Its ongoing evolution will help consolidate and enhance the healthcare experience for more effective, personalized, and user-friendly modern healthcare. This continuous evolution re-emphasizes the importance of cooperative efforts by all stakeholders – healthcare providers, technology developers, policymakers, and patients to further unlock the opportunities and mitigate the challenges comprising the HealthTech ecosystem.

Relevance and its repercussions on modern healthcare HealthTech have reshaped the face of the healthcare industry, paving the path for multiple advantages like enhanced patient outcomes, greater efficiency, and lower costs. Its impact on modern healthcare includes:

- **Improved Patient Care:** HealthTech makes it possible to deliver more accurate and efficient health services through innovative diagnostic equipment, individualized treatment strategies, and real-time health monitoring.
- **Increase in Efficiency:** On the productive end, the use of automation and digitization pacifies administrative tasks and lessens the burden on healthcare providers, offering more time for focusing on patient care. EHRs and HIT systems improve the exchange and collaboration of information among healthcare teams.
- **Cost Reduction:** Telemedicine and other remote monitoring technologies make it easier for patients to take care of themselves and their caregivers, thus allowing medical costs to remain low.
- **Rise of Patient Empowerment:** HealthTech tools allow patients to manage their health, because of more and more health management applications and access to personal health data.
- **Public Health:** Better data analytics and real-time monitoring of diseases will make it easier to detect sophisticated public health issues, enabling the public health authorities to respond promptly and efficiently in case of a health crisis.

11.2 HISTORICAL CONTEXT AND EVOLUTION

The historical perspective and progress of the HealthTech landscape underscore a palpable metamorphosis in the ways of delivering and managing healthcare inspired by advancements in technology over the last few decades. In the beginning, healthcare was labor intensive using simple tools with everything being written on paper and few choices in diagnosis tools with the basic imaging and laboratory tests. The digital era began in the late 20th century, and with it EHRs emerged as a groundbreaking data solution that recently redefined various processes of patient data management granting a more accessible way of managing data, storing, and sharing data. There has been a significant increase in HealthTech innovations in the 21st century with the rise of advanced diagnostic tools, telemedicine platforms, and wearable health devices. This evolution was further activated due to the advances made in AI and ML, which gave way to predictive analytics, personalized medicine, and more accurate diagnostics [4]. For example, AI-powered algorithms are now helping to decipher intricate medical images, thus promoting the diagnosis of diseases like cancer and cardiovascular conditions at an earlier stage. Telemedicine Application Telecom has enabled patients to interact with doctors and get patients to consult and heal without regard to geographical boundaries in remote areas and places. The use of the IoT in the healthcare sector makes it easy to enable continuous monitoring of health, enabling the provision of real-time data that helps in improving disease management and in preventative care. This technological evolution is also coupled with important regulatory and ethical issues, as the importance of privacy and patient confidentiality takes on an increasingly central role. Nevertheless, the trajectory of HealthTech innovation from the past to the present and the future offers hope for the success of changing healthcare for the better, making it more efficient, more convenient, and more patient-focused. This evolution is still never-ending, and it helps to determine how healthcare will shape our future with improved innovations, patient outcomes, and process efficiency.

11.2.1 Milestones in Medical Technology

HealthTech has evolved over time as shown in Figure 11.2, and there have been some key milestones that have changed how we access healthcare.

11.2.1.1 19th-Century Innovations

- **Stethoscope (Laennec; 1816):** Invented by Rene Laennec, the stethoscope changed the way doctors could listen to a patient's internal sounds, which was a vital tool in beginning to diagnose.
- **X-Ray** (1895): Wilhelm Conrad Roentgen discovered X-rays, which made it possible to view the interior of the body without invasive measures and hence revolutionized diagnosis.

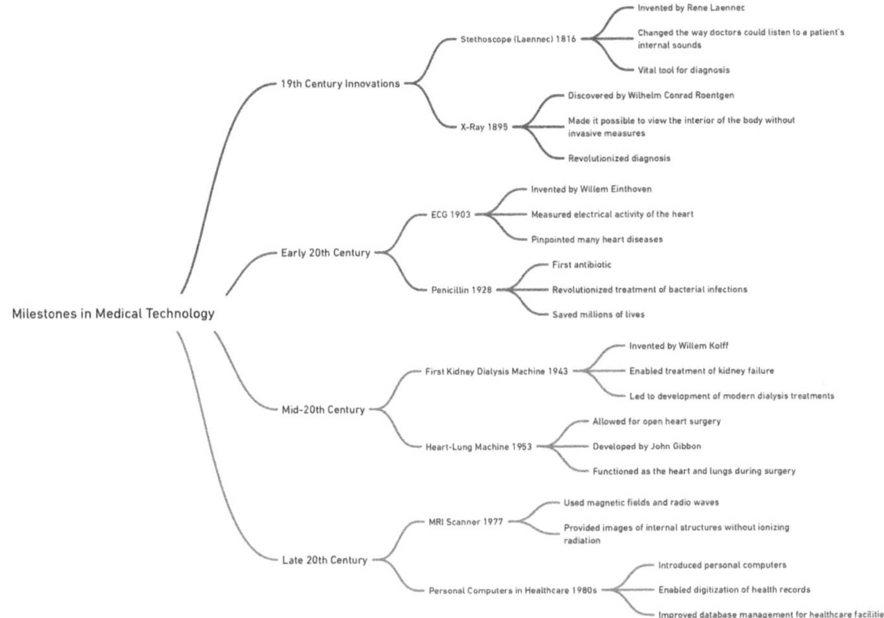

FIGURE 11.2 Background of Medical Technology.

11.2.1.2 Early 20th Century

- Electrocardiogram (ECG; 1903): Invented by Willem Einthoven, the ECG offered a new method of measuring the electrical activity of the heart and pinpointing many heart diseases.
- Penicillin (1928): The first antibiotic and the one that revolutionized all bacterial infection treatments, saving millions of lives.

11.2.1.3 Mid-20th Century

- First Kidney Dialysis Machine (1943): Invented by Willem Kolff, this machine enabled the treatment of kidney failure, leading to the development of modern dialysis treatments.
- Heart–Lung Machine (1953): This machine allowed for open heart surgery and was developed to function as the heart and lungs of a patient during surgery by John Gibbon.

11.2.1.4 Late 20th Century

- MRI Scanner (1977): Magnetic resonance imaging (MRI) uses magnetic fields and radio waves to provide images of the internal structures of the body, but without using ionizing radiation.
- Personal Computers in Healthcare (1980s): In the 1980s, personal computers were introduced, along with the ability to digitize health records providing primarily a better database management solution for healthcare facilities.

11.2.2 Transition from Traditional to Digital Health Solutions

Traditional health solutions, as shown in Figure 11.3, are transitioning into their digital counterparts and this shift defines a new era in healthcare, where technology is incorporated into nearly every process to both administer care to patients and make operations more efficient, further improving patient experience. Healthcare has, traditionally, depended heavily on face-to-face interactions, physical records, manual diagnostics, etc. All patient information was in paper records, and the responsibility to handle them was quite a headache; these records were hardly accurate, and many times lost [5]. The diagnostics and treatments were mostly done manually with very less technological interventions, and therefore the journey was tiring, prolonged, and often resulted in inaccuracies.

The digital revolution in healthcare started by storing patient information in electronic paper records, known as electronic health records, that contain demographic information, medical history, medication history, and laboratory test results. This move helped in doing data entry more accurately and efficiently, making fewer mistakes and ensuring better healthcare continuity. The advent of EHRs was just the beginning of the digital transition; it helped set the stage for more technology changes to come.

Telemedicine is a powerful digital solution that helps transition practices to remote care. The technology became of even greater importance following the COVID-19 pandemic, as its global adoption accelerated. Telemedicine reduces geographical limitations and allows patients from remote and underprivileged locations to avail themselves of quality healthcare facilities. It is also more convenient for patients and relieves the burden on healthcare facilities by cutting down on the number of in-person visits needed.

Wearable and mobile health (mHealth) devices are also an important step up in digital health solutions. These technologies enable patients to track their health and also their vital signs, physical activity, and other health metrics. It is possible to combine data obtained from these wearables into the healthcare systems which will

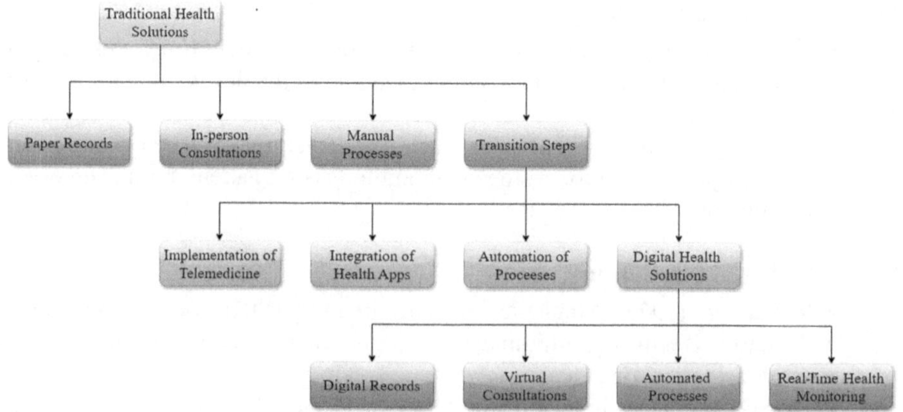

FIGURE 11.3 Healthcare Solutions.

enable continuous monitoring and early diagnosis of potential health problems. By taking a more patient-centric proactive health management approach, these measures helped with preventative care and ensuring proper management of chronic diseases, leading to higher patient outcomes.

With AI and ML – which power sophisticated data analytics, predictive modeling, and personalized medicine – digital health solutions take on a life of their own. Consumers too understand that AI algorithms are now capable of processing enormous sets of health data, enabling them to more quickly recognize global patterns, predict future outbreaks of disease, and help clinicians in decision-making as well as personalize treatment for each patient as per their genetic and health system. According to results published in the *Journal of Medical Internet Research,* traditional methods could not achieve this precision in the past and stood as a proof-of-concept for the disruptive force of digital health solutions.

In addition, the implementation of the IoT has transformed patient monitoring and care coordination. A system named XINHU enables real-time monitoring and sharing of health data through IoT devices such as smart home health systems, medical sensors, etc. This connectivity allows healthcare providers to monitor the health status of their patients continuously, respond in an emergency, and adjust treatments as necessary.

The move toward digital health can provide a plethora of advantages, but it nevertheless presents challenges in the form of data privacy and security, interoperability, and regulatory frameworks, which must be addressed. Security around sensitive health data must not be compromised due to patient safety and privacy concerns. Moreover, seamless interoperability between a multitude of health systems and devices is required to truly operationalize the use of digital health technologies.

11.2.3 Current Trends

- **Telemedicine:** Involves the use of digital communication technologies to deliver healthcare services remotely. Key trends include the following:
  - **Virtual Consultations:** Patients can consult with healthcare providers via video calls, reducing the need for in-person visits.
  - **Remote Monitoring:** Devices and apps that monitor patient health metrics (e.g., blood pressure, glucose levels) and transmit data to healthcare providers for ongoing management of chronic conditions.
  - **Telehealth Platforms:** Comprehensive systems that integrate various telemedicine services, including virtual visits, remote monitoring, and patient education.
- **AI in Healthcare:** AI is transforming healthcare with applications such as:
  - **Diagnostic Tools**: AI algorithms analyze medical images (e.g., X-rays, MRIs) to identify abnormalities with high accuracy, assisting radiologists in diagnosis.
  - **Predictive Analytics**: AI models predict patient outcomes, readmission risks, and disease outbreaks, enabling proactive and preventive care.
  - **Personalized Medicine**: AI analyzes genetic and clinical data to recommend personalized treatment plans tailored to individual patients.

- **Wearable Technology:** Wearable devices are becoming increasingly prevalent in healthcare, offering benefits such as:
  - **Health Monitoring**: Devices like smartwatches track vital signs, physical activity, sleep patterns, and more, providing continuous health data.
  - **Chronic Disease Management**: Wearables help manage conditions such as diabetes and hypertension by monitoring relevant health metrics and alerting users to potential issues.
  - **Fitness and Wellness**: Fitness trackers motivate users to stay active and adopt healthier lifestyles by setting goals and tracking progress.
- **Digital Health Records**: Digital health records, including EHRs and PHRs, streamline healthcare data management by:
  - **Improving Data Accessibility**: Digital health records are easily accessible to authorized healthcare providers, facilitating better-coordinated care.
  - **Enhancing Patient Engagement**: PHRs allow patients to access and manage their health information, empowering them to take an active role in their healthcare.
  - **Data Integration**: EHRs integrate data from various sources (e.g., lab results, imaging studies, clinical notes), providing a comprehensive view of a patient's health.

11.3 GLOBAL REGULATORY BODIES AND THEIR ROLES

The HealthTech ecosystem is shaped by a multitude of regulatory authorities worldwide, each with distinct mandates and requirements. The U.S. Food and Drug Administration (FDA) is one of the most influential bodies, regulating medical devices, software as medical devices (SaMD), and other health technologies. The FDA's main responsibility is to secure the safety, efficacy, and security of all these products before being offered. In Europe, the European Medicines Agency (EMA) is a similar product regulation arm of the European Union and is responsible for the extraordinary authority over the approval of medicines and medical devices. The Pharmaceuticals and Medical Devices Agency (PMDA) in Japan and the National Medical Products Administration (NMPA) in China are also major influencer agencies in regulating HealthTech products in their respective countries. These regulatory bodies set the standards of what manufacturers must comply with – in everything from clinical trials to post-market surveillance – to ensure the safety of the public.

11.3.1 Key Regulations in Major Markets

Federal Regulatory Environment: FDA in the United States has jurisdiction over various laws and guidelines pertaining to HealthTech products For instance, the 21st Century Cures Act is meant to facilitate the development of medical products and bring novel innovations to patients quicker by cutting down on regulatory processes. Another major initiative is the Digital Health Innovation Action Plan, which emphasizes a streamlined process for the regulation of software-based medical technologies. The European Union with the Medical Device Regulation (MDR) and the In Vitro Diagnostic Regulation (IVDR) offer unified frameworks that overhauled the previous Medical Device Directive (MDD) and In Vitro Diagnostic Directive (IVDD). These rules involve increased demands with respect to clinical data, identification, and monitoring in the post-market phase, underlining the result in the field and patient portrayal [6]. Detailed technical documentation and conformity assessments are now required by the MDR and IVDR, which has been recognized as one of the most difficult aspects for manufacturers.

11.3.2 Variations and Harmonization Efforts

With differing regulatory needs, the global regulatory ecosystem faces a significant obstacle as each jurisdiction comes with different requirements. For example, the determination of classification criteria for medical devices may be vastly different between the United States, EU, and other such regions, with differing regulatory pathways as a result. Yet, these variations mean that any successful compliance strategy varies directly with each market, further complicating and increasing the price of getting regulatory approval. Nevertheless, moves for harmonization are underway, as regulatory requirements are evolving to be more in sync with each other to help enable smoother global business. Initiatives such as the International Medical Device Regulators Forum (IMDRF) have been developed to encourage convergence on regulatory principles and practices. The IMDRF aims to decrease regulatory burden and enhance predictability for HealthTech companies by creating globally recognized guidelines [7]. Furthermore, the Global Harmonisation Task Force (GHTF) based on significant efforts to harmonize standards and procedures has helped improve global collaboration and efficiency.

11.3.3 Compliance Issues

11.3.3.1 Data Privacy (Health Insurance Portability and Accountability Act, General Data Protection Regulation)

Because health data is especially sensitive, data privacy is a key pillar in HealthTech regulatory compliance. In the United States, the HIPAA imposes regulatory requirements developed to ensure the confidentiality and privacy of medical records. Specifically, HIPAA requires a set of concrete steps to keep data confidential, intact, and safe subject to administrative, physical, and technical safeguards. HIPAA compliance includes defined policy implementation to limit who can access data also audit controls, data is encrypted at rest and in motion along with recurring risk assessments. As the strictest data protection and privacy legal regulation, GDPR is very challenging to comply with within the EU. GDPR applies to all companies processing the personal data of subjects residing in the EU, even if the company is not based in the EU. Notable concepts in GDPR are data minimization, purpose limitation, and the right to access and control data by individuals. Penalties for not satisfying GDPR can be severe, with fines as high as 4% of annual global turnover, meaning strict compliance is essential.

11.3.3.2 Security Standards and Protocols

Apart from the requirement for data privacy, HealthTech companies have to comply with robust cybersecurity measures as well, and their data systems are constantly challenged by data breaches and cyber-threats. ISO/IEC 27001 is a framework of organizational information security controls centered on the specification for an information security management system (ISMS). The policy includes risk management, security policies, asset management, and incident response as the most important measures. The National Institute of Standards and Technology (NIST) Cybersecurity Framework provides standards for critical infrastructure in the United States to improve their ability to prevent, detect, and respond to cyber-attacks. Compliance with these frameworks includes periodic penetration testing, educating employees on best security practices, deploying security controls like encryption and intrusion detection systems, and establishing an incident response team. Trust and regulatory compliance depend on the institutions having strong cybersecurity in place, as a breach can have significant legal, financial, and reputational implications.

11.4 TECHNOLOGICAL CHALLENGES IN HEALTHTECH

Several technological challenges in HealthTech are as follows.

11.4.1 Interoperability

11.4.1.1 Issues with Integrating Diverse Systems and Platforms

The key and biggest challenge in the HealthTech ecosystem is interoperability. This can be applied across disparate systems within healthcare systems like EHRs, Laboratory Information Systems (LIS), Radiology Information Systems (RIS), and other clinical and administrative systems. Each of these systems may have been developed by different vendors, at different times, meaning differences in architecture, data format, and communication protocols.

Another key problem is marrying legacy systems and modern digital health offerings. Most of the known legacy systems, which were developed many years ago, were not built to dialogue with digital platforms that contemporarily most company businesses experience today. They tend to use outdated data formats and communication protocols, meaning that interconnecting with newer systems is slow, difficult, and costly. Also, because proprietary systems do not work natively together with each other that they tend to establish what is called "data silos," where information is locked behind in its system and cannot intermix across the organization or with external parties easily.

There are additional complexities because this diversity of systems serves a dynamic healthcare delivery environment where the workflows are complex and quite different between organizations. The integration scenarios are rendered complex and cost more owing to the customization and configuration mandates. In the absence of this seamless integration, healthcare providers have to deal with inefficiencies such as lack of access to comprehensive patient records, duplicated tests, and delayed care delivery.

11.4.1.2 Standards and Frameworks for Interoperability

There are many standards and frameworks to help tackle these integration problems, including the Health Level Seven International (HL7) – the globally accepted organization for standards for the exchange of electronic health information. One of the more significant standards is the web-based Fast Healthcare Interoperability Resources (FHIR) standard from HL7. FHIR uses a set of resources that each represents a particular type of clinical data, for example, patient, observation, medication, and other resources using RESTful Application Programming Interfaces (APIs) to facilitate data exchange and accessibility between systems.

Similarly important are the Digital Imaging and Communications in Medicine (DICOM) standard and the Systematized Nomenclature of Medicine Clinical Terms (SNOMED CT) clinical terminology. The objectives of these standards are to ensure that heterogeneous systems can communicate, understand, and act based on data being exchanged.

However, the adherence to these standards does not come without its difficulties. Upgrading or replacing non-compliant systems frequently requires substantial investment, with a drawn-out and potentially complicated implementation process. Moreover, the bar keeps rising for quality standards; they need to be always maintained. Uphill battles aside, interoperability standards are indispensable for the smooth flow of health information that patient care and operational efficacies depend on.

11.4.2 Data Management

11.4.2.1 Big Data Handling and Analytics

This has resulted in an exponential increase in health data due to the ready availability of digital health tools like EHR systems, wearables, and mHealth applications [8]. This data sprawl comes in the form of everything from clinical data and genomic data to patient-generated health data and social determinants of health, while analysis, storage, and processing of this big data is one of the challenges to overcome.

Big data: For the sake of consolidating the huge amount of data, you need to have the infrastructure to store it in a well-maintained way that is secure and reliable This is how cloud computing is playing an important role in delivering storage solutions that are scalable and flexible. Managing large datasets is efficiently done with the help of distributed databases like Hadoop and NoSQL databases.

After your data is stored, you process and analyze it to turn it into valuable insight. This requires advanced analytics techniques such as ML and AI. These technologies help us to analyze large datasets, find patterns, predict outcomes based on existing datasets or real-time data, and support decision-making processes. This includes, for example, the identification of patients at risk for readmission, the detection of infectious disease outbreaks, and the personalization of treatment decisions based on patient information.

However, using big data analytics in healthcare would need considerable investment in technology and human resources. Aside from providing access to data, most of us would not know where to begin,; healthcare organizations also need data scientists and data analysts with a certain level of skill to design and run these types of algorithms on the healthcare data. On top of this, many sources of health data are siloed and come with poor data quality and integration due to variabilities in accuracy and completeness.

11.4.2.2 Ensuring Data Accuracy and Integrity

It is essential to maintain accurate and secure data in this vast ocean of healthcare data for reaching out and delivering the best possible healthcare to patients. Data accuracy is related to the correctness and precision of the data, whereas data integrity is associated with data integrity about keeping data in the lifecycle consistent and reliable.

Unreliable or missing data places lives at risk with incidents found that medication errors can be anywhere from 100 to 10,000 times greater. Human error in manual data entry, nonuniform data formatting, and inconsistencies between disparate data sources are common culprits. One example: a patient's medication history may be documented in one way within their primary care EHR and a different way within their hospital EHR, and this could result in medication errors.

Healthcare organizations need strong data governance approaches to tackle these challenges. At a high level, data governance means to set rules and practices for managing data during each step of its lifecycle This includes creating data quality standards, verification and validation of data regularly, and data cleaning techniques to address inaccuracies.

Other technologies such as blockchain are also being studied to ensure data integrity. Because of its tamper-proof ledger, recorded and verified transactions guarantee that health records maintain their original and correct version through time. It allows the system to continue to operate accurately and optimally. In the context of health, blockchain can assure the accuracy and integrity of health data by creating both a transparent and an immutable ledger of data transactions.

11.4.3 Cybersecurity

11.4.3.1 Threats and Vulnerabilities

With the healthcare industry going digital, it is also the most common attack case in point. Ransomware, phishing, and data breaches of the like are serious cyber-threats that healthcare organizations face. This can put patient care at risk, breach patient privacy, and cause financial loss.

Ransomware recently surpassed HIPAA violations as the number one cause of healthcare data breaches troubling reality for a trade that can access incredibly sensitive information. You can even imagine that these attacks could shut down the hospital, and get all your physicians called out, causing a backup in patient care that could lead to a patient who is waiting that likely could have a life-threatening situation. The threat of phishing attacks, in which attackers exploit an employee to steal sensitive information or click on a malicious link, is common as well. These attacks usually pave the way for more exploits like dropping malware or credential stealing.

Several factors make healthcare organizations especially susceptible to cyber-attacks. One, the complexity of systems in healthcare is vast with a plethora of devices and platforms jostling with each other for real estate and creating a fairly sizable attack surface. Two, most healthcare organizations have been relying on outdated software and systems that do not come with updated security features. Additionally, the sector is heavily reliant on third-party vendors and partners which opens the door to further threats as these vendors may not adhere to the same security practices.

11.5 BEST PRACTICES FOR SECURING HEALTHTECH SOLUTIONS

HealthTech must work equally to brick-and-mortar healthcare to ensure its solutions are protected from cyber-threats by applying comprehensive cybersecurity best practices as health organizations do normally. Such practices include the use of access control including multi-factor authentication and clear role-based access, ensuring that only specific individuals can access the pertinent information. For instance, by default, access controls prevent unauthorized access to systems and data, thereby decreasing the likelihood of insider threats and external attacks.

HealthTech solutions advise anyone who has been a victim of ransomware in the past to vigilantly install updates to software and systems when they appear, as most of the ransomware attacks are due to exploits of new vulnerabilities. Most cyber-attacks leverage well-known weaknesses in obsolete software, so system updates must be done on time to preserve security [9]. A good practice for healthcare organizations is to have a patch management process in place to update all systems and applications to the most current level with the latest security patches applied.

Encryption: One more elementary building block of robust security is the encryption of data during its motion or at rest. Encrypting data ensures that even if data is intercepted and stolen, it still unreadable and unusable to any unauthorized parties. All sensitive data, containing patient records, financial information, and communications, should be encrypted.

Regular security assessments and penetration tests help to find and eliminate system and network vulnerabilities. These are essentially a recon technique to identify vulnerabilities and provide a best-efforts approach to remediation. These assessments should be conducted with the guidance of cybersecurity experts and security levels must be provided as per the requirements of healthcare organizations.

Lastly, reinforcing a culture of cybersecurity awareness among your employees is vital to achieving comprehensive security. Traditional programs to train and educate employees can include how to identify and defend against different cyber-threats like phishing attacks and social engineering ploys. Foster a security-first mentality – health organizations that start to think security-first rather than security-later suffer from fewer human error risks and overall improved cybersecurity postures.

To sum it up, the challenges posed by technology for the HealthTech sector need more than an AI, ML, and Natural Language Processing (NLP) solution for better interoperability achievements, managing the quantum of big data efficiently, ensuring data authenticity, accuracy, and integrity, and for secure cybersecurity attacks as shown in Figure 11.4. Healthcare organizations that can address these challenges are better equipped to improve both the quality of care and operational efficiency, as well as secure patient data amid the digital revolution.

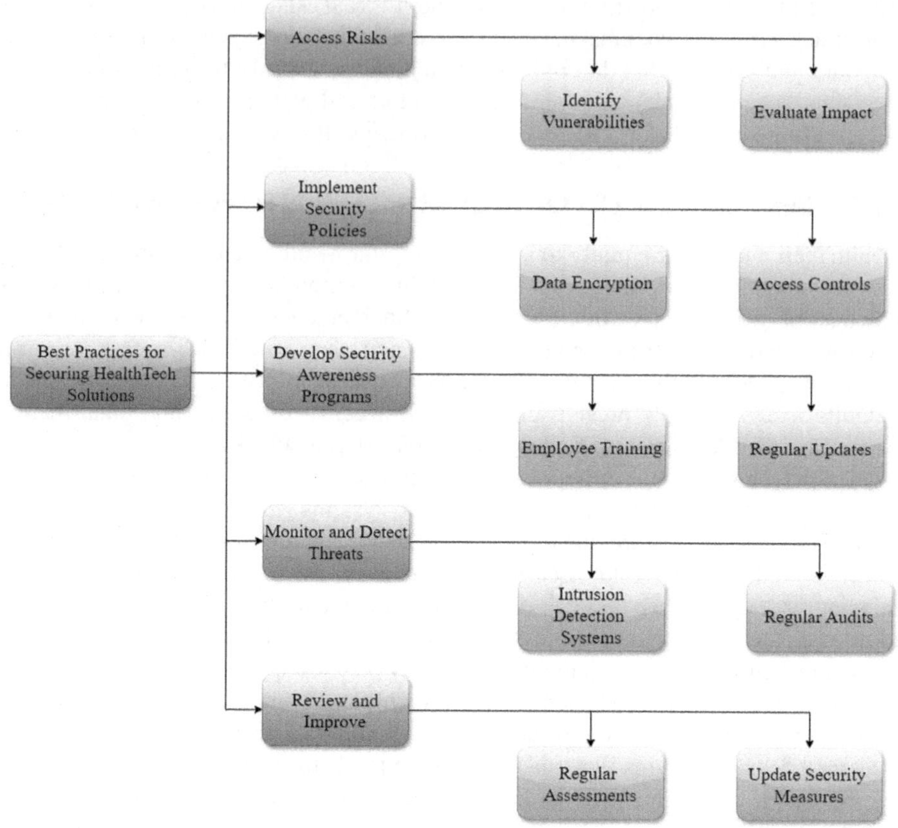

FIGURE 11.4 Securing HealthTech Solutions.

11.6. FINANCIAL AND ECONOMIC BARRIERS IN HEALTHTECH

11.6.1 Funding and Investment

11.6.1.1 Venture Capital and Private Equity Landscape

HealthTech Venture Capital (VC) and Private Equity (PE) Landscape: Dynamic and challenged ecosystem startups in HealthTech are known to rely on VC and PE funding to accelerate growth and scale their innovations in the early stages of their development. HealthTech also attracts long-term investors as the sector generates substantial returns on the proliferation of digital health solutions and the development of technologies such as AI, telemedicine, and wearable health devices. However, funding has a ton of competition. When a startup raises capital, it goes through an intense due diligence process where investors review the startup on anything from business models to technology to market potential and scalability. Furthermore, with the healthcare sector the unique regulatory environment only adds to the complexity; often however insurers and hospitals validate HealthTech features on a whim, but investors are wary of the long timelines and steep costs of bringing HealthTech products to market as a result. At the same time, the "valley of death" is often experienced by startups during their development phases when they need to have enough funding to advance from the developing stage to the commercial scale.

11.6.1.2 Public Funding and Grants

HealthTech innovations require public funding and grant support, especially during the early stages of research and development (R&D). HealthTech is the answer for governments and public institutions worldwide, as they see potential in adopting this new way of delivering diagnosis and treatment faster, more efficiently, and more effectively in treating public health challenges while reducing the cost of medical care while improving patient outcomes. There is significant financial support from initiatives such as the National Institutes of Health (NIH) grants in the United States, the Horizon Europe funding of the European Union, and various national health innovation funds. But it is very competitive to get this fund, and they are difficult to access, requiring to submit detailed proposals describing the impact, feasibility, and innovation of the proposed project. The time-consuming application process coupled with stringent terms and reporting requires patient and time-consuming steps. Also, the bureaucratic way of obtaining public money has allowed it to take time, but for small startups and small businesses looking for liquidity, this time of liquidation of funds is essential.

11.6.2 Cost of Implementation

11.6.2.1 High Initial Costs and Return on Investment Concerns

A major hurdle for many other healthcare organizations is the fact that numerous great HealthTech solutions necessitate large upfront investments. These costs involve the acquisition of new technology, its integration into existing systems, the education of healthcare professionals, as well as the maintenance of said technology over time. For instance, in large healthcare facilities, the implementation of EHR systems can easily cost millions of dollars if you sum up the price of hardware, new software, training, and ongoing maintenance [10]. Such high initial investment leaves the clients with questions regarding ROI. Healthcare organizations will need to balance the long-term benefits of improved patient outcomes, more efficient operations, and fewer hospital readmissions (which can help to reduce costs) with the immediate financial strain this solution may place on their budgets. Showing a tangible ROI that is appealing to stakeholders is a must. Moreover, the uncertainty of technological progress and changing regulations may further complicate the ROI calculation as future costs and benefits arise which are hard to quantify.

11.6.3 Economic Impact

11.6.3.1 Cost–Benefit Analysis of HealthTech Adoption

It is also important that the economic impact of the introduction of HealthTech solutions be evaluated through a detailed cost–benefit analysis. That means, it is a way of reviewing all the costs associated with a project, or product, to determine whether the total amounts should outweigh the total benefits. The direct cost includes all expenses related to technology procurement, deployment, integration, and training. Indirect costs could encompass a disruption in existing workflows, new cybersecurity measures required, and a loss of productivity as the change process takes place. There are huge benefits of patient outcomes improving, operations becoming more efficient, and, of course, hospital readmissions falling to result in cost savings in the long term. Also, it should have some numbers: shorter hospitalizations, fewer mistakes, and better care, as well as patient satisfaction. Impact reports through in-depth cost–benefit analysis facilitate healthcare providers and stakeholders to take informed decisions by elucidating the economic value of HealthTech investments. This is accomplished by extrapolating the savings and benefits into the future, accounting for risk and uncertainty, and justifying that the benefits exceed the costs.

11.6.3.2 Socio-Economic Disparities in Access to Technology

Socio-economic disparities are increasingly becoming a big challenge for equal health adoption. Impoverished populations – including rural and low-income demographics – often encounter obstacles related to restricted access to broadband internet, financial shortcomings, and ineptitude to navigate proficiently through all things digital. Something that would enable HealthTech services like telemedicine, remote monitoring, and digital health platforms to reach them. Telemedicine, for example, is largely dependent on being able to connect to the internet, which rural areas lack. Moreover, significant costs of HealthTech solutions hamstring healthcare providers that serve low-income populations contributing to broader health disparities. To rectify this, it calls for targeted interventions. It can reduce financial barriers through state-subsidized technology programs and support the improvement of digital infrastructure to better access essential services [11]. It is also important to undertake efforts to improve digital literacy among at-risk people as they may not have the ability to use HealthTech tools correctly. Policymakers and stakeholders need to work together to develop holistic strategies that account for these socio-economic gaps and support equal opportunities for accessing health technologies.

11.7 ORGANIZATIONAL AND CULTURAL ROADBLOCKS IN HEALTHTECH

11.7.1 Change Management

11.7.1.1 Resistance to Change within Healthcare Organizations

Resisting changes is something that most healthcare organizations deal with, simply because healthcare is such a conservative industry by nature. Healthcare providers follow long-established protocols and understandably are sometimes slow to shed the old skin of what we do every day. This resistance can stem from any number of psychological and logistical factors. This fear of the unknown is one of the biggest reasons as new technologies can feel overwhelming, or even deceivably complex, mostly for those who are completely unfamiliar with them. Furthermore, professionals worry that these technologies and automated systems may take some jobs away or cheapen their skills.

Resistance also could be magnified by the hierarchical structure seen in various healthcare organizations. Such decisions on new technologies are generally taken by senior management or local IT groups and have excessive reliance on staff who are not directly impacted by day-to-day changes to the traditional methods. A few end up with people who feel left out of the decision-making, resulting in no buy-in with a top-down approach. Also, the breakneck speed of the tech evolution can be daunting for already hard-pressed healthcare providers who are trying to ensure that patient care is of the highest quality.

11.7.1.2 Strategies for Effective Change Management

It requires managing transitions and resistance at numerous levels of the institutional hierarchy – implementation of HT solutions demands effective change management to sync them in healthcare organizations. Executives should utilize an effective communication strategy to start a structured change management plan. This includes describing a clear vision of the change, outlining how the change will be positive for patients and staff, and clearing up any misunderstandings and concerns. Transparency can also improve with frequent updates and open forms where staff can air grievances or queries.

Inclusiveness in its development among all stakeholders helps to create ownership and thereby resistance can be minimized. This can be done by including healthcare workers in the design and implementation of solutions that work for them – as well as recognizing their work. Implementing change management policies and imparting training and education are all part of change management as well [12]. Even staff interactions with technology differ widely and thus need design training programs tailored so that everyone feels confident in interacting with new tools. Some effective methods include hands-on workshops, online tutorials, and simulation-based training.

Another important strategy is to provide ongoing support in the transition period. That may involve setting up helpdesks, providing one-to-one coaching, and creating easy-to-read manuals and FAQs. Change management starts with a leader acting as a role model and demonstrating both a personal commitment to the new tools, along with ongoing encouragement and support. These tactics can help create a nurturing atmosphere for healthcare organizations that promote comfort with change in their successful transition.

11.7.2 Workforce Challenges

11.7.2.1 Training and Skill Development

With the constant evolution of HealthTech, healthcare workers have to continue training and up-skilling. The problem is that traditional medical education is slow to adapt to new technology, and that is why training programs are so essential. The scope of such programs needs to be expansive and all-inclusive, spanning EHRs, telemedicine platforms, AI applications, and more.

Training needs to be equipped for a variety of different professions and necessarily to fit the landscape of the various professional territories within the healthcare system. For example, clinicians may need more extensive training to learn to use AI-driven diagnostic tools, whereas administrative staff may need to become proficient at managing new scheduling software or patient management systems. For these types of experiences, hands-on workshops can be the most effective, as having the opportunity to use the tools in a safe, guided setting helps employees see first-hand how a solution enables their work to be less stressful, more efficient, or otherwise more effective in their work. Online courses and webinars may be helpful sources as well, and they can be a flexible alternative that allows staff to learn when they have time.

The continuous advancements in HealthTech mean that ongoing professional development opportunities are essential. This may require retraining and/or refresher training, and/or advanced training for individuals interested in building on their knowledge. Through investing in extensive training and development programs, healthcare providers can empower their employees to confidently adopt new technologies to improve productivity and quality of patient care.

11.7.2.2 Addressing the Digital Divide among Healthcare Professionals

One of the most pronounced hurdles to the successful embrace of HealthTech is the digital intermediation within healthcare professionals. One example is the digital divide, which can exist along several dimensions, such as access to technology, one's skills and knowledge of digital tools, and a person's willingness to embrace them. One possible complication is that, on one hand, experienced healthcare professionals who have relied on a paper-based care approach for the bulk of their career may struggle to use digital solutions, while, on the other, younger staff may be tech-savvy but less familiar with how tech integrates into healthcare.

Faced with this digital divide, targeted and inclusive measures are needed to address this challenge. In the first place, equal access to technological resources as necessary is necessary. This could include hardware, like laptops or tablets for staff who may not have them, while all facilities should have strong IT systems and secure internet connectivity. Professional development programs must incorporate digital literacy training, to develop foundational and advanced digital skills for all healthcare professionals.

That said, a mentorship program is a solid strategy to bridge the divide. Match less tech-savvy people with tech-savvy individuals so they can learn from one another – peer technology learning. This will not only boost his/her confidence but also develop a team culture in the organization. Focus on a culture of learning and the adaptability to that learning. One major corrective action an organization needs to take is to build a culture of continuous learning and provide resources for employees to learn the new technologies [13]. If healthcare organizations work to bridge the divide, they can operate under the assumption all their staff has the means to access HealthTech tools deliver quality patient care and optimize operations.

11.7.3 Cultural Considerations

11.7.3.1 Varied Acceptance and Trust Levels Across Different Cultures

Acceptance and trust of HealthTech innovations are highly dependent on cultural (behavioral) factors. Cultural differences change the trust they have in technology and the institutions who use it, in historical, social, and economic circumstances. There may be other cases where there is high trust in medical authorities on one end of the spectrum and ready adoption of eHealth technologies on the other. In contrast to this, others may have a history of mistrust about technological interventions, or government action more generally, and therefore have lower levels of acceptance.

These cultural nuances could be the key to the creation of sticky HealthTech solutions. This includes connecting with communities to listen to their needs and experiences. Additionally, the acceptance can be improved by customizing communication strategies according to cultural values and beliefs. In contrast, cultures that stress personal relationships may benefit from highlighting the human dimension of healthcare professionals administering and providing support for the use of new technologies. Clear, culturally appropriate messaging regarding the potential benefits, convenience, and safety of digital certificates will be critical [14]. This could involve communication in local languages, reinforcing messages from trusted community leaders, and making sure that communication materials are widely available and easy to understand.

Trust takes time to build and you need long-term effort and work for people to start trusting you. Working with community leaders and other stakeholders in the planning and implementation of new technologies can improve legitimacy and acceptance. Pilot programs as well as case studies that showcase the results on the ground are a good way to demonstrate some concrete benefits of HealthTech solutions. Accessibility is also key to ensuring technologies are culturally appropriate and equitable for migrant and refugee groups. This entails solving for affordability, health literacy, language, and digital literacy, making these the health technology solutions that are accessible and amenable to every stratum of the population. That said, when HealthTech businesses respect and address cultural differences in their business approaches, they can drive acceptance and trust within these audiences, ultimately driving the wider adoption of innovative healthcare solutions and inspiring those around them to do the same.

11.8 ETHICAL AND SOCIAL CONSIDERATIONS IN HEALTHTECH

11.8.1 Patient Privacy and Consent

For HealthTech, patient privacy consists of the protection of sensitive health information from disclosure, unauthorized access, or use. The collection of healthcare data in digital form has opened another avenue of vulnerability over data security and privacy breaches. HealthTech companies also follow strict regulatory guidelines such as the HIPAA (in the United States) or GDPR (in the EU) to keep patient data safe and compliant. Key capability upload summary file, uberized access, and strengthened compliance encryption, access controls, and frequent audits are all measures that must be put into place to protect a patient's data.

Although compliance is important, the patient needs to trust you. Patients will be much more likely to trust companies that make it transparent how data is collected, stored, and used. Transparency regarding privacy policies, data-sharing practices, and the design of consent forms allows patients to make informed choices about their health data. In addition to this, accessible consent management tools empower patients to handle their privacy preferences and their data.

11.8.2 Informed Consent in the Digital Age

The critical issue of informed consent is at the heart of ethical healthcare practice, ensuring that patients understand that their data is being used and that they are agreeing (or not!) to be treated or participate in research. HealthTech is much more complicated – consent processes need to be adapted to the digital age. Permission slips can include whether the patient's information will be used and stored, what information will be shared, and potential risks or benefits.

Modes of interactive consent, including videos and decision aids, facilitate patient comprehension and engagement. They guide patients through complicated information in a manageable way, which supports the decision-making process [15]. In addition, digital platforms should enable continuous consent management: patients must be able to update their consent or withdraw it at any time as circumstances change.

For consent processes to be equitable, the issue of digital literacy disparities must be addressed. Some patients may lack the technical competence required to navigate digital interfaces or to appreciatively comprehend complex data use policies. Hence, consent processes should be designed to be universal and easy to understand by all categories of patients and should be implemented by healthcare providers as well as HealthTech developers.

11.8.3 Addressing Health Disparities

HealthTech can decrease healthcare disparities over the globe by increasing people's access to care and services, but it may also serve to worsen inequities if it is not implemented carefully. To combat health disparities, we need to be more proactive to ensure digital health is available and equitable for all and imposes a minimum burden on any group.

Access to technology and internet connectivity is still a major hurdle – especially in underserved communities – as the digital divide remains a stark reality. This is where HealthTech can help, by providing health solutions that are created with these populations in mind and using mobile health technology and community health partners to reach healthcare to them.

Cultural and language considerations are paramount as well. For instance, HealthTech solutions need to be culturally aware and offer translation services in different languages to offer support to diverse patient populations [16]. From involving community stakeholders in the development process to implementing inclusive design practices, there are several critical steps to support the development of technologies that better reflect the unique lifestyles and preferences of all of its users.

There is a need to monitor and evaluate whether HealthTech has any effect on health disparities. Metrics must be used for the level of access, usability, and health outcomes among different population groups. This means that HealthTech has the potential to enable healthcare to become more inclusive and accessible when design and deployment strategies are also prioritizing equity.

11.8.4 Ensuring Inclusive Design and Deployment of HealthTech

Inclusive design principles focus on designing products and services that can be accessed and used by as many people as possible, whatever their age, ability, or background. Within the world of HealthTech, inclusive design is essential to ensuring that digital health access meets the needs of all patients and healthcare providers.

The process of engaging end-users in the development process is called user-centered design approaches. The objective is to keep products user-friendly and responsive to genuine needs. For instance, you can create interfaces that are friendly to different levels of digital literacy and incorporate accessibility features for people with disabilities, which will contribute greatly to the usability of your projects and the adoption of these technologies.

Access metrics belong to monitoring and evaluation of continuous feedback from users via HealthTech facilitate a better understanding of room for improvement and guarantee the development of solutions that adapt to evolving needs. Embracing inclusive design principles and moving toward this type of product design help HealthTech to design more just and effective solutions that promote healthy outcomes for all.

11.8.5 Balancing Technology and Human Touch

HealthTech innovations have revolutionized the way healthcare provision is delivered, introducing new remote diagnostics, monitoring, and remote patient care capabilities. As these technologies get increasingly powerful, the way people approach healthcare is transforming from direct patient-to-professional interaction to a relationship that relies less and less on physical presence and direct human contact.

Ensuring that the human element remains in healthcare is critical to establishing its efficacy and improving the quality of care for patients [17]. While technologies such as telemedicine allow for remote consultations, they practically dehumanize the interaction. Healthcare providers will need to find ways to use technology for clinical activities, all while maintaining communication and empathy with patients.

HealthTech has a place in clinical practice, but proper training and education are essential to ensure it is used safely and in the best interests of patients. Providers should develop skills in both technology and communication, meeting a patient virtually or in person, utilizing that same active listening, empathetic, and shared decision-making approach.

11.9 STRATEGIES FOR OVERCOMING CHALLENGES

11.9.1 Collaborative Approaches

The HealthTech ecosystem operates through collaboration by different stakeholders to solve complex problems. Typically, these collaborations will include healthcare providers, technology developers, regulatory bodies, academics, and patient advocacy groups [18], thereby breaking down barriers, ranging from interoperability challenges and data privacy issues to aligning new technologies in the clinical workflow, that are not so simple to overcome.

Advanced technologies are found frequently too technical for many healthcare providers to create or to afford to be creative beyond some of the same that pork. This will enable them to better access innovative solutions (e.g. telemedicine platforms, remote monitoring devices, AI-powered diagnostic tools) offered through technology firms. These partnerships allow those technologies to be tailored to individual clinical needs and regulatory demands, which in turn boost their uptake and functionality in healthcare.

Academic centers are central to this model, by researching new technology and validating clinical utility in stringent scientific trials. Research is translated to practice in healthcare driven by evidence-based, clinically adept discovery through the collaboration of academia and industry.

Regulatory bodies too see the benefits of such a collaborative approach by learning from technological advancements and their implications on patient safety and data privacy. Partnerships allow for the creation of informed public health policies, keeping the public at the center of innovation.

At a macro level, collaborative approaches engender a culture of innovation and cooperation within the HealthTech ecosystem, thus encouraging the coming together of minds to combine resources, share learnings, and tackle mutual problems that are industrywide.

11.9.2 Public–Private Partnerships

In the healthcare innovation space, the procurement of public services is undertaken in public–private partnerships (PPPs) – strategic alliances between public institutions and private sector entities. PPPs can be vital in eliminating economic obstacles and negotiating complex regulatory systems that hinder the emergence and adoption of HealthTech solutions.

Public health departments and bureaus also partner with the private sector to share costs on R&D and infrastructure support as well as pilot tests. By combining government funding and expertise with the innovation and market-driven discipline of private sector partners, these partnerships substantially hasten the development and deployment of healthcare technologies.

PPPs can also support regulatory harmonization by aligning the interests of the parties in negotiating complex regulatory systems and lobbying for policy reforms in favor of the encouragement of HealthTech innovation [19]. For example, joint proceedings involving regulatory bodies and industry players can simplify and speed up digital health product approval, and take them to market faster, without compromising on product efficacy and safety.

In addition, PPPs facilitate the sharing of knowledge and build capacity in various sectors which create an enabling environment for entrepreneurship and investment in HealthTech. PPPs help to build collaboration between public and private players, thus offering scalable as well as sustainable solutions to healthcare challenges, and mandatory to improve the outcomes of patients.

11.9.3 Industry Consortiums and Alliances

An industry consortium or alliance is a gathering of several organizations in the HealthTech space officially organized to achieve common goals – generally, the task includes defining industry standards, commissioning regulatory changes, and other forms of industry innovation. These consortia unite competitors, startups, incumbents, and industry stakeholders to jointly tackle industry-level problems that cannot be solved by single units alone.

Most industry consortiums can create interoperability standards and guidelines with healthcare actors and technology platforms that make it easy for data to move. One type of consortia, such as HL7 and FHIR, which focus on interoperability standards, develop technical specifications and protocols that allow various HIT systems to communicate with one another.

Lobbying for regulation changes that facilitate HealthTech innovation and protect patient safety and data privacy is another key function of consortiums. Through healthy dialogs with legislators and regulatory bodies, business groups will have some impact on how adaptive regulatory frameworks evolve and how the approval processes should be shortened to digital health solutions.

In addition, consortia offer a path to R&D collaboration, providing members a method to pool resources, learn from one another, and make investments in game-changing technologies, together [20]. Industry consortia stimulate innovation, drive progress, and improve the competitiveness of their constituents in the global HealthTech market by enabling pre-competitive, open innovation in a real-time, collaborative pre-competitive environment.

11.9.4 Innovative Solutions

In the HealthTech space, the introduction of emerging technologies based on AI, blockchain, and IoT can provide new ways to solve longstanding problems. They have the potential to transform healthcare delivery by enhancing care efficiency, accuracy, and patient outcomes, and reduce costs and administrative burden.

Through AI-powered analytics and ML algorithms, the data can be analyzed to find patterns, predict patient outcomes, and improve patient care. For instance, AI-based diagnostics tools can help in making better and more timely clinical decisions for healthcare providers, which will result in better patient care and resource optimization.

Blockchain-Enabled Health Records: Blockchain technology ensures data security and privacy by allowing a decentralized and immutable ledger to store health records, thus ensuring tamper-proof data integrity. Due to the secure and decentralized nature of blockchain transactions, health institutions can use the technology to help protect themselves, their patients, and the data they share against breaches and unauthorized access with secure sharing of data among authorized participants.

Continuous real-time data capture and monitoring outside of traditional healthcare settings can be facilitated using connected IoT devices such as health monitoring wearables and remote patient monitoring systems [10, 11]. They empower patients to engage in managing their healthcare, as well as making it possible for healthcare providers to deliver individualized, proactive care interventions.

Integrating these disruptive technologies into legacy healthcare systems will help institutions to break down technological silos and improve interconnect ability of HealthTech innovations [21]. In addition, these capabilities empower healthcare organizations to use data-driven insights and predictive analytics to streamline clinical workflows, better population health outcomes, and foster digital transformation in delivering care.

11.9.5 Adaptive Regulatory and Business Models

To sail through the HealthTech sector, the players will need adaptive regulatory and business models. However, traditional frameworks are rarely designed to handle the rapid pace of technological advancement; they find it to be inhibiting to innovate and difficult to approve new healthcare technologies to enter the market.

Adaptive regulatory approaches (e.g. regulatory sandboxes, fast-track approvals) develop a safe space for testing and validating innovative solutions while ensuring patient safety and data privacy. A regulatory sandbox allows startups and innovators working in the digital health and wellness space to work with regulators in real-world scenarios to allow iterative testing and improvement of their digital health solutions before a complete roll-out to the market.

Equally important to fostering HealthTech innovation and scalability is flexible business models. By using subscription-based services, pay-for-performance arrangements, and outcome-based reimbursement models, financial incentives can be more closely aligned with healthcare outcomes, motivating stakeholders to invest in innovative solutions that deliver clear clinical and economic advantages.

In addition, adaptive regulatory and business models support market entry by startups and small-to-medium enterprises (SMEs) by reducing the traditional onerous regulatory requirements, lowering barriers to entry, and creating a competitive market for healthcare innovation. This will be important for supporting the growth of entrepreneurship, investment, and continuous innovation in the HealthTech sector by allowing for regulatory agility and business model flexibility.

11.9.6 Policy Recommendations

Policy recommendations for promoting an enabling environment.

A supportive policy ecosystem by policymakers is critical to HealthTech innovation. It enables such an environment through relevant policy intervention for collaboration, investment, and regulatory certainty.

Key policy recommendations:

1. **Mainstreaming Regulation:** Adopting an establishing-in and going-in framework for regulation to design inclusively and engage innovative healthcare technologies to ensure rapid market access.
2. **Supporting Interoperability Standards:** Defining interoperability standards and data exchange protocols of medical information to enable digital health products to work with healthcare systems and foster better coordination of care.
3. **Incentivizing Investments in Digital Health:** Providing tax rebates, grants, and funding for R&D investments for digital health technologies with a special focus on startups and SMEs.
4. **Establishing Regulatory Sandboxes and Pilot Programs to Test and Validate in a Controlled Environment:** Sandboxes and pilot programs will allow innovators to test new digital health products under scenarios that are approved and controlled by regulators (e.g., states, and federal agencies), and allow innovation to move forward while also protecting patients.
5. **Support Public-Private Partnerships:** The incentives will be directed from the public agency to the private sector online businesses, and educational institutes on the funding programs and incentives, aimed at the PPPs with emphasis on healthcare innovation.
6. **Dealing with Data Privacy:** We need to create a way to protect patient data, and in a fast-growing system like digital health, we need to set a standard of security if we want to gain trust in this technology.

Adoption of these policy recommendations will establish a supportive environment that drives entrepreneurship, sparks innovation, and enhances healthcare delivery for people across the globe. The collaborative effort of stakeholders and adaptations to regulatory as well as business innovations will be vital to address barriers to the transformative power of HealthTech on the global healthcare delivery landscape.

11.10 CONCLUSION

The chapter deems HealthTech transformation promising but challenging, offering improved patient care, operational efficiency, and personalized health monitoring. Challenges include data security, regulatory compliance, financial constraints, and systems interoperability. Moreover, the implementation of new technologies is usually challenged by high costs and necessary workforce training. However, the promise and opportunity for HealthTech to disrupt healthcare delivery are so evident. Neither of these predictions is inevitable, but the route that HealthTech will take is cooperation from healthcare providers, policymakers, and developers to navigate these issues and ensure any implementation is secure, ethical, and universal.

REFERENCES

[1] K. Honda, K. Takakura, and Y. Otsubo, "Smart Gateway for Healthcare Networks Based on Beam Steering Technology," *Sensors*, vol. 23, no. 6, p. 2959, 2023, doi: 10.3390/s23062959.

[2] H. Herman, S. S. Grobbelaar, and C. Pistorius, "The design and development of technology platforms in a developing country healthcare context from an ecosystem perspective," *BMC Medical Informatics and Decision Making*, vol. 20, no. 1, pp. 1–24, 2020, doi: 10.1186/s12911-020-1028-0.

[3] S. Hermes, T. Riasanow, E. K. Clemons, M. Böhm, and H. Krcmar, "The digital transformation of the healthcare industry: Exploring the rise of emerging platform ecosystems and their influence on the role of patients," *Business Research*, vol. 13, no. 3, pp. 1033–1069, 2020, doi: 10.1007/s40685-020-00125-x.

[4] R. Sebastiani and A. Anzivino, "The long and winding road of eHealth. The service ecosystem perspective," *Journal of Business and Industrial Marketing*, vol. 37, no. 10, pp. 2036–2049, 2022, doi: 10.1108/JBIM-02-2021-0107.

[5] I. Y. Chen, E. Pierson, S. Rose, S. Joshi, K. Ferryman, and M. Ghassemi, "Ethical machine learning in healthcare," *Annual Review of Biomedical Data Science*, vol. 4, pp. 123–144, 2021.

[6] Y. Park, S. Park, and M. Lee, "Digital Health Care Industry Ecosystem: Network Analysis," *Journal of Medical Internet Research*, vol. 24, no. 8, p. e37622, 2022, doi: 10.2196/37622.

[7] P. Moss, R. O'callaghan, A. Fisher, C. Kennedy, and F. Tracey, "Navigate your health: A case study of organisational learnings from an integrated care pilot for children and young people in care," *International Journal of Integrated Care*, vol. 21, no. 3, pp. 1–11, 2021, doi: 10.5334/ijic.5659.

[8] Y. Zurynski, et al., "Engagement with healthcare providers and healthcare system navigation among Australians with chronic conditions: A descriptive survey study," *BMJ Open*, vol. 12, no. 12, pp. 1–9, 2022, doi: 10.1136/bmjopen-2022-061623.

[9] C. Saunders, D. Currie, S. Virani, and J. De Grood, "Navigating the systemic conditions of a digital health ecosystem in Alberta, Canada: Embedded case study," *JMIR Formative Research*, vol. 6, no. 12, 2022, doi: 10.2196/36265.

[10] H. J. Schünemann, *et al.*, "The ecosystem of health decision making: From fragmentation to synergy," *Lancet Public Health*, vol. 7, no. 4, pp. e378–e390, 2022, doi: 10.1016/S2468-2667(22)00057-3.

[11] T. Manyazewal, *et al.*, "Mapping digital health ecosystems in Africa in the context of endemic infectious and non-communicable diseases," *NPJ Digital Medicine*, vol. 6, no. 1, 2023, doi: 10.1038/s41746-023-00839-2.

[12] K. Teggart, *et al.*, "Effectiveness of system navigation programs linking primary care with community-based health and social services: A systematic review," *BMC Health Services Research*, vol. 23, no. 1, pp. 1–35, 2023, doi: 10.1186/s12913-023-09424-5.

[13] V. Yellapa, *et al.*, "How patients navigate the diagnostic ecosystem in a fragmented health system: A qualitative study from India," *Global Health Action*, vol. 10, no. 1, p. 1350452, 2017, doi: 10.1080/16549716.2017.1350452.

[14] K. Cresswell, *et al.*, "Interorganizational knowledge sharing to establish digital health learning ecosystems: Qualitative evaluation of a national digital health transformation program in England," *Journal of Medical Internet Research*, vol. 23, no. 8, p. e23372, 2021, doi: 10.2196/23372.

[15] N. González-Gálvez, *et al.*, "Impact and Learner Experience of a Technology Ecosystem as an Approach to Healthy Lifestyles: Erasmus+ SUGAPAS Project," *Sustainability (Switzerland)*, vol. 14, no. 23, pp. 1–10, 2022, doi: 10.3390/su142315849.

[16] P. Ruotsalainen and B. Blobel, "Transformed health ecosystems – challenges for security, privacy, and trust," *Frontiers in Medicine*, vol. 9, no. 8, pp. 1–10, 2022, doi: 10.3389/fmed.2022.827253.

[17] S. N. Weimar, R. S. Martjan, and O. Terzidis, "Conceptualizing the landscape of digital health entrepreneurship: A systematic review and research agenda," *Management Review Quarterly*, 2024. doi: 10.1007/s11301-024-00417-0.

[18] C. Gjellebæk, A. Svensson, C. Bjørkquist, N. Fladeby, and K. Grundén, "Management challenges for future digitalization of healthcare services," *Futures*, vol. 124, no. November, p. 102636, 2020, doi: 10.1016/j.futures.2020.102636.

[19] G. E. Iyawa, M. Herselman, and A. Botha, "Digital health innovation ecosystems: From systematic literature review to conceptual framework," *Procedia Computer Science*, vol. 100, pp. 244–252, 2016, doi: 10.1016/j.procs.2016.09.149.

[20] B. Van Winkle, Y. Solad, N. Vaswani, and B. I. Rosner, "Navigating the digital health ecosystem to bridge the gap from innovation to transformation: A NODE. Health perspective on digital evidence," *Digital Biomarkers*, vol. 3, no. 2, pp. 83–91, 2019, doi: 10.1159/000500194.

[21] A. I. Stoumpos, F. Kitsios, and M. A. Talias, "Digital transformation in healthcare: Technology acceptance and its applications," *International Journal of Environmental Research and Public Health*, vol. 20, no. 4, p. 3407, 2023, doi: 10.3390/ijerph20043407.

12 Real-World Examples of HealthTech Empowerment

Sridhar Raj S., Ashok R., and Robert Cep

12.1 INTRODUCTION

The healthcare sector is experiencing a substantial transformation due to emerging technologies. CB Insights' recent report reveals that HealthTech startups worldwide secured a staggering $31.6 billion in funding through 1,538 deals in 2022, setting a new annual record. Although the HealthTech market experienced a decline in 2022 and early 2023 due to macroeconomic conditions affecting the United States, venture capital funding for the sector dropped approximately 30% compared to 2021, decreasing from $39.3 billion to $27.5 billion. Nonetheless, investments in 2022 remained approximately 30% higher than in 2020 and more than doubled compared to 2019. The current increase in interest and investment indicates that traditional healthcare delivery models are insufficient to address the changing needs of our global population. Given the pandemic's emphasis on these difficulties and the rapid implementation of digital health technologies, this sector is poised to redefine healthcare features.

Precedence research predicts that the worldwide healthcare information systems market would increase from $309.2 billion in 2023 to an anticipated $528.5 billion in 2030. Additionally, the global healthcare services market is growing, with its value increasing from $7.4 trillion in 2022 to $7.9 trillion in 2023. Projections indicate that the value will rise to $9.8 trillion by 2027, and by 2030, home healthcare alone is expected to reach $666.9 billion [1]. Every aspect of healthcare, including laboratories, dental care, home healthcare, mental health, and hospitals, is experiencing growth. Figure 12.1 discusses the market size of the healthcare system.

Information technology in the healthcare sector encompasses not only enhancing patient care but also transforming the entire healthcare system [2]. Technological advancements, such as hospital information systems, pharmaceutical track-and-trace systems, big data analytics (BDA), and artificial intelligence applications [3], are improving the efficiency, cost-effectiveness, and accessibility of healthcare. With the help of these innovations, healthcare providers can assess patients' needs, make intelligent choices, and reduce the occurrence of medical mistakes. Personal health records (PHR), Central e-Prescription, and DrugXafe are practical implementations of the pharmaceutical track-and-trace system. The incredible power of technology to

DOI: 10.1201/9781003516163-12

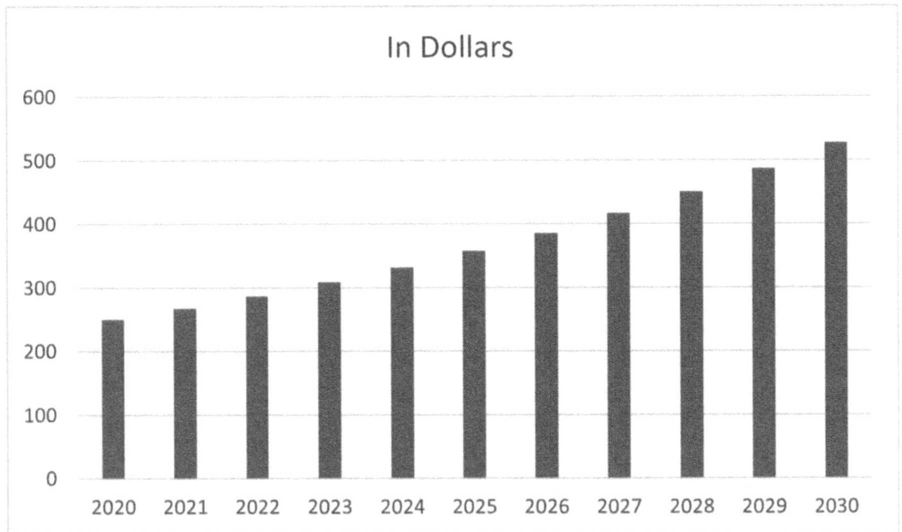

FIGURE 12.1 Market Size of Healthcare Information System .

improve healthcare delivery and quality is the main motivator here, with the ultimate goal of making healthcare more accessible in the future, tailored to individual needs, and highly efficient. The use of information technology (IT) in healthcare is a significant and impactful force that is transforming management and healthcare settings from the ground up.

HealthTech uses technology to address the intricate problems that the healthcare industry faces. With benefits like telemedicine, electronic health records (EHRs), and remote patient monitoring, it makes it easier to integrate digital solutions into conventional healthcare systems [4]. One day, these technological advancements might make healthcare delivery more efficient, saving costs and improving patient happiness. The continuous advancement of health technology is expected to primarily impact medical devices by introducing novel solutions that will ultimately improve overall healthcare outcomes, improve patient care, and increase diagnostic accuracy [5]. A significant benefit of IT in healthcare is that it enhances patient care by offering a comprehensive.

12.2 TELEMEDICINE AND REMOTE PATIENT MONITORING

Telemedicine employs video conferencing and home health checks to give online medical visits and care. Patients can get health advice, detect ailments, and receive medical care without the need to go anywhere else. Medication safety is the primary goal of DrugXafe, which fights counterfeit pharmaceuticals. Patients' health is jeopardized when they take counterfeit pharmaceuticals, which can have devastating consequences on the body and even cause death in rare cases. DrugXafe eliminates this problem by employing cutting-edge 2D Data Matrix technology to track medications during their whole distribution cycle.

As a result, customers are guaranteed to receive safe and authentic medications, which strengthen trust in the drug manufacturing industry. DrugXafe's capacity to thwart fraudulent payments and illegal transactions is a significant advantage.

This incident exemplifies the effective reinforcement and utilization of authority in such circumstances. The report presents concerning data, indicating that approximately 72,000 to 169,000 children perish each year from pneumonia as a result of counterfeit medications. Similarly, an estimated 116,000 children die annually from counterfeit anti-malarial medications. Immediate and decisive action is necessary to protect health and save lives due to the devastating consequences.

Because of its user-friendly design, DrugXafe is useful for patients, healthcare providers, and government organizations. With its reliable features, scalability, and compliance with international standards, it is an excellent choice. Through the DrugXafe mobile app, users have access to up-to-date information on medication prices, can verify their medical records, and can assist in improving patient safety. This app is indispensable for effectively managing healthcare and public health. The distinctive characteristics of **Telemedicine and Remote Patient Monitoring** are listed below.

- **Remote consultations:** Patients can engage with their doctors via video conferencing, avoiding the necessity for face-to-face appointments, their valuable time, and the cost of traveling.
- **Accessibility and convenience:** Telemedicine overcomes geographical limitations, enhancing the accessibility of healthcare services to remote or underserved regions.
- **Improved patient outcomes:** Prompt remote consultations can result in timely identification, improved control of persistent ailments, and decreased hospital admissions.

12.3 ARTIFICIAL INTELLIGENCE AND MACHINE LEARNING IN HEALTHCARE

Software developers will utilize AI and machine learning (ML) algorithms to examine extensive quantities of health data, assisting in the identification of medical conditions, planning treatment strategies, and forecasting patient results. These technologies will enable personalized and data-driven healthcare approaches. AI and ML are crucial technologies that have the power to bring about significant changes in various fields, especially in healthcare [6].

Figure 12.2 illustrates significant developments in ML and AI that have recently improved patient care and the precision of disease diagnosis. AI systems that rely on lifestyle, medical, and genetic data can pinpoint individual risk factors. The Lancet digi-health demonstrated how ML can reliably predict when sepsis will manifest in hospitalized patients. By starting treatments quickly, our forecasting technique contributes to a 24% decrease in death rates.

Research demonstrates the efficacy of AI-driven predictive analytics in detecting outbreaks of the disease and developing focused plans to reduce risks to public health.

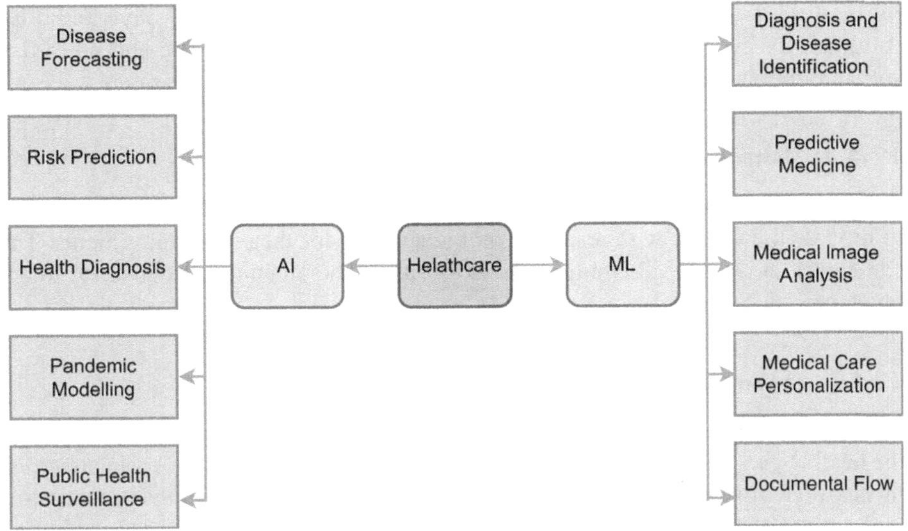

FIGURE 12.2 Healthcare Applications of Machine Learning and Artificial Intelligence.

To illustrate this, Fittkau and colleagues used machine learning (ML) techniques to analyze data and predict outcomes accurately [7].

12.4 WEARABLE MEDICAL DEVICES

Nowadays, people can track their vitals and health in real time with wearable medical devices, which are essentially sensor-based gadgets.

12.4.1 Blood Pressure Monitors

The blood pressure monitor is positioned on either the right or left arm and precisely delivers the user's blood pressure measurement directly to their mobile device. The home blood pressure monitor can be linked to a smartphone to save blood pressure and pulse information.

12.4.2 Glucose Meters

Diabetic glucose monitoring utilizes a phone sensor to measure the readings obtained from the device placed on the upper arm. It reduces the necessity for patients to puncture their fingers.

12.4.3 Electrocardiogram Monitors and Fitness Trackers

This smartwatch is renowned for its exceptional accuracy and user-friendly interface, making it one of the most precise and effortless fitness trackers on the market. This streamlined and condensed design precisely tracks various metrics, including heart rate and steps, and boasts a battery life that can endure for up to 7 days. Fitbit has continuously evolved its technology and now boasts highly precise and up-to-date software for accurately monitoring and storing your health and fitness data.

12.4.4 Integrated Activewear

Activewear utilizes subtle vibrations generated by sensors embedded in the garments to provide the wearer with feedback on the accuracy of their yoga movements. This can contribute to overall equilibrium and result in the attainment of superior fitness objectives.

12.4.5 Smart Bandages

The smart bandage, which combines stimulation and sensing capabilities, accelerates the healing process while also monitoring the progress of the wound. A thin electronic layer with temperature sensors is integrated into the bandage, allowing for continuous monitoring of the wound's status. If deemed essential, they can initiate additional electrical stimulation to expedite the process of tissue closure. Before entering mass production, the device must address cost and data storage challenges. Nevertheless, it has the potential to provide substantial assistance to individuals with compromised immune systems and conditions such as diabetes, who frequently experience delayed wound healing.

Researchers in the United States have developed a bandage equipped with sensors to monitor the process of wound healing. According to the Stanford University team, it accelerates wound healing, improves blood circulation to damaged tissue, and reduces the formation of scars, leading to faster skin recovery.

The distinctive characteristics of **Wearable Medical Devices** are listed below.

- Wearables offer users practical suggestions and notifications derived from gathered data.
- Healthcare providers can monitor patients' health conditions from a distance and take action when needed.

12.5 ELECTRONIC HEALTH RECORDS AND HEALTH INFORMATION SYSTEMS

Leaders may access a wide range of information on their tablets or smartphones, which generate reports automatically. Based on these reports, decisions are made about expanding testing capacity, dividing patients, and monitoring adherence to screening guidelines. UPHO (Urban Public Health Observatory) is established with the use of EHRs [8] to analyze and monitor COVID-19 data, as described in detail by Brakefield and colleagues [9, 10]. EHR data exchange has been proposed by numerous additional researchers to promote collaborative studies or public health initiatives. As a result, COVID-19 patient data is often contained in EHRs and Health Information Systems [11].

Memora Health is a complex care delivery platform that can empower care teams to better monitor and support patients by automating clinical and administrative workflows. Memora Health's platform integrates with electronic health records, embeds into existing workflows, and offers tools such as remote patient monitoring, scheduling, virtual care, and outcomes management, to help enhance the patient and clinician experience. The platform uses natural language processing to automate follow-up communication with enrolled patients and categorize care management tasks. The intelligent, scalable platform enables clinicians to focus on serving patients throughout the entire care journey in areas including cancer, surgical, gastrointestinal, chronic, maternal, population health, and more. It can reduce clinician burnout by reducing repetitive, manual administrative tasks and decreasing the number of patient portal messages that need to be answered. According to Memora Health, the platform has diminished inbox messages by 40.5% Furthermore, it has reduced emergency department visits, increased patient education and screening rates, and improved medication adherence [5].

12.6 MOBILE HEALTH APPS

EHRs are digital representations of storing the patient's medical records. Laboratories store patient data which includes test findings, diagnoses, treatments, and medical records. San Diego Health used analytics and reporting tools based on EHRs, to address the challenges posed by COVID-19 [12]. With the help of data collection, the system aids in patient segregation, screening adherence, and test capacity development. In their analysis of COVID-19 data and surveillance using EHRs, Brakefield et al. [9, 10] highlighted the role of the Urban Public Health Observatory [13] in monitoring and addressing public health challenges effectively.

With the help of healthcare services through mobile phones, it promotes healthy lifestyle choices. When patients and doctors make decisions together, it gives a fruitful result. Patient–provider communication, better information sharing, and more seamless healthcare delivery is the PHR [14]. The ability of the PHR to give patients full control and visibility into their health records is a major benefit [15].

The distinctive characteristics of **Mobile Health Apps** are listed below.

- Mobile health applications and wearable devices allow individuals to monitor essential signs, physical activity, and sleep patterns, as well as control chronic illnesses.
- Mobile applications offer health information, preventative measures, and medication adherence reminders.
- Healthcare professionals can keep an eye on the health of their patients remotely and step in when necessary.
- EHRs include medical standards and alerts, helping medical staff make choices for care that are backed by solid proof.

12.7 ROBOTICS AND AUTOMATION IN HEALTHCARE

Healthcare robots are built to perform various activities within medical settings. They are present in hospitals, medical clinics, and ambulances. They encompass a variety of robotic tools that are crucial in aiding surgeons during surgeries, as well as autonomous surgical systems that are capable of performing entire procedures independently. Worldwide, a significant quantity of robot-assisted minimally invasive surgeries was conducted in 2007.

Medical robots are specifically engineered to enhance the efficiency, speed, and precision of medical procedures, including applications in surgical procedures, such as excising tumors, performing needle biopsies, and conducting endoscopic operations. Medical robots are capable of conducting routine tests that human doctors may find monotonous or challenging to accomplish. Some examples of medical tests are blood cell analysis, eye exams, and mammograms.

The da Vinci Surgical System is a medical robot. By creating tiny openings in the patient's body, surgeons can perform invasive surgery with the help of the robotic system. Surgeons manipulate and operate the gadget using the remote and control the robot arms. The main and the secondary arms are used to hold and control the surgical tools, and to control the movement of lights and cameras. In addition to lowering costs and increasing recovery time for patients, these kinds of medical robots limit invasive surgery and bleeding.

12.8 GENOMICS AND PERSONALIZED MEDICINE

The examination of a genetic composition to develop an individualized medical treatment plan is known as genomics or precision medicine. Healthcare planning should take into account each person's characteristics, which is the fundamental concept of IT healthcare development. Precision and patient-specific care are ensured through the use of genetic data and large datasets. Genomics is the scientific study of human genetics with the goal of identifying disease-related genetic markers. By utilizing this data, doctors can tailor treatment regimens to fit each patient's DNA, reducing the likelihood of side effects while maximizing the chances of success. Genomic technology makes it possible to diagnose diseases accurately, to tailor treatment plans, and to take preventative measures.

12.9 ENHANCING PRESCRIPTION MANAGEMENT AND ENSURING PATIENT SAFETY: CENTRALIZED ELECTRONIC PRESCRIPTION SYSTEM

This system greatly enhances prescription handling and distribution within the healthcare system, which leads to better patient care and safety. Thus, it results in lower costs, reduces prescription errors, and reduces the risk of negative drug side effects. To ensure its effectiveness, the system must maintain connections with medical professionals and pharmacies across the country. This connection ensures a seamless, continuous flow that makes sure drugs are provided exactly when needed. Additionally, the system helps doctors create more successful treatment strategies by offering in-depth and up-to-date details on drugs, along with alerts for guidance in medical decisions. The main feature of Central e-Prescription is its sophisticated integration with an extensive drug database.

12.10 BLOCKCHAIN TECHNOLOGY IN HEALTHCARE

Blockchain technology is becoming an innovator in the field of healthcare, with genuine applications already having a significant impact. These applications are revolutionizing how healthcare organizations handle patient data, clinical trials, pharmaceutical supply chains, telemedicine, and health data exchange. This will examine the five primary practical applications of blockchain technology in healthcare organizations, supported by specific illustrations.

12.10.1 Enhanced Patient Data Management

BurstIQ is leading the way in utilizing blockchain technology to transform the management of patient data. It offers a highly secure and decentralized setting for the storage, sharing, and management of confidential health data. This encompasses patients' medical records, social security numbers, and banking information.

LifeGraph is an advanced digital platform that utilizes a Web3-ready blockchain to revolutionize the management of sensitive data. It provides businesses with reliable, secure, and data-driven ecosystems. LifeGraph provides businesses with a streamlined operation, facilitates compliance, and enables hyper-personalization. LifeGraph has the future to transform data management and utilization across a wide range of industries, including digital health. This transformation could offer advantages to both businesses and individuals. By integrating advanced technologies like blockchain into healthcare networks, benefits such as enhanced security, an immutable feature, and seamless integration are achieved.

12.10.2 Optimizing Clinical Trial Records

Clinical trial records are being protected and managed by Guard time with the help of BC technology. In its development, the company plays a critical role in solving real-world business problems, and it offers a comprehensive and adaptable solution. Medical systems are embracing BC technology to improve data accuracy and create a system of shared agreements. These results in clinical trials are genuine and unaltered [16, 17].

12.10.3 Efficient Pharmaceutical Supply Chain Management

Chronicled uses BC technology to manage the pharmaceutical supply chain and combat fake drugs. MediLedger is a new cutting-edge technology that simplifies pharmaceutical life sciences transactions. MediLedger hopes to recover $4 billion in lost revenue through industry-wide agreements and streamlined settlements. This technology allows third-party data for eligibility verification and party connections to improve transaction accuracy. Automating tedious tasks simplifies data collection and transfer, and this promotes business ideas to be adopted by many firms. BC technology records every drug distribution step to ensure medication safety and integrity. It detects and eliminates fakes and also so tracks these products in real time, improving supply chain management. This function allows medications to be closely monitored from manufacture to delivery, ensuring that all parties have access to current pharmaceuticals.

12.10.4 Empowering Telemedicine and Remote Monitoring

With the help of AI and BC technology, the Robomed Network changed the way for telemedicine and remote monitoring. Internet of Things (IoT) device connection is possible because the integrated systems have greater levels of security. Because of these changes, sending data over telemedicine can now be done with full confidence, as it is safer than ever. With these features working together, doctors can use smart, safe IoT objects to keep an eye on their patients.

12.10.5 Interoperable Health Data Exchange

To simplify the transfer of patient records, Avaneer Health has created a BC-based, transparent information recording system. The Avaneer Health platform is a complete answer for healthcare organizations looking to update their application development processes. This platform offers a variety of services and tools to help developers save time.

12.11 VIRTUAL REALITY (VR) AND AUGMENTED REALITY (AR)

Healthcare professionals are finding new ways to teach and prepare students without cadavers or live patients. Augmented reality (AR), virtual reality (VR), and mixed reality (XR) train nurses, doctors, and surgeons for real-world procedures. The healthcare metaverse includes new technologies: AR superimposes virtual images in the real world using digital elements. VR medical training is a VR-exclusive experience. Virtual headsets and controllers provide haptic feedback to healthcare students. XR incorporates all immersive learning methods, including AR and VR. The global VR and AR market is expanding as healthcare applications become more prevalent. The technology can be applied to complex surgeries, pain management, and mental health issues.

12.11.1 Augmented Reality for 3D Body Mapping

There is an inherent risk in any surgical operation. A lack of unique perspectives on patients' internal organs is a common cause of problems. X-rays and magnetic resonance imaging (MRI) assist doctors in planning their operations, but surgery reveals clear illustrations. Occasionally, this can result in surgical errors that impede the recuperation process and potentially result in fatalities for patients. Healthcare facilities are confronted with legal disputes, fines, and damage to their reputation.

To prevent such a situation, technology startups develop AR tools that generate virtual 3D representations of patients along with anatomical maps. Initially, the solution examines MRI scans. They can analyze even the tiniest 3D anatomical segments like bones, arteries, and veins. In addition, they can detect tumors, areas of inflammation, and other sites that require medical intervention. These instruments facilitate precise surgical procedures and enhance physicians' ability to make informed judgments.

Iowa Spencer Hospital aimed to enhance the safety of medical procedures and improve the precision of surgery and diagnostics. To accomplish this, they implemented an AR solution in their routine treatment activities. The AR tool utilizes simultaneous localization and mapping (SLAM) technology. Healthcare providers can see inside the body by simply pointing their smartphones at a specific area of the patient. They can generate a digital model of the body that includes a thorough examination of its arteries and any existing or absent tumors.

These advanced scans lead to precise medical treatment. These innovations increased biopsy success rates by 50% and aneurysm surgeries were 30% more accurate. These technologies allow healthcare professionals to perform procedures more carefully by offering clear and detailed body maps. Surgeons benefit substantially from 3D anatomy, as it allows them to visualize the inside of the frame in a huge element, allowing diagnosis and planning of surgery.

12.11.2 Augmented Reality for Maintenance in Medical Labs

Modern clinical laboratories are equipped with cellular counts, new microscopes, and other necessary tools. However, laboratory equipment is susceptible to malfunction, just like any other advanced technical gadget. Due to its inherent issues, the intricacy of this technology often requires outside specialists to be involved to restore it. This could be a lengthy process that takes days or even weeks to finish, which would be quite expensive.

Hospitals encounter a variety of difficulties as a result of unplanned disruptions in the operation of laboratory equipment. For doctors to correctly identify patients and create treatment regimens that work, test results are essential. Engineers can use AR helmets and eyewear to communicate in real time via video chat with professionals who are located remotely.

Professionals assist an engineer in navigating the repair procedure, offering precise instructions that ensure a seamless and efficient process. Additionally, the technology can assist technicians in independently repairing the equipment by providing them with AR instructions. Technicians follow AR instructions to directly target malfunctioning pieces of equipment, prompting instant display of 3D visual representations of its internal structure. Then, it overlays straightforward and precise maintenance and repair manuals, providing step-by-step instructions. These tools enable technicians to troubleshoot equipment even in the absence of remote assistance. Consequently, their technicians who work at the physical location are now capable of independently resolving nearly any malfunction within a few hours, rather than taking several days. The advantages are

- Minimizing the time and expenses associated with maintenance
- Closing the knowledge and experience disparity between on-site engineers and typically more experienced remote technicians.

12.11.3 Virtual Reality for Mental Health Treatment

Mental Health America raises a warning: 20% of the adult American population experiences a form of mental illness. Sixty percent of individuals do not seek treatment or medication due to their disregard for their symptoms. Some intentionally delay their visit to the doctor due to their apprehension of the unfamiliar. In addition, a significant number of individuals are apprehensive about consuming medication because of the potential for developing dependence without experiencing any beneficial outcomes.

VR has brought significant and profound changes to this place. Primarily, it enables treatment without the use of drugs. Empirical evidence has demonstrated the efficacy, comfort, and convenience of this approach, to the extent that patients may not be required to physically depart from their residences.

This technology facilitates the practice of breathing and meditation exercises in immersive environments. Additionally, it provides individuals with the chance to directly face their fears. For instance, individuals with arachnophobia or thalassophobia can confront and address their fears through immersion in a simulated environment. Additionally, there are games available that individuals can utilize as a means of diversion. These are effective for managing and alleviating anxiety.

XRHealth's solution is utilized by a healthcare provider in the United States to provide treatment for patients suffering from phobias. For instance, if a patient experiences a phobia of large crowds, the VR tool generates a secure simulation that replicates the sensation of being encompassed by a multitude of individuals. Once the patient demonstrates improvement, they can advance to more challenging circumstances. The advantage is to enhance the efficacy of drug-free therapy administered in a home setting.

12.11.4 Virtual Reality for Pain Management

Analgesics not only alleviate pain. The statistics are disheartening: on a daily basis, 40 individuals in the United States succumb to fatal overdoses caused by prescription opioids. The number of deaths resulting from this cause exceeds the combined number of deaths caused by heroin and cocaine. Individuals frequently abuse analgesics due to their rapid efficacy and inclusion of highly addictive compounds. To amplify the impact, individuals surpass the recommended dosage and develop a dependency.

VR functions as a non-pharmacological substitute for conventional anesthetic techniques in pain management. The technology has the potential to decrease the utilization of detrimental painkillers and potentially prevent fatalities. VR applications provide a range of interactive games that offer cognitive distraction as a means to alleviate pain. Put simply, VR allows patients to be fully engaged in a captivating virtual environment, which could be an interactive gamified experience or a lifelike and calming setting.

St. Jude Research Hospital aimed to provide its patients with a non-pharmaceutical approach to managing chronic pain. Their objective was to reduce the utilization of addictive opioids and assist patients for whom sedation is not recommended. The solution provides a range of programs, such as pain diversion through immersive games and retreats in tranquil environments. After a duration of 6 months, the hospital acknowledged that they had successfully achieved a 50% reduction in pain scores. In addition, they managed to reduce their monthly expenditure on pain-relieving medications by $200,000. The advantages are

- Minimizing the utilization of highly addictive opioids in medical care
- Decreasing hospital admissions because of the efficacy of VR treatment
- Offering a secure treatment option for individuals who are unable to tolerate analgesics.

12.12 DIGITAL THERAPEUTICS

Digital therapeutics provides scientifically supported solutions to manage and enhance health conditions using software and other digital health technologies that supplement traditional treatment methods. The quantity of current DTx(Digital therapeutics) solutions is continuously increasing. The Alliance possesses a product library, although they acknowledge that the inventory is not comprehensive. Currently, several healthcare sectors appear to be making the most use of their potential. Diabetes care and mental health apps are particularly prominent in this regard, with some of them operating on a subscription-only basis, similar to certain medications.

12.12.1 Real-world Examples

Evidence from the real world shows that data-driven methods can revolutionize health communication. Here are a few examples of successful implementations and case studies: According to Fiordelli et al. [18], one mobile health effort called Text4Baby targets pregnant women and new moms with individualized health messages that are based on their specific stage of pregnancy or motherhood. To provide real-time illness surveillance and communication alerts, HealthMap compiles and analyzes data from several sources regarding disease outbreaks. According to Fiordelli et al. [18], Project RedDot uses data-driven methods to create individualized strategies for diabetes treatment, which improves health outcomes and makes patients happier. As an end result of the individualized recommendations made feasible by mPower Heart's use of sophisticated analytics and gadget learning algorithms, customers' cardiovascular outcomes are substantially improved. Healthcare providers, records scientists, and tech professionals need to work together across disciplines to create information-pushed strategies that efficiently address the complex demands of assorted populations through the improvement of comprehensive conversation strategies.

Health services have demonstrated that SMS text message reminders are an effective means of enhancing service delivery, leading to positive health outcomes for patients [18]. Furthermore, GPS and heart rate monitors are used to track players' movements and provide coaches with data on how much effort their players are putting in during games [19]. In addition, subspecialized hospital treatment delivery has been efficiently implemented through the systematic distribution of tele-training curricula [20].

Research conducted by Kempf et al. [21] and Massimo et al. [22] has confirmed that telemedical interventions and schooling can assist caregivers of people with frontotemporal degeneration to improve their self-care and lead more healthy lives. These methods can provide excellent weight loss and protection. According to research, coaching can improve academic performance in diabetic pupils and boost physical activity in those with chronic neurological illnesses [23, 24]. Additionally, patients with sarcoidosis have stated less weariness and better exercise performance after the usage of pastime trackers [25].

McGuigan et al. [26] encourage athletes to use training monitoring strategies such as exercise heart rate and resting coronary heart rate to improve their overall performance in sports. Furthermore, Janssen et al. [27] and Costa et al. [28] discovered that athletes can benefit from smart swimming analytics and personalized training plans that incorporate wearable sensors.

12.13 CHALLENGES AND LIMITATIONS

Ethical data collection and analysis is a must for the safeguarding of people's rights and liberties, in particular, when sensitive health information disclosure is involved. Safety, permission, honesty, and privacy are the main considerations in studies dealing with human beings. Open-access research articles are a great alternative, as many of the advantages of science communication through open access are also advantages of publications. Ethical issues are usually not considered when making selections in sampling techniques even though the design, analysis, and selection of the sample may lead to the imposition of moral issues. In an ever-dynamic data environment characterized by data exploitation in the course of its collection, analysis, and sharing, the pressing issue of the privacy of health records is raised. Online qualitative data collection should be approached carefully, and ethical considerations should be taken into account as well due to the recent COVID-19 catastrophe.

Despite the rules that have been put in place to keep the on-time research and the practice in the right direction, we are fully aware that these rules will obstruct the way of major studies if they are to be imposed all around the world regardless of the circumstances. Issues of low response rates and limited costs can be lumped together with issues of bias and lack of transparency across the studies. The research faker makes a big deal of it. Challenges in the current methods and the need for ethical standards are not mutually exclusive. The ethical quandaries in using web scraping technology to collect personal information are immediately confronted by issues of secrecy, blocking of services, and the monetary cost, which should be adduced that all cases must be treated with serious human consideration.

12.14 FUTURE DIRECTIONS

It is necessary to investigate how different sectors may cooperate in advocacy, policy, and communication when it comes to the development of activities aimed at the reduction of neglected tropical diseases. In such a way, leads can go from underserved populations to primary care through community connectors. Nowadays, fair health communication is an essential part of public health data collection, and evidence-based intervention studies are becoming increasingly necessary.

The period of inequalities in health is the time for the use of recruitment strategies with principles taking inspiration from community-partnered participatory research to engage the target groups. These methods can be used to decrease the health disparities that affect the Hispanic and African American communities. These results display the importance of community involvement as a technique and of policies that have their roots in research knowledge for the implementation of fair health communication. Partnerships in research and practice are expected to be valuable; public health professionals must examine the opportunities that are so critical; and lawmakers must develop new funding opportunities to improve public health. The recommendations made in these studies can lead to greater benefits for partnerships, addressing health disparities, and promoting health equity.

12.15 CONCLUSION

HealthTech empowerment is fundamentally transforming healthcare by promoting patient-centered approaches that prioritize prevention, accessibility, and personalized care. The integration of pervasive health devices, telemedicine technologies, and AI-driven personalized medicine illustrates the potential of technology to enhance patient outcomes significantly. As digital health platforms and mobile applications further engage individuals in their healthcare journey, the sector moves toward more proactive and inclusive healthcare models. These advancements not only improve health outcomes but also elevate the overall quality of life for people globally, heralding a new era where technology and healthcare work hand in hand to deliver optimal care and empower individuals in their health decisions.

REFERENCES

[1] Menachemi, N., & Brooks, R.G. (2006). *Reviewing the benefits and costs of electronic health records and associated patient safety technologies. Journal of Medical Systems*, 30(3), 159–168.

[2] Bates, D.W. (2000). *Using information technology to reduce rates of medication errors in hospitals. BMJ*, 320(7237), 788–791.

[3] Garg, A., & Garg, S. (2020). *A review on artificial intelligence in cybersecurity*. In *2020 4th International Conference on Intelligent Computing and Control Systems (ICICCS)* (pp. 693–698). IEEE.

[4] Davis, S., Roudsari, A., Raworth, R., Courtney, K.L., & MacKay, L. (2017). *Shared decision-making using personal health record technology: a scoping review at the crossroads. Journal of the American Medical Informatics Association*, 24(4), 857–866.

[5] Deloitte Insights. (2023). Health tech investment trends: Technology and platform-enabled ecosystems could change health care. Available from www.deloitte.com/us/en/insights/industry/health-care/healthcare-technology-trends.html

[6] Ogunjobi, O.A., Eyo-Udo, N.L., Egbokhaebho, B.A., Daraojimba, C., Ikwue, U., & Banso, A.A., (2023). *Analyzing historical trade dynamics and contemporary impacts of emerging materials technologies on international exchange and US strategy. Engineering Science & Technology Journal*, 4(3), 101–119.

[7] Fittkau, F., Obermeier, S., Rossi, A., Maglio, P. P., & Yigitbas, E. (2019). *Challenges and opportunities of artificial intelligence in cybersecurity. Business & Information Systems Engineering*, 61(5), 531–537.

[8] Brat, G.A., Weber, G.M., Gehlenborg, N., Avillach, P., Palmer, N.P., Chiovato, L., … & Kohane, I.S. (2020). *International electronic health record-derived COVID-19 clinical course profiles: the 4CE consortium. npj Digital Medicine*, 3, 109. https://doi.org/10.1038/s41746-020-00308-0

[9] Brakefield, W.S., Ammar, N., Olusanya, O., Ozdenerol, E., Thomas, F., Stewart, A.J., … & Shaban-Nejad, A. (2020). *Implementing an urban public health observatory for (near) real-time surveillance for the COVID-19 pandemic. Studies in Health Technology and Informatics*, 275, 22–26.

[10] Brakefield, W.S., Ammar, N., Olusanya, O.A., & Shaban-Nejad, A. (2021). *An urban population health observatory system to support covid-19 pandemic preparedness, response, and management: design and development study. JMIR Public Health and Surveillance*, 7(6), e28269.

[11] Melissa, H., Christopher, C., & Kenneth, G. (2020). *The National COVID Cohort Collaborative (N3C): rationale, design, infrastructure, and deployment. Journal of American Medical Informatics Association*, 28(3), 427–443.

[12] Wissel, B.D., Van Camp, P.J., Kouril, M., Weis, C., Glauser, T.A., White, P.S., … & Dexheimer, J.W. (2020*). An interactive online dashboard for tracking COVID-19 in U.S. Counties, cities, and states in real time. Journal of the American Medical Informatics Association*, 27(7), 1121–1125. https://doi.org/10.1093/jamia/ocaa071

[13] Madhavan, S., Bastarache, L., Brown, J.S., Butte, A.J., Dorr, D.A., Embi, P.J., … & Ohno-Machado, L. (2021). *Use of electronic health records to support a public health response to the COVID-19 pandemic in the United States: a perspective from 15 academic medical centers.* I 28(2), 393–401.

[14] Morris, M. (2022). *Striving toward equity in health care for people with communication disabilities. Journal of Speech Language and Hearing Research*, 65(10), 3623–3632.

[15] Raliphaswa, N., Ramathuba, D., Luhalima, T., Mulondo, S., Malwela, T., Tshililo, A., … & Netshikweta, M. et al. (2023*). Barriers to effective communication between patients, relatives, and health care professionals in the era of COVID-19 pandemic at public hospitals in Limpopo Province. Journal of Respiration*, 3(1), 29–39.

[16] Dagliati, A., Malovini, A., Tibollo, V., & Bellazzi, R. (2021). *Health informatics and EHR to support clinical research in the COVID-19 pandemic: an overview. Briefings in Bioinformatics*, 22(2), 812–822.

[17] Ibe, C., Hickman, D., & Cooper, L. (2021). *To advance health equity during COVID-19 and beyond, elevate and support community health workers. JAMA Health Forum*, 2(7), e212724.

[18] Fiordelli, M., Diviani, N., & Schulz, P. (2013). *Mapping mHealth research: a decade of evolution. Journal of Medical Internet Research*, 15(5), e95. https://doi.org/10.2196/jmir.2430

[19] Lim, J., Sim, A., & Kong, P. (2021). *Wearable technologies in field hockey competitions: a scoping review. Sensors*, 21(15), 5242. https://doi.org/10.3390/s21155242

[20] Addala, A., Filipp, S., Figg, L., Anez-Zabala, C., Lal, R., Gurka, M., … & Walker, A. (2022). *Tele-education model for primary care providers to advance diabetes equity: findings from project echo diabetes. Frontiers in Endocrinology*, 13, 1066521. https://doi.org/10.3389/fendo.2022.1066521

[21] Kempf, K., Röhling, M., Stichert, M., Fischer, G., Boschem, E., Könner, J., … & Martin, S. (2018). *Telemedical coaching improves long-term weight loss in overweight persons: a randomized controlled trial. International Journal of Telemedicine and Applications*, 2018, 1–8. https://doi.org/10.1155/2018/7530602

[22] Massimo, L., Hirschman, K., Aryal, S., Quinn, R., Fisher, L., Sharkey, M., … & Riegel, B. (2023). *Icare4me for FTD: a pilot randomized study to improve self-care in caregivers of persons with frontotemporal degeneration. Alzheimer's & Dementia: Translational Research & Clinical Interventions*, 9(2), e12381. https://doi.org/10.1002/trc2.12381

[23] Garbin, A., Diaz, J., Bui, V., Morrison, J., Fisher, B., Palacios, C., … & Petzinger, G. (2022). *Promoting physical activity in a Spanish-speaking Latina population of low socioeconomic status with chronic neurological disorders: proof-of-concept study. JMIR Formative Research*, 6(4), e34312. https://doi.org/10.2196/34312

[24] Chinnici, D., Middlehurst, A., Tandon, N., Arora, M., Belton, A., Franco, D., … & Cavan, D. (2019). *Improving the school experience of children with diabetes: evaluation of the kids project. Journal of Clinical & Translational Endocrinology*, 15, 70–75. https://doi.org/10.1016/j.jcte.2018.12.001

[25] Drent, M., Elfferich, M., Breedveld, E., Vries, J., & Strookappe, B. (2020). *Benefit of wearing an activity tracker in sarcoidosis. Journal of Personalized Medicine*, 10(3), 97. https://doi.org/10.3390/jpm10030097

[26] McGuigan, H., Hassmén, P., Rosic, N., & Stevens, C. (2020). *Training monitoring methods used in the field by coaches and practitioners: a systematic review. International Journal of Sports Science & Coaching*, 15(3), 439–451. https://doi.org/10.1177/1747954120913172

[27] Janssen, M., Goudsmit, J., Lauwerijssen, C., Brombacher, A., Lallemand, C., & Vos, S. (2020). *How do runners experience personalization of their training scheme: the inspirun e-coach? Sensors*, 20(16), 4590. https://doi.org/10.3390/s20164590

[28] Costa, J., Silva, C., Santos, M., Fernandes, T., & Faria, S. (2021). *Framework for intelligent swimming analytics with wearable sensors for stroke classification. Sensors*, 21(15), 5162. https://doi.org/10.3390/s21155162

13 Revolutionizing Healthcare

The Impact of Wearable Health Technology on Proactive and Preventative Care

S. Prasanth, M. Robinson Joel, V. Ebenezer, K. Martin Sagayam, E. Bijolin Edwin, M. Roshni Thanka, S. Stewart Kirubakaran, and Belfin Robinson

13.1 INTRODUCTION

Healthcare tracking and administration are changing as an outcome of the emergence of artificial intelligence (AI) in wearable technology. These days, martwatches and activity trackers come with complex AI technologies that improve performance and offer prognostic health information [1]. These AI-powered gadgets can detect minute changes in health, provide personalized guidance, and spot possible health problems before they get worse. By identifying trends in health information that human researchers might overlook, AI has greatly improved the management of chronic health disorders, enabled early identification, and contributed to illness prevention [2]. These smart gadgets also provide distant monitoring and e-health, which promotes a more dynamic and networked strategy in healthcare services. Healthcare organizations will become even more streamlined and more individually tailored as wearable technology and AI advance.

The field of medical research is changing because of wearable health technologies. Smartwatches, fitness trackers, and elegant biometric apparatus are examples of a new wave of technological advancement that puts an emphasis on sensitive and protective healthcare [3]. Using these innovations, people gain the ability to regularly monitor and control their health, moving away from traditional methods that mostly focus on treating ailments after they arise. The capacity to monitor in immediate form makes it easier to identify any health issues early, create customized wellness plans, and take appropriate action [4]. This has a significant impact on how medical care is delivered and received.

DOI: 10.1201/9781003516163-13

In addition to enhancing patient consequences, wearable health technology is also changing the structure of the larger healthcare system. These gadgets help medical professionals make better choices, advance the field of precision medicine, and improve the effectiveness of healthcare delivery by providing continuous data on a range of health parameters [5]. These advancements are anticipated to have a major role in mitigating the effects of chronic diseases, increasing patient involvement, and eventually changing medical treatment into a more assertive and safeguarding framework as they develop and develop increasingly commonly used, especially through integration with AI [6].

The term "wearables," which is short for "handy wellness technological advancement," describes a variety of intelligent technological devices intended to track and enhance individual health [7]. These gadgets are a component of the Internet of Things (IoT) ecosystem and tend to be worn by humans. Wearable technology gathers and evaluates medical information by fusing hardware, software, and mobile apps [8]. This information is then sent to the servers of the cloud for additional processing. People can adopt a more proactive approach to their health and fitness by using the data produced by cutting-edge medical devices. These cutting-edge gadgets are designed to provide all-encompassing wellness tracking, gathering a variety of information from users through biosensors, such as cardiovascular health, blood pressure, sleep patterns, and daily activity levels. People get vital information about their general health via the continuous evaluation of these indicators, which empowers them to make decisions about their habits and medical treatment. Fusing routine wellness workouts with standard healthcare procedures, wearable clinical innovation is revolutionizing the way we check for and manage wellness [9]. Devices such as electronic watches, biometric detectors, and welfare displays provide continuous, reliable tracking of many health metrics, such as blood pressure, heart rate, real-world employment, sleep patterns, and vital indications, including blood sugar and blood pressure. By employing these components, which offer users both quick observations and substantial medical information over a period of time, people can take greater control over their health and make more educated clinical recommendations through AI technologies [10].

13.2 RELATED WORKS

The transformation of wellness from an emergency response to a more ongoing preventative and strategic perspective is being partially facilitated by recent developments in smart health technologies. Analysis shows that wearables such as trainers, smartwatches, and portable devices can be biased as they continuously monitor vital health parameters, including blood pressure, glucose levels, and heart rate. This allows for the early identification of implicit health enterprises [11]. Through virtual surveillance of health, these devices have shown promise in improving patient adherence to medication regimens, managing persistent illnesses, and reducing demand for hospital stays [12]. Prophecy analytics has been further transformed by the combination of computational intelligence and machine learning (ML) with these developments, enabling more personalized and swift treatments for patients [13]. A major movement into a more reactive and active pharmaceutical paradigm is being brought about by this refinement of the healthcare sector, which is enabling physicians and cases alike to make data-driven choices that improve the welfare of patients and alleviate their impact on healthcare organizations.

Featuring practical applications from everyday life and the accompanying difficulties, Table 13.1 offers an organized summary that covers the various facets of wearable health technology and its revolutionary influence on healthcare services.

TABLE 13.1
Overview of Wearable Technology

Class	Contributing Components	Implications on Healthcare	Illustrations
Handles of smart technology	Biometric technology indicators, clinical handheld devices, health monitors, and intelligent watches	Constant monitoring of well-being, prompt diagnosis of problems, and customized healthcare knowledge	The fitness tracker fit the Dexcom G6 device, watch from Apple, Firebolt, and ECG screens
Preventive surveillance of health	Healthcare alerts, individualized wellness approaches, and instant information acquisition	Increased clinical effects, superior defensive diligence, and expanded way of life maintenance	Observing of cardiovascular activity and blood sugar reliably
Augmented AI fusion	ML simulations, taking decisions assistance, and intelligent insights	Prognostic concerns unique therapy regimens, and the rapid identification of illnesses	AI-driven predictive modeling and heath informatics for hazard evaluation
Applications for conservative healthcare	Persistent condition managing, behavioral change, and virtual Gesundheit tracking	Reduced stays in hospital, timely assistance, and better handling of complex conditions	Diabetic management and surveillance of antihypertensive
Barriers and moral concerns	Ethics aspects, availability, consistency, and confidentiality of information	Guaranteeing safe information handling procedures, fair accessibility, and seamless integration wellness approaches	Privacy adherence, database security, and equitable accessibility on devices

TABLE 13.1 (Continued)
Overview of Wearable Technology

Class	Contributing Components	Implications on Healthcare	Illustrations
Novel scenario research findings	AI-powered evaluation, online evaluation, and health system connectivity	Achievement in lowering hospitalization rates and increasing client interaction	AI in identifying severe disorders and noninvasive evaluation of ECGs
Prospective trends and improvements	Modern medical facilities, precise biometrics and surveillance, and ubiquitous solutions	New methods of the provision of care as well as linked, individualized treatment	Removable modifications, intelligent textiles and clothing, and IoT connectivity
Influence on wellness services	Reduced expenses, better clinical results, better service provision	Reduced medical expenditures, increased satisfaction with care, and efficient utilization of resources	Simplified crisis care consultations and more efficient long-term condition treatment

13.3 TECHNOLOGIES BEHIND THE WEARABLE SENSOR DEVICES

Smart health technology has a substantial impact on the healthcare system as a whole that extends and transcends individual well-being advice. By using the data that these devices capture, medical professionals may grow better informed about an individual's wellness habits and provide more timely, tailored care [14]. Furthermore, wearable technology, as mentioned in Figure 13.1, combined with AI and ML, is opening up new possibilities for predictive analytics, early diagnosis, and remote patient tracking [15]. As they evolve, these gadgets have the ability to considerably enhance patient outcomes and the efficiency of health services transmission [16], which renders them essential in the setting of advanced health care system [17]. Wearable health technologies are often constructed with certain components.

13.3.1 Monitoring Device of Sensor

It is the type of GPS devices that incorporate degree-specific wellness indicators into wearable technology [18]. Cardiac monitors, heat gauges, gyroscopes, acceleration detectors, and implanted pacemakers are a few instances of these devices. Every sensor combines a specific task and gathers information on indicators of health such as rest schedules, exercise habits, heart rate variability, and pressure intensities [19].

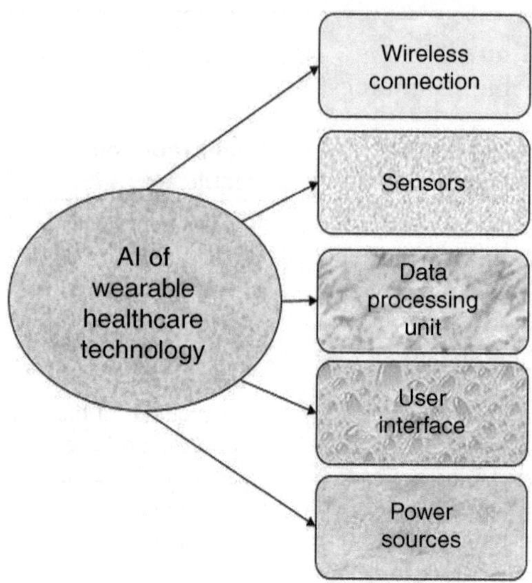

FIGURE 13.1 General Framework of Wearable Healthcare Technology.

13.3.2 Data Managing Device

An information examination framework, which is integrated into devices and often takes the form of a small computer or chip, analyzes the first data collected by the sensor arrays. Additionally, techniques for quickly interpreting and evaluating input can be coordinated into this computational component [20].

13.3.3 Wireless Communication

These gadgets frequently feature cellular interaction, Bluetooth connections, and Wi-Fi for communication via the internet. Relatively, with the assistance of these capabilities, medical information may be synchronized and transferred with ease to handheld devices and cloud-based devices, where it can be kept and examined more thoroughly.

13.3.4 User Interface

These devices provide an easy-to-use approach that lets individuals navigate the device, monitor information about their health, and access a variety of functions [21]. This user experience usually takes the shape of a touchscreen display or LED signals.

13.3.5 Power Source

Wearable devices come with a means of power as they are meant to be used continuously. This power source can be battery packs or, in certain situations, technology that harvests energy that can draw energy from the user's movement or body heat.

Portable electronics, called wearable health devices, are worn on the body by users to constantly track different health indicators. Such devices are made to track and log

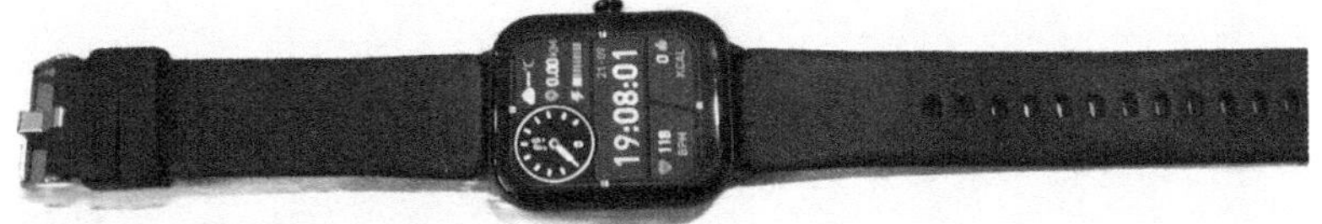

FIGURE 13.2 Digital Wearable Technology.

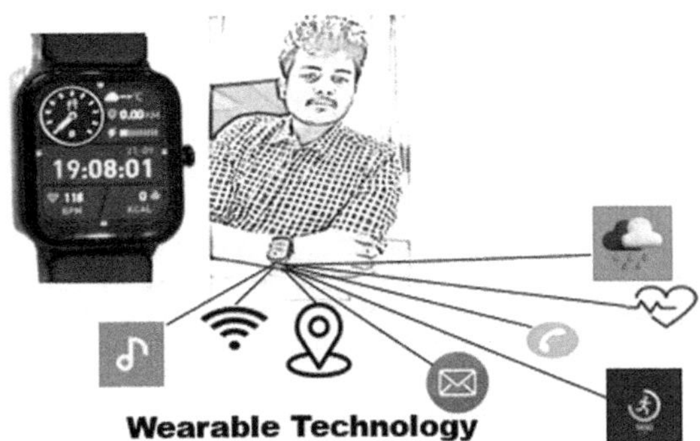

FIGURE 13.3 Overview of Wearable Technology.

information on symptoms, workouts, and other medical-related behaviors. They frequently offer ongoing wellness tracking, as in Figure 13.2, as well as instant commentary. Healthcare that is more preventive and individualized is made possible by the devices' combination of detectors, wireless connection, and imposing intelligence.

Modern digital sensors, known as wearable health gadgets, are used by people who constantly track a variety of physiological factors. Continuous tracking and data collecting made possible by these gadgets, as we shown in Figure 13.3, have transformed healthcare. AI may be used to evaluate information and produce predictive analytics and customized healthcare recommendations [22]. Smart AI technology improves peripheral healthcare technologies' functioning and increases their efficacy in diagnosis, preventative treatment, and health monitoring.

13.4 TYPES OF WEARABLE HEALTH DEVICES AND THEIR FUNCTIONS

13.4.1 Fitness Trackers

Fitness trackers are one type of wearable health device. Their features encompass assessing several aspects of being active, including your heart rate, steps taken, distance traveled, and calories burned; Figure 13.4 shows the general framework of fitness trackers.

They frequently have functions like lethargic alarms and monitoring your sleep. Figure 13.5 shows the real-time smart device. By establishing objectives and offering encouragement through data visualization and alerts, these gadgets encourage users to keep healthy [23].

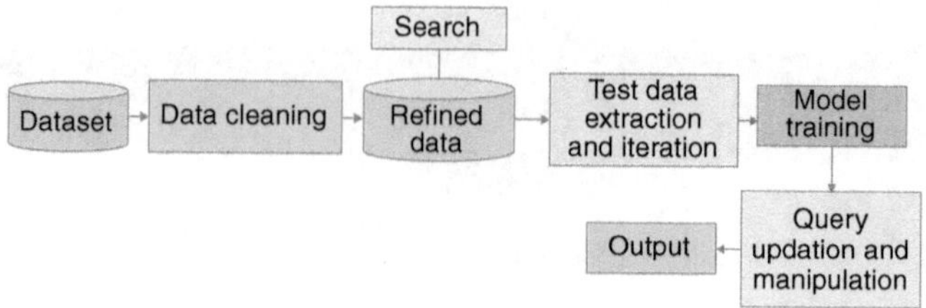

FIGURE 13.4 General Architecture of Fitness Trackers.

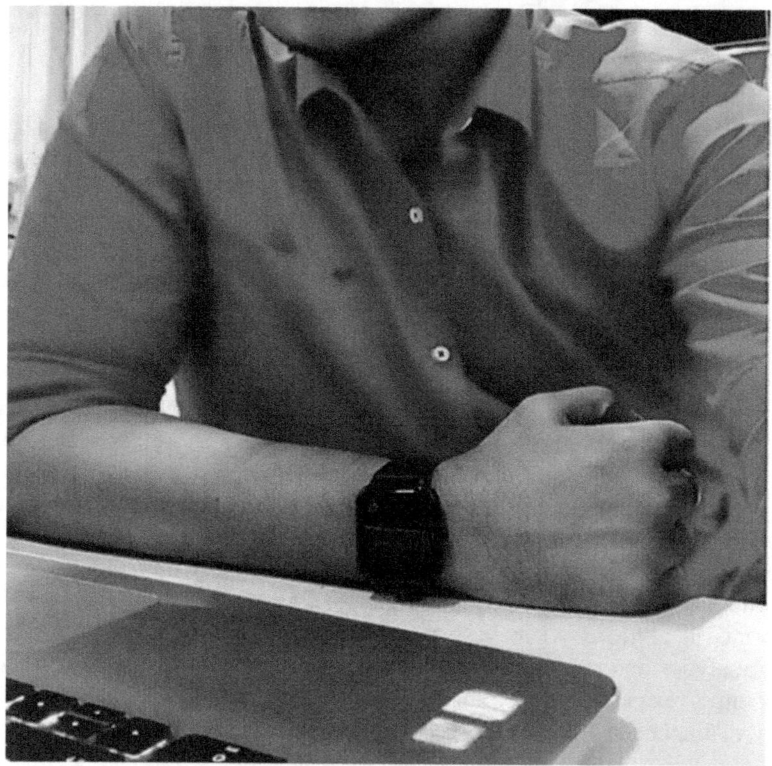

FIGURE 13.5 Real-Time Wearable Technology.

13.4.2 Smartwatches

Along with extra capabilities like notifications, phone calls, and mobile applications, smartwatches incorporate the functions of health monitors, as shown in Figure 13.6.

In addition to cardiac beat and sleeping routines, they occasionally track more complex parameters like saturation levels of oxygen and electrocardiograms (ECGs) [24].

Wearable devices are multipurpose gadgets that can be used in conjunction with other health apps to provide a complete wellness management solution, and as shown in Figure 13.7, the outlook of wearable smart watches is designed.

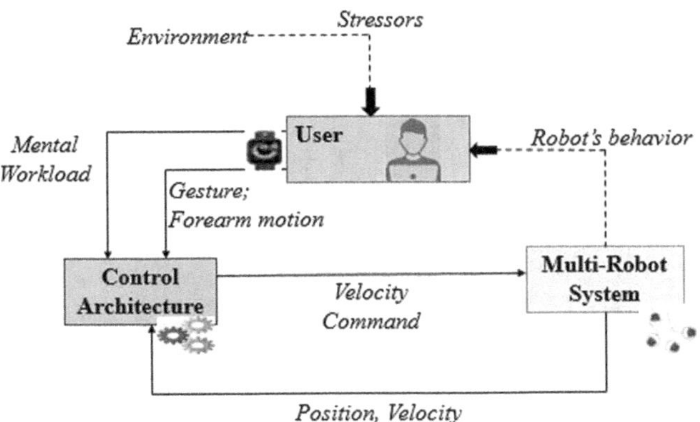

FIGURE 13.6 General Architecture of Smart Watches.

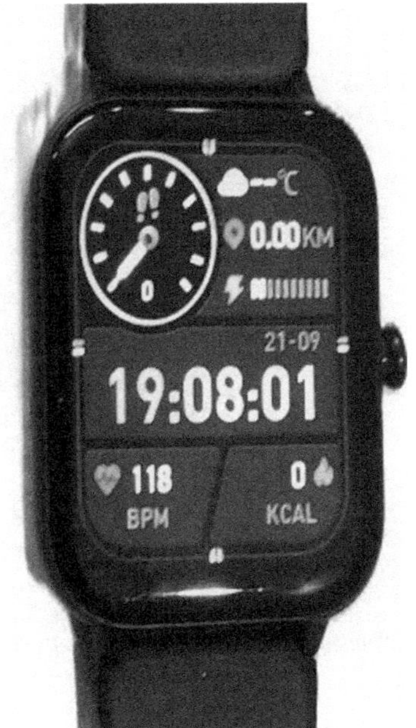

FIGURE 13.7 Overview of Smart Watch.

13.4.3 Wearable Electrocardiogram Monitors

Particularly designed to keep an eye on the heart rate, these pieces of equipment can identify abnormal heartbeats such as ventricular fibrillation. For people with cardiac issues, external ECG monitoring offers vital information that enables the early identification of possible heart attacks [25]. The general framework of wearable ECG monitors is shown in Figure 13.8.

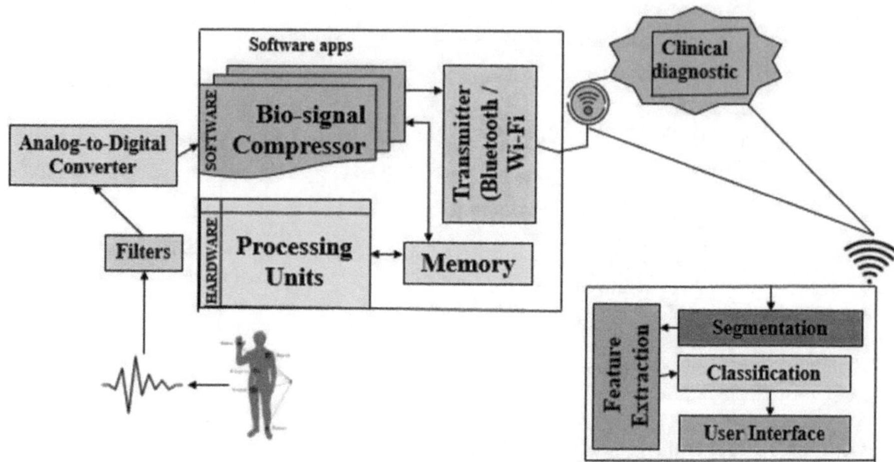

FIGURE 13.8 General Architecture of Wearable ECG Monitors.

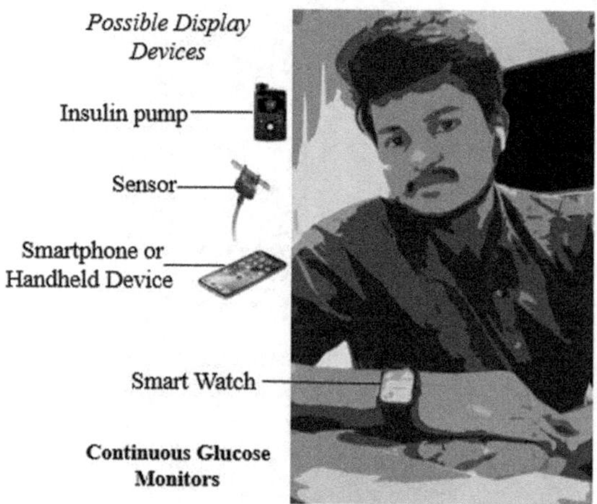

FIGURE 13.9 View of Wearable Continuous Glucose Monitors.

13.4.4 Continuous Glucose Monitors

Individuals who have type II diabetes are the main users of continuous glucose monitors (CGMs) for ongoing blood sugar monitoring, as shown n Figure 13.9.

Through the provision of precise data and real-time glucose readings, trends, and alerts, these devices enable better management of the condition by enabling patients to make informed nutritional or behavioral changes [26].

13.4.5 Astute Clothing

Skillfully incorporate locators into the fabric that record biological information , such as respiration, pulse, and movements of the muscles [27]. These attires are especially

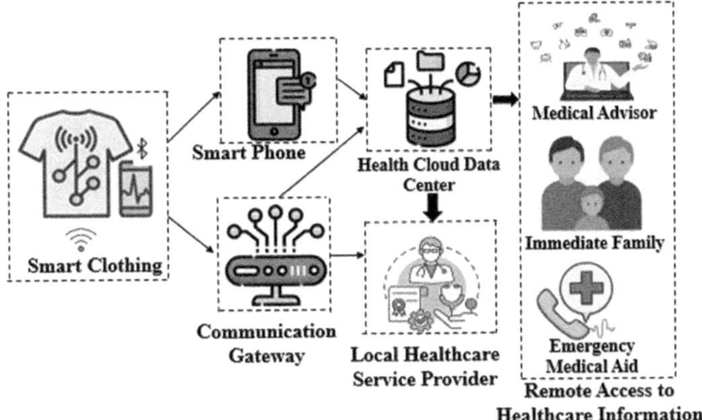

FIGURE 13.10 General Architecture of Smart Clothing.

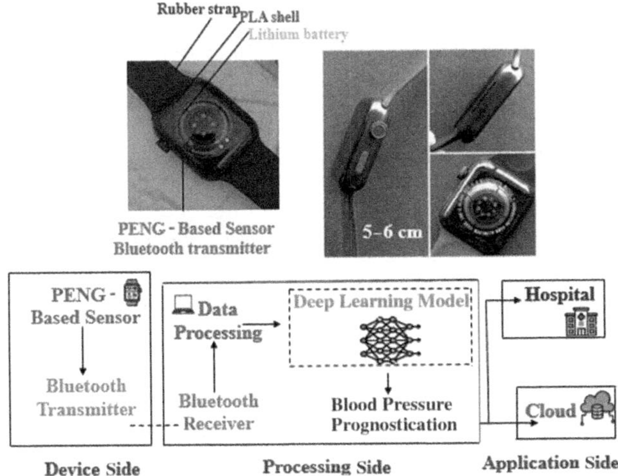

FIGURE 13.11 General Architecture of Wearable Blood Pressure Monitors.

useful for competitors andpatients undergoing physiological rehabilitation as they provide a comprehensive picture of continued preparation and recuperation [28]. Figure 13.10 shows the framework of smart clothing.

13.4.6 Wearable Technology Arterial Pressure Tracks

These are specialized gadgets that you can wear to examine the health of your blood vessels and heart, as shown in Figure 13.11. Physicians can periodically check your blood levels or throughout the day as needed to ensure optimal health [29]. It additionally lets you monitor the quality of your blood pressure and the effectiveness of any medications you may be taking.

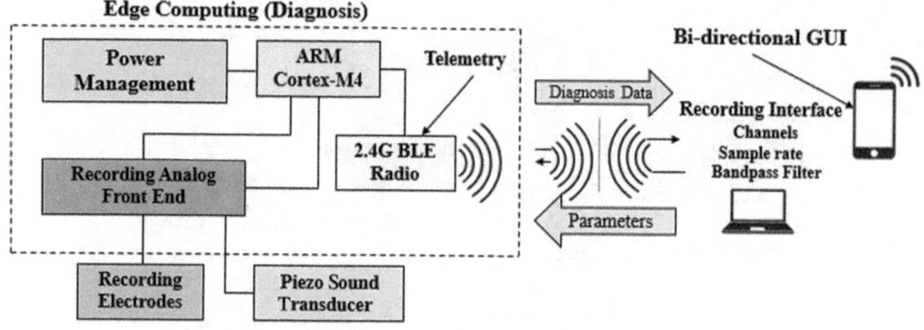

FIGURE 13.12 General Architecture of Wearable Respiratory Monitors.

Specialized equipment called peripheral pulmonary sensors allow people to track their breathing while they are completely asleep. The framework of this device is shown in Figure 13.12. Devices detect vital signs, including heart rate and oxygen saturation levels in the human organism [30]. For those with respiratory conditions, such as asthma, this equipment is extremely beneficial as it enables medical professionals to promptly diagnose and treat patients.

13.5 FUNCTIONS OF WEARABLE HEALTH DEVICES

Through routinely monitoring indicators of health such as blood pressure, blood sugar levels, and other vital signs, medical professionals and pharmacists can obtain crucial data that aids in the management of patients' ailments and preventive measures for future health concerns. The activity monitoring widgets assist users in preserving or enhancing their current level of physical and psychological well-being by tracking exercise metrics such as route, distance traveled, calories burned, and intensity [31].

1. Research of Sleep: Wearable technology monitors the quantity and caliber of sleep, offering information on sleeping habits and assisting in the treatment of issues related to sleep [32].

2. Medical Notifications: Certain gadgets allow for prompt medical action by providing instantaneous notifications for abnormal readings, such as dangerously high blood sugar levels or rapid heart rates.

3. Integration with Health Apps: Wearable health devices can exchange information with doctors and other healthcare professionals [33], assess long-term trends, and make individualized wellness recommendations by syncing with cloud-based systems or applications for smartphones [34].

13.5.1 Artificial Intelligence-Enhanced Attributes of Wearable Health Devices

13.5.1.1 Personalized Health Insights

Users examine wearable information from devices to generate food suggestions, workout schedules, and health regimens that are specific to each user. Predictive analytics is a technique that uses patterns and trends in the gathered data [35]; AI can identify possible health problems in advance, facilitating early detection and precautionary treatment. AI-driven algorithms, known as an anomalous endorsement, search for odd patterns in real-world instances or health indicators and send out alerts when an emergency arises. The use of AI in persistent healthcare regulation enhances smart tech's ability to keep track of chronic illnesses , such as coronary artery disease, diabetes, and hypertension. Providing viewpoints enables drug users to take better care of their fitness.

13.5.1.2 Data Linkage and Interpretation

Multifunctional AI technology may estimate and aggregate data from several sources, providing an in-depth understanding of the stoner's health and assisting medical practitioners in making more informed decisions [36].

Contemporary technical devices known as wearable healthcare sensors allow individuals to monitor and measure a range of health-related variables. Health services have changed because of the continuous surveillance and data collection made possible by these widgets [37]. AI can be used to estimate data, generate predictive prognostications, and generate customized heartiness suggestions. Mounted AI technology enhances the functionality of auxiliary wellness icons and boosts their effectiveness in diagnosis, wellness prevention, and heart health conservation. In summary, wearable medical technology is a vital utility for modern healthcare, and the likelihood of it happening grows when it is combined with AI. AI enables these artificial biases to behave better by providing basic medical data, improved conditional operations, and apocalyptic analysis [38]. With the advancement of AI, wearable healthcare technology is expected to become increasingly significant in personalized and innovative healthcare.

The integration of AI innovation and digital health analytics has the potential to completely transform the medical industry by providing more elegant, aggressive, and customized health tracking. Wearable AI health bias will impact several domains, including predictive healthcare, remote surveillance, customized therapy, information extraction, and many more.

13.6 WEARABLE HEALTH DEVICES' FUTURE PROSPECTS USE IN ARTIFICIAL INTELLIGENCE

13.6.1 Personalized Health Care and Expertise

AI-Powered Customized Health and Human Services Plans leverage advancements in AI-driven computations, enabling wearable healthcare devices to deliver highly customized medical guidance [39]. These personalized care plans and treatment guidelines will be derived from everyone's unique biometric data, genetic composition, daily decisions, and lifestyle circumstances of tailored healthcare. The use of AI in healthcare will be critically important for validated treatment by providing constant and thorough medical knowledge. Through customizing treatments to the particular needs of each patient, practitioners will be able to improve patient outcomes and reduce side effects. For instance, artificial neural networks may be able to assist with real-time treatment adjustments based on continuous analysis of tracking Signs.

13.6.2 Rapid Detection and Improved Perspectives

Disease vaticinator and its initial development of personal diagnostic sensors with AI capabilities will go beyond basic observation to predict illnesses beforehand. AI will eventually look at patterns in medical data to identify microsecond variations that could indicate early signs of diseases like dementia or myocardial heart disease. This will enable early intervention , which could prevent the full development of some illnesses [40]. AI-Based Contextual Biomarker Recognition suggests that Smart watches may eventually use AI to discover novel diagnostic markers for various illnesses. Intelligent technology, AI, has the inherent ability to uncover previously unknown labels that may be tracked via connected bias through extensive investigation of data, improving early assessment and personalized care decisions [41].

13.6.3 Blending Consolidated Health Data with the Internet of Medical Things

13.6.3.1 Sleek Interfaces and Data Cooperation

The Internet of Medical Things will make it simpler to connect health monitoring devices with other medical devices, electronic health records (EHRs), and health services. AI will enable effective system-to-system collaboration , creating a continuous, exhaustive ecosystem for monitoring health conditions. Increased patient outcomes, heightened dependability, and more integrated care will ensue from innovation [42].

13.6.3.2 Live Digital Observing and Actual E-Health

Wearable technologies will be used increasingly frequently in online medical care to enable medical practitioners to monitor patients remotely in real-time. AI will play a crucial role in assessing the data and alerting clinicians to any issues that require to be resolved to improve the efficacy and accessibility of medical products or services [43].

13.6.4 Artificial Intelligence-Driven Self-Sustained Medical Technologies

Future sensors will be able to track themselves autonomously. Machines with the use of AI will be able to calculate data tediously and issue warnings immediately without human intervention [44–51]. For example, AI could identify and alert pharmaceutical users of irregular pulses, signs of potential hypoglycemia or breathing problems, urging them to seek medical attention or take necessary steps [52]. Automation of Healthcare Selection Assistance: Smart AI will help consumers and medical professionals make recommendations by utilizing real-time data to provide insightful analysis [53]. This can entail digital recommendations for changing one's diet, prescribing medications, or even scheduling hospital stays in response to recognized advancements in healthcare services [54].

13.6.5 Artificial Intelligence-Powered Analytics for Intellectual and Behavioral Wellness

13.6.5.1 Analysis of Cognitive Health

In the future, alongside monitoring physical health, pervasive devices will monitor behaviors, including stress, activity level, and sleep hygiene [55]. AI will analyze this data to provide insights into the emotional well-being of an individual, identifying signs of conditions like anxiety, depression, or exhaustion and recommending appropriate interventions.

13.6.5.2 Evaluating Intellectual Description

Future technology could employ AI to monitor brain activity and potentially spot early signs of Alzheimer's or other neurological diseases [56]. By examining movement, pattern of speech, and other characteristics, AI may be able to identify cognitive health issues and recommend preventative actions [57].

13.6.6 Artificial Intelligence-Driven Research and Clinical Trials Expedited Development

By supplying enormous databases of present-day medical information, wearable AI will speed up and improve the research process [58]. The information gathered will help inquirers understand how diseases advance, how well cures work, and how changing one's lifestyle affects health. This will hasten the discovery of novel medicines and measures.

13.6.6.1 Virtual Clinical Trials

Wearable technology and AI will make it possible to conduct remote participant monitoring in simulated research studies. AI will guarantee that the information gathered is trustworthy and capable of yielding insights comparable to those obtained from conventional clinical trials, streamlining the procedure and lowering costs while opening it up to a wider audience [59].

13.6.7 Data Protection, Confidentiality, and Morality

13.6.7.1 Artificial Intelligence-Powered Security Remedies

As wearable technology gathers enormous volumes of individual health information, protecting privacy and security will become critical. Upcoming AI algorithms will be built with data anonymization, breach protection, and individuals having control over who can access their personal information in mind [60].

13.6.7.2 Ethical Artificial Intelligence Innovation

To make sure that AI systems are impartial, open, and do not promote prejudices, practical AI production will place a greater emphasis on issues of ethics [61]. This shall grow increasingly important when these gadgets are included in routine practice.

AI-enabled personal healthcare gadgets have a promising and revolutionary future. These devices will advance to offer extremely individualized health information, make early identification of diseases possible, and support self-managed health [62]. Smartphones and tablets will be essential for distant surveillance, accurate healthcare, and treatment for mental illnesses as AI advances [63]. Their function in contemporary treatment will be further enhanced by their ongoing integration with Internet of Medical Things (IoMT) and advancements in confidentiality and ethics. Connected medical research will become increasingly essential as AI technology develops, serving as a tailored and adaptive approach to managing well-being and health [64].

13.6.8 Algorithm

13.6.8.1 Transforming Healthcare with Wearable Health Technology

By using wearable health technologies for proactive and preventative care, you may improve healthcare.

Aim: The objective is to utilize wearable health technology, as shown in Figure 13.13, reduce the effect of persistent ailments, and improve general healthcare consequences, thus revolutionizing healthcare by providing patients with proactive health management resources [65].

Step 1: Gathering Information

Information, such as heart rate, physical activity, sleep habits, and vital indicators, via gadgets that are worn, is continuously inputted instantaneously.

Procedure: Compile information and keep it safe in a cloud-based system.

Results: Unprocessed medical information flows prepared for additional handling.

Step 2: Raw Health Data Streams Are the Input for the Processing of Information

Procedure: Remove distortion from the data and fill in any unfilled values.

To ensure uniformity between many devices and individuals, baseline the data.

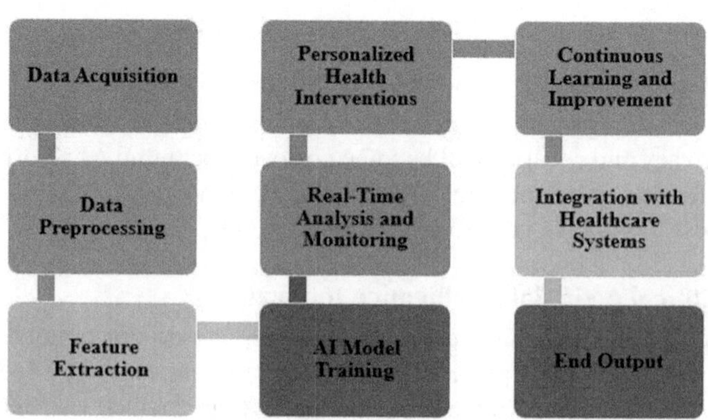

FIGURE 13.13 Process Flow Chart of Anticipated Wearable Health Technology.

Divide up the data according to time periods or particular health-related occurrences.

Results: Health information that has been sorted and analyzed.

Step 3: Characterization of Features

Translated wellness information was entered.

Procedure: Determine the most important health indicators (heart rate variability, length of sleep, activity levels, etc.).

Examine the data for trends and patterns (such as daily activity cycles and sleep quality).

Results: Analysis-ready pertinent health features.

Step 4: AI Model Building: Recognized Health Characteristics and Past Medical Records as Input

Procedure: Utilize ML techniques (such as decision tree structures and artificial neural networks) to create prediction models.

Utilize AI to find relationships between characteristics and possible health hazards.

Output: Trained AI models with the ability to recognize hazards and forecast health outcomes.

Step 5: Analyzing and Monitoring in Real Time

Source: Created AI models and instantaneous fashion medical information.

Procedure: Use AI models to actively examine data that comes in.

Look for trends or irregularities that could point to health problems.

Give users real-time information and notifications.

Results: Quick health insights, warnings, and suggestions.

Step 6: Customized Health Care Plans

Personal wellness profiles and evaluation results are the input.

Procedure: Tailor health advice (such as workout recommendations and dietary guidance) based on personal information.

Put individualized healthcare plans into action, emphasizing early detection and prevention.

Results: Proactive care prescriptions and personalized health programs.

Step 7: Ongoing Modeling Enhancement

Assistance from users and continual information on health are inputted.

Procedure: To improve precision, add updated information to AI models on an ongoing basis.

Modify health programs in response to feedback from consumers and outcomes.

Results: Enhanced AI models and progressively more potent health advice.

Step 8: Synchronization of Gesundheit Systems: Reports and consumer health data are input.

Procedure: Use safe ways to communicate pertinent health information with healthcare practitioners.

Encourage online consultations and remote surveillance.

Results: Improved linking of patient care with healthcare services and integration of care.

13.7 HEALTHCARE REVOLUTION'S PROSPECTIVE POTENTIAL: WEARABLE HEALTH TECHNOLOGY'S EFFECT ON PROACTIVE AND PREVENTIVE CARE

By increasing the integration of AI, enhancing information accuracy, and bringing its advantages to a larger spectrum of people, ubiquitous health innovation is poised to radically transform healthcare. Wearable technology will provide more precise wellness tracking and prediction capabilities as AI develops, allowing for earlier interventions and more individualized treatment and possibly delaying the onset of chronic illnesses. The future of customized healthcare will be ushered in by the development of sophisticated predictive analytics systems that can identify ailments based on unique profiles and activities.

It is anticipated that gadgets that are worn will become increasingly popular and reach a wide range of demographics, including the elderly and residents of neglected or distant areas. The creation of more accessible and reasonably priced medical equipment will fuel this growth and improve treatment for all [66]. Additionally, as wearable technology develops further, it will interface more with other health technologies – such as electronic health records and telemedicine – promoting a broader and integrated healthcare environment. Decision-making and outcomes for patients will be enhanced by this integration's ability to support ongoing health monitoring and real-time data exchange with healthcare professionals. In the end, personal health technology holds the promise of transforming healthcare into an individualized, proactive, and preventive approach that will improve wellness and save costs for everyone on the planet [67].

13.7.1 MATH'S BEHIND THESE TECHNOLOGY

The complex ideas that underpin the revolutionary effects of wearable health technology on preventive and curative care involve numerous models, algorithms, and rational approaches.

The hypothesis for Signal Processing and Data Filtering suggests that Worn sensors collect signals, such as glucose levels and heart rate, at regular intervals. The NYquist–Shannon principle is used to ensure that these indications are sufficiently tested to record all relevant data [68]. The Fourier transform transforms time-domain information into frequency-domain data, making it easier to analyze periodic components in bodily signals collected by ubiquitous monitors [69]. The Identification of Trends and Statistics Analysis of Time Series involves Time-series mathematical models, such as ARIMA, to detect developments, variations in the seasons, and predict future healthcare occurrences based on actual data, as wearable device data is time -dependent. Similarly, the evaluation of regression model, such as those predicting blood sugar levels based on physical activity and nutrition [70], reveals relationships between dynamic metabolic parameters and health problems [71]. Predictive Modeling and Machine Learning Bracket Algorithms, such as Neural networks, logistic regress, and support vector machines (SVMs) categorize information about health into directives, such as determining whether a patient poses a risk of developing a particular ailment. Grouping algorithms, such as K-means and hierarchy clustering, combine similar patient histories to help identify similarities between individuals and personalize treatment [72]. A High level of literacy Convolutional Neural Networks(CNNs) and Recurrent Neural Networks(RNNs)or, is used to analyze and interpret complicated health data, such as continuous ECG rhythms, to identify anomalies [73].

Predictive Analytics Bayesian Inference: A probabilistic method that is advantageous in predicting the evolution of complaints in healthcare, which modifies the probability estimate for a hypothesis when fresh information becomes accessible [74]. Evaluation of Life: To estimate the threat across time, tools such as the Cox commensurable hazards model and the Kaplan–Meier estimator predict when an important health event, such as the commencement of a protest, occurs [75]. By optimizing and making decisions similar to balancing side goods with treatment efficacy, linear modeling enhances therapies by taking limits into account. Dynamic software is used in supported wellness services planning, where decisions at every stage (e.g., daily doses of medication) influence chronic medical conditions. Management and Distance Observation involve Smartwatch technology that regulates glucose levels using regulation methodssimilar to insulin pumps do. These methods employ feedback loop to maintain equilibrium. Kalman filters are used for real-time information processing and prediction, essential for biases that provide ongoing input, like diabetes or heart rate monitors.

The Division and Handling Risks: Risk ratings comparable to the Framingham threat score, which estimates the threat associated with cardiovascular complaints based on variables like aging and levels of cholesterol; computational models calculate threat ratings based on several parameters. Markov processes are used to simulate the evolution of complaints over time and calculate the value for money of solutions in health economics and making decisions. Data compression and privacy are supported by digital encryption techniques such as Rivest-Shamir-Adleman (RSA) and Advanced Encryption Standard (AES), which ensure the security of delicate healthcare information transferred through smart technology. By creating distinct hash coefficients for each piece of data, hashing functions ensure data integrity by rendering illegal modifications logical. These exquisite textiles play a crucial role in the development, functionality, and efficacy of wearable health technology, which is transforming healthcare from a reactive to a proactive and forward-thinking paradigm. The use of statistics in improving problems with healthcare will become increasingly important as cognitive technology continues to develop.

13.8 CONCLUSION

Proactive and preventative care is becoming increasingly important in healthcare as portable technology is being used to replace responsive care. These electronic devices enable people to consciously regulate their health by providing continuous, real-time monitoring and data collecting. This enables advanced diagnosis of any issues and the development of more individualized care plans. By enabling precision medicine, improving the results for patients, and reducing the overall burden on medical facilities, smartphone and tablet technology is positioned to substantially improve medical care as it evolves, particularly with the inclusion of AI. As an inspiration for a more informed, involved, and healthcare-conscious society, visible wellness equipment eventually transforms our approach to healthcare and goes beyond simply being a means of tracking.

REFERENCES

[1] Adeghe, E.P., Okolo, C.A., & Ojeyinka, O.T. (2024). A review of wearable technology in healthcare: Monitoring patient health and enhancing outcomes. *OARJ of Multidisciplinary Studies*, 7(01), 142–148.

[2] Rustamov, S. (2024). Wearable fitness and health monitoring devices: Revolutionizing personal health management. *Modern Education and Development*, 6(1), 314–319.

[3] Tariq, M.U. (2024). Advanced Wearable Medical Devices and Their Role in Transformative Remote Health Monitoring. In *Transformative Approaches to Patient Literacy and Healthcare Innovation* (pp. 308–326). IGI Global.

[4] Babu, M., Lautman, Z., Lin, X., Sobota, M.H., & Snyder, M.P. (2024). Wearable devices: Implications for precision medicine and the future of health care. *Annual Review of Medicine*, 75(1), 401–413.

[5] Siva, S.R., Sudha, K., Pooja, E., Maheswari, B., & Girija, P. (2024). Revolutionizing Healthcare Delivery: Applications and Impact of Cutting-Edge Technologies. In *AI and IoT Technology and Applications for Smart Healthcare Systems* (pp. 75–91), Taylor and Francis

[6] Das, S. (2024). Applications of Sensor Technology in Healthcare. In *Revolutionizing Healthcare Treatment with Sensor Technology* (pp. 79–99). IGI Global.

[7] Rawat, B.S., Srivastava, A., & Garg, N. (2024, February). Health Monitoring Transforming Using IoT: A Review. In *2024 IEEE International Conference on Computing, Power and Communication Technologies (IC2PCT)* (Vol. 5, pp. 17–22). IEEE.

[8] Ranjan, R., & Ch, B. (2024). A comprehensive roadmap for transforming healthcare from hospital-centric to patient-centric through healthcare Internet of Things (IoT). *Engineered Science*, 30, 1175.

[9] Nissar, G., Khan, R.A., Mushtaq, S., Lone, S.A., & Moon, A.H. (2024). IoT in healthcare: A review of services, applications, key technologies, security concerns, and emerging trends. *Multimedia Tools and Applications*, 1–62.

[10] Bangash, S.H., Khan, I., Husnain, G., Irfan, M.A., & Iqbal, A. (2024). Revolutionizing healthcare with smarter AI: In-depth exploration of advancements, challenges, and future directions. *VFAST Transactions on Software Engineering*, 12(1), 132–168.

[11] Mishra, G. (2024). A comprehensive review of smart healthcare systems: Architecture, applications, challenges, and future directions. *International Journal of Innovative Research in Technology and Science*, 12(2), 210–218.

[12] Ogundipe, D.O. (2024). The impact of big data on healthcare product development: A theoretical and analytical review. *International Medical Science Research Journal*, 4(3), 341–360.

[13] Arowoogun, J.O., Babawarun, O., Chidi, R., Adeniyi, A.O., & Okolo, C.A. (2024). A comprehensive review of data analytics in healthcare management: Leveraging big data for decision-making. *World Journal of Advanced Research and Reviews*, 21(2), 1810–1821.

[14] Shastry, K.A., & Shastry, A. (2024). E-Health Services and Applications: A Technological Paradigm Shift. In *Digital Transformation in Healthcare 5.0: Volume 1: IoT, AI and Digital Twin* (pp. 101–110).

[15] Adekunle, J.J., Abiodun, W.O., Sodipe, A.O., Igweh, J.C., & Kenechukwu, N.M. (2024). Exploring the transformative effects of data science in healthcare. *Journal of Advanced Science and Optimization Research*, 5(1), 23–33
[16] Kamble, P.C., & Ragha, L.K. (2024, February). Sensing Health: Exploring Issues, Scope, and Future of Smart Wearable Sensors in Healthcare. In *2024 11th International Conference on Computing for Sustainable Global Development (INDIACom)* (pp. 223–228). IEEE.
[17] Bhambri, P. (2025). Artificial Intelligence Enabled Internet of Medical Things for Enhanced Healthcare Systems. In *Smart Healthcare Systems* (pp. 1–17). CRC Press.
[18] Singh, B., & Kaunert, C. (2024). Integration of cutting-edge technologies such as Internet of Things (IoT) and 5G in health monitoring systems: a comprehensive legal analysis and futuristic outcomes. *GLS Law Journal*, 6(1), 13–20.
[19] Ramalingam, V., & Eraiarasan, A. (2023). The future of wearable technology and its impact on healthcare. *Quing: International Journal of Innovative Research in Science and Engineering*, 2(2), 110–116.
[20] Ebenezer, V., Falicica, U., Baskaran, R., Celesty, A., & Eden, S. R. (2023). IoT-based wristband for women safety. *Journal of Artificial Intelligence and Technology*, 3(2), 69–74.
[21] Katoch, O.R. (2024), *Reshaping Public Health through Technology: Exploring Innovations, Challenges, and Future Avenues*Journal of Policies and Recommendations, 3(1), 412–422.
[22] Gabrani, G., Gupta, S., Vyas, S., & Arya, P. (2024). Revolutionizing Healthcare: Impact of Artificial Intelligence in Disease Diagnosis, Treatment, and Patient Care. In *Handbook on Augmenting Telehealth Services* (pp. 17–31). CRC Press.
[23] Joel, M., Ebenezer, V., Jenefa, A., Martin Sagayam, K., Jerlin Rajan, J., & Deepak Medali. (2024). Designing a Secure and Lightweight Ecosystem for Internet of Medical Things (IoMT) in Healthcare. In *Lightweight Digital Trust Architectures in the Internet of Medical Things* (pp. 84–105). IGI Global.
[24] Yadav, S. (2024). Transformative frontiers: A comprehensive review of emerging technologies in modern healthcare. *Cureus*, 16(3). doi: 10.7759/cureus.56538.
[25] Aruna, R., Vani, V., Roopa, H., Reshma, J., Shankar, B.B., & Patil, H. (2024). Leveraging IoT and Wearable Devices in Smart Hospitals and Medical Applications for Smart Cities. In *Applying Internet of Things and Blockchain in Smart Cities: Industry and Healthcare Perspectives* (pp. 267–292). IGI Global.
[26] Piwek, L., Ellis, D.A., Andrews, S., & Joinson, A. (2016). The rise of consumer health wearables: Promises and barriers. *PLOS Medicine*, 13(2), e1001953. doi: 10.1371/journal.pmed.1001953.
[27] Patel, M.S., Asch, D.A., & Volpp, K.G. (2013). Wearable devices as facilitators, not drivers, of health behavior change. *JAMA*, 313(5), 459–460. doi: 10.1001/jama.2014.14781.
[28] Cadario, R., Longoni, C., & Morewedge, C. K. (2021). Understanding, explaining, and utilizing medical artificial intelligence. *Nature Human Behaviour*, 5(12), 1636–1642. .
[29] Paglialonga, A., Polo, E., & Caprino, M. (2020). Wearable devices in health care: Narrative systematic review. *JMIR mHealth and uHealth*, 8(2), e16911. doi: 10.2196/16911.
[30] Esteva, A., Robicquet, A., Ramsundar, B., Kuleshov, V., DePristo, M., Chou, K., … & Dean, J. (2019). A guide to deep learning in healthcare. *Nature Medicine*, 25(1), 24–29. doi: 10.1038/s41391-018-0316-z.
[31] Jiang, F., Jiang, Y., Zhi, H., Dong, Y., Li, H., Ma, S., … & Wang, Y. (2017). Artificial intelligence in healthcare: Past, present and future. *Stroke and Vascular Neurology*, 2(4), 230–243. doi: 10.1136/svn-2017-000101.

[32] Kheterpal, S., & Mohammadi, B. (2020). The role of wearables in personalized medicine. *Digital Medicine*, 3, 64. doi: 10.1038/s41746-020-0277-7.

[33] Ashley, E.A. (2013). The precision medicine initiative: A new national effort. *JAMA*, 313(21), 2119–2120. doi: 10.1001/jama.2013.3595.

[34] Omisore, A.G. (2018). The role of health literacy in self-management and the prevention of chronic diseases: A quick review. *Journal of Education and Health Promotion*, 7, 2. doi: 10.4103/jehp.jehp_26_17.

[35] World Health Organization. (2021). *Global Status Report on Noncommunicable Diseases*. Geneva: WHO. Available at: WHO NCD Report.

[36] Evenson, K.R., Goto, M.M., & Furberg, R.D. (2013). Systematic review of the validity and reliability of consumer-wearable activity trackers. *International Journal of Behavioral Nutrition and Physical Activity*, 12, 139. doi: 10.1186/s12966-013-0314-1.

[37] Piwek, L., Ellis, D.A., & Joinson, A. (2016). The influence of mobile health technologies on self-management and engagement: An analysis of real-world data. *Journal of Medical Internet Research*, 18(1), e52. doi: 10.2196/jmir.4224.

[38] Boulos, M.N.K., Brewer, A.C., Karimkhani, C., Buller, D.B., & Dellavalle, R.P. (2014). Mobile medical and health apps: State of the art, concerns, regulatory control, and certification. *Online Journal of Public Health Informatics*, 5(3), e229. doi: 10.5210/ojphi.v5i3.4814.

[39] Izu, L., Scholtz, B., & Fashoro, I. (2024). Wearables and Their Potential to Transform Health Management: A Step towards Sustainable Development Goal 3. *Sustainability*, 16(5), 1850, 1–22. doi: 10.3390/su16051850. (.

[40] Ching, T., Halevy, A., & Blumberg, S. (2021). Smartwatches in health monitoring: A comprehensive guide to best practices. *Journal of Health & Biomedical Informatics*, 8(2), 245–267. doi: 10.1002/hbi.12345.

[41] Lee, J.M., Kim, Y., & Welk, G.J. (2014). Validity of consumer-based physical activity monitors. *Medicine & Science in Sports & Exercise*, 46(9), 1840–1848. doi: 10.1249/MSS.0000000000000287.

[42] Tarassenko, L., Villarroel, M., Guazzi, A., Jorge, J., Clifton, D.A., & Pugh, C.W. (2014). Non-contact monitoring of respiratory function using photoplethysmography. *Computer Methods and Programs in Biomedicine*, 113(1), 44–53. doi: 10.1016/j.cmpb.2014.04.013.

[43] Bumgarner, J.M., & Knight, B.P. (2020). Overview of wearable ECG devices and recent advancements in technology. *Current Cardiology Reports*, 22, 111. doi: 10.1007/s11886-020-01338-z.

[44] Heinemann, L. (2018). Continuous glucose monitoring (CGM) technology – introduction. *Diabetologia*, 61(1), 2–10. doi: 10.1007/s00125-017-4465-8.

[45] Rodbard, D. (2016). Continuous glucose monitoring: A review of recent studies demonstrating improved glycemic outcomes. *Diabetes Technology & Therapeutics*, 18(S2), S3–

[46] Pantelopoulos, A., & Bourbakis, N.G. (2010). A survey on wearable sensor-based systems for health monitoring and prognosis. *IEEE Transactions on Systems, Man, and Cybernetics, Part C (Applications and Reviews)*, 40(1), 1–12. doi: 10.1109/TSMCC.2009.2032660.

[47] Axisa, F., Schmitt, P.M., Gehin, C., Delhomme, G., McAdams, E., & Dittmar, A. (2005). Flexible technologies and smart clothing for citizen medicine, home healthcare, and disease prevention. *IEEE Transactions on Information Technology in Biomedicine*, 9(3), 325–336. doi: 10.1109/TITB.2005.854507.

[48] Picone, D.S., Schultz, M.G., Otahal, P., Aakhus, S., Al-Jumaily, A.M., Black, J.A., & Sharman, J.E. (2017). Accuracy of wearable devices for measuring blood pressure: A systematic review and meta-analysis. *Journal of Hypertension*, 35(7), 1355–1366. doi: 10.1097/HJH.0000000000001351.

[49] Bilo, G., Parati, G., & Kario, K. (2020). Blood pressure telemonitoring in the 21st century: New evidence and perspectives. *Hypertension*, 76(3), 674–677. doi: 10.1161/HYPERTENSIONAHA.120.14659.
[50] Liu, H., Li, X., & Chen, Z. (2018). Wearable devices for respiratory monitoring: From clinical to daily healthcare. *Journal of Breath Research*, 12(3), 034002. doi: 10.1088/1752-7163/aaa53e.
[51] Baker, J., & Byrne, R. (2020). Wearable technologies in respiratory medicine. *Respiratory Care*, 65(5), 718–723. doi: 10.4187/respcare.07642.
[52] Topol, E.J. (2019). *Deep Medicine: How Artificial Intelligence Can Make Healthcare Human Again*. Basic Books.
[53] Patel, S., Park, H., Bonato, P., Chan, L., & Rodgers, M. (2012). A review of wearable sensors and systems with application in rehabilitation. *Journal of NeuroEngineering and Rehabilitation*, 9(1), 21. doi: 10.1186/1743-0003-9-21.
[54] Esteva, A., Kuprel, B., Novoa, R.A., Ko, J., Swetter, S.M., Blau, H.M., & Thrun, S. (2017). Dermatologist-level classification of skin cancer with deep neural networks. *Nature*, 542(7639), 113–118. doi: 10.1038/nature21056.
[55] Obermeyer, Z., & Emanuel, E.J. (2016). Predicting the future – big data, machine learning, and clinical medicine. *The New England Journal of Medicine*, 375, 1216–1219. doi: 10.1056/NEJMp1606181.
[56] Islam, S.M.R., Kwak, D., Kabir, M.H., Hossain, M., & Kwak, K.S. (2013). The Internet of Things for health care: A comprehensive survey. *IEEE Access*, 3, 678–708. doi: 10.1109/ACCESS.2013.2437951.
[57] Gubbi, J., Buyya, R., Marusic, S., & Palaniswami, M. (2013). Internet of Things (IoT): A vision, architectural elements, and future directions. *Future Generation Computer Systems*, 29(7), 1645–1660. doi: 10.1016/j.future.2013.01.010.
[58] Jarraya, Y., Youssef, H., & Ammar, A. (2020). Wearable Devices for the Internet of Medical Things (IoMT) and Healthcare Monitoring. In S.M.A. Alaoui (Ed.), *Advanced Intelligent Systems for Sustainable Development* (pp. 29–43). Springer. doi: 10.1007/978-3-030-22135-2_3.
[59] Shah, P., Kendall, F., Khozin, S., Goosen, R., Hu, J., Laramie, J., Ringel, M., & Schork, N.J. (2019). Artificial intelligence and machine learning in clinical development: A translational perspective. *npj Digital Medicine*, 2, 69. doi: 10.1038/s41746-019-0148-3.
[60] Cornet, V.P., & Holden, R.J. (2018). Systematic review of smartphone-based passive sensing for health and wellbeing. *Journal of Biomedical Informatics*, 77, 120–132. doi: 10.1016/j.jbi.2017.12.008.
[61] Mohr, D.C., Zhang, M., & Schueller, S.M. (2017). Personal sensing: Understanding mental health using ubiquitous sensors and machine learning. *Annual Review of Clinical Psychology*, 13, 23–47. doi: 10.1146/annurev-clinpsy-032816-044949.
[62] Casey, R., Milton, S., & Albers, D.J. (2019). The impact of wearable devices on research and clinical trials: Applications and outlook. *Journal of Clinical Investigation*, 129(9), 3626–3634. doi: 10.1172/JCI130436.
[63] Izmailova, E.S., Wagner, J.A., & Perakslis, E.D. (2018). Wearable devices in clinical trials: Hype and hypothesis. *Clinical Pharmacology & Therapeutics*, 104(1), 42–52. doi: 10.1002/cpt.996.
[64] Price, W.N., & Cohen, I.G. (2019). Privacy in the age of medical big data. *Nature Medicine*, 25(1), 37–43. doi: 10.1038/s41391-018-0272-7.
[65] Mittelstadt, B.D., Allo, P., Taddeo, M., Wachter, S., & Floridi, L. (2016). The ethics of algorithms: Mapping the debate. *Big Data & Society*, 3(2), 2053951716679679. doi: 10.1177/2053951716679679.

[66] Indrakumari, R., Poongodi, T., Suresh, P., & Balamurugan, B. (2020). The Growing Role of Internet of Things in Healthcare Wearables. In *Emergence of Pharmaceutical Industry Growth with Industrial IoT Approach* (pp. 163–194). Academic Press.

[67] Topol, E.J. (2019). High-performance medicine: The convergence of human and artificial intelligence. *Nature Medicine*, 25(1), 44–56. doi: 10.1038/s41391-018-0300-7.

[68] Oppenheim, A.V., & Schafer, R.W. (2009). *Discrete-Time Signal Processing*. Pearson Education.

[69] Proakis, J.G., & Manolakis, D.G. (2006). *Digital Signal Processing: Principles, Algorithms, and Applications*. Pearson Prentice Hall.

[70] Box, G.E.P., Jenkins, G.M., Reinsel, G.C., & Ljung, G.M. (2013). *Time Series Analysis: Forecasting and Control*. Wiley.

[71] Shumway, R.H., & Stoffer, D.S. (2017). *Time Series Analysis and Its Applications: With R Examples*. Springer.

[72] Bishop, C.M. (2006). *Pattern Recognition and Machine Learning*. Springer.

[73] Goodfellow, I., Bengio, Y., & Courville, A. (2016). *Deep Learning*. MIT Press.

[74] Gelman, A., Carlin, J.B., Stern, H.S., Dunson, D.B., Vehtari, A., & Rubin, D.B. (2013). *Bayesian Data Analysis*. CRC Press.

[75] Hastie, T., Tibshirani, R., & Friedman, J. (2009). *The Elements of Statistical Learning: Data Mining, Inference, and Prediction*. Springer.

14 Artificial Intelligence in Healthcare

From Diagnosis to Treatment

Manoj Kumar, Vishal Kumar, and Ritesh Kumar

14.1 INTRODUCTION

Artificial intelligence (AI) is the term used to describe computer systems that mimic human intelligence. AI process includes steps like data collection, protocol development for various uses, provides general or specialized inference from collected data, and makes necessary changes. The enormous volume of digital data and the quick increase in processing power have sparked a great deal of interest in advancements of AI applications in medical field. AI is gradually changing the medical industry, by improving many aspects of patient care, diagnosis of diseases, rehabilitation, surgery, and result prediction. Clinical decision-making and disease identification are two critical areas where AI is making notable strides [1].

Large-scale data analysis and clinical decision-making are being made easy by AI techniques such as machine learning (ML), deep learning (DL), and natural language processing (NLP). ML is a branch of AI which includes supervised learning for outcome prediction, unsupervised learning for the identification of new disease subtypes, and reinforcement learning (RL) for result optimization. DL is a subfield of ML which includes use of neural networks to find patterns in big datasets. NLP makes it possible for computers to understand and produce human language, as well as helps recognize speech, mine text, and translate languages [2].

Introduction of AI into healthcare, especially since the 1950s, has helped medical field primarily in terms of disease diagnosis, treatment personalization which has led to increased healthcare precision and quality of patient care. AI is being used in many different fields, such as the creation of innovative teaching methods and the automation of corporate processes.

14.2 OVERVIEW OF ARTIFICIAL INTELLIGENCE TECHNIQUES AND TECHNOLOGIES

AI technology can identify diseases and can help in guiding clinical decisions by processing, analyzing, and interpreting large amount of data from many sources. The enormous volumes of data generated in the medical industry can be easily handled by AI techniques, which later can provide insightful information regarding various

DOI: 10.1201/9781003516163-14

disease diagnosis and treatment modifications [3]. NLP, DL, and ML are the subfields that are included in AI. Large language models (LLMs) are AI systems that use DL techniques and massive volumes of data to understand, generate, and predict text-based content [4, 5]. ML is one of the essential aspects of AI which enables the system to learn from data without the need for explicit programming. Three main categories of ML are supervised learning, unsupervised learning, and RL which are explained below:

- Supervised learning includes developing models which predicts the results based on the input information. For practical purpose, this subfield can be utilized to identify diseases or anticipate the efficacy of a medication and the possible adverse reactions of that medication.
- Unsupervised learning can analyze the data and cash categories it in the absence of predetermined classifications. That is why this subfield can be useful for the detection of novel disease. This can also help in recognition of prospective candidates for innovative therapies.
- RL focuses on improving results in a particular context and making calculated decisions. Using ultramodern modeling techniques and quantum chemistry concepts, it can be used to create new drugs or plan studies.

DL is a branch of ML, which uses artificial neural networks to extract insights from vast amounts of experimental data, thereby significantly amplifying AI's potential and uses across diverse domains. Another subfield of AI is NLP, which enables computer system to grasp and communicate in human language. This includes methods such as sentiment analysis, speech recognition, text mining, and machine translation to generate, analyze, and understand spoken and written language. In summary:

- AI is a broad field that includes anything related to making machines smart.
- NLP is the branch of AI focused on teaching machines to understand, interpret, and generate human language.
- ML is a subset of AI that involves systems that can learn by themselves.
- DL is a subset of ML that uses models built on deep neural networks to detect patterns with minimal human involvement.

14.3 HISTORICAL PERSPECTIVE: EVOLUTION OF ARTIFICIAL INTELLIGENCE IN HEALTHCARE

AI has achieved significant growth in the field of medicine since its introduction in the 1950s. The drawbacks in the early models of AI initially limited AI's application in the field of medicine, but the origin of DL in the early 2000s marked a turning point. The development of AI in healthcare sector over time has been marked by significant innovations and transformative possibilities. The journey of AI in the field of healthcare started as rule-based systems which later continued as ML and DL techniques. These applications help medical personnel to diagnosing a disease and suggesting the treatment.

Revolutionary chapter of AI in medical field began when AI techniques learned to analyze complex formulas and adjust on their own. These developments in AI have helped to improve healthcare by improving the diagnostic accuracy of various diseases and increasing operational effectiveness [6].

Alan Turing laid the foundation of AI in 1950 in the field of healthcare when he proposed the idea of using computers to mimic human intelligence. The first industrial

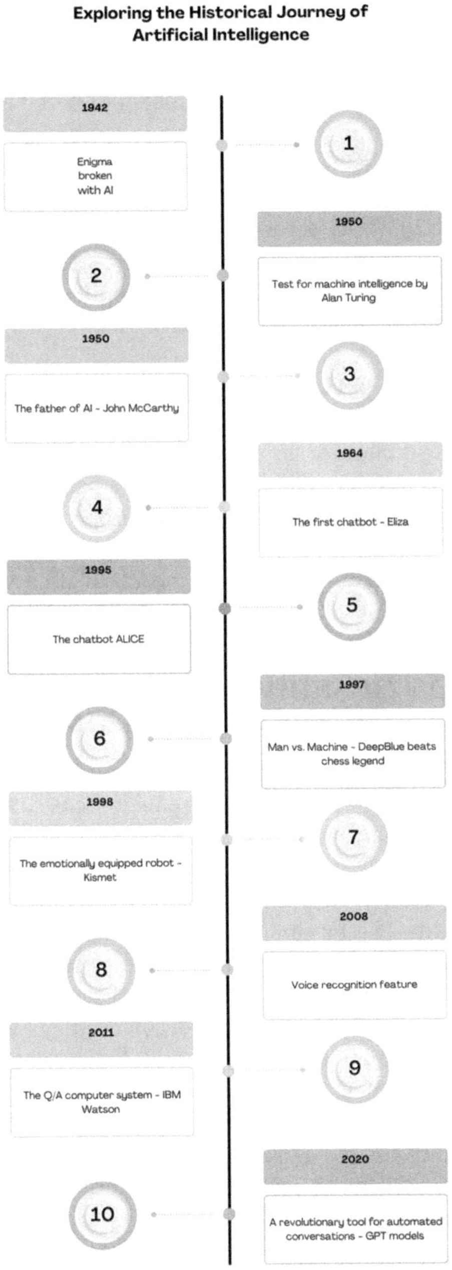

FIGURE 14.1 Chronological Path of Machine Intelligence.

robot arm and Eliza, a program that could mimic human speech, was introduced in 1960s which, proved AI's potential in medical field. However, throughout this period, the healthcare industry was slow and resistant to adopt these technologies. Nevertheless, the development of medical record systems and digital repositories in the 1960s and 1970s helped AI to gain popularity in the field of healthcare.

The period from the 1970s to the 2000s is known as the "AI winter" because this period saw a drop in the funding and interest in AI research. However, many significant advancements took place during this period, for example, the MYCIN system for treatment recommendations for bacterial infections and the Casual Associational Network (CASNET) model for glaucoma diagnosis. The introduction of ML in the late 1990s and early 2000s led to the considerable advancement of AI in the field of medicine [7].

Between 2000 and 2020, AI achieved some groundbreaking developments like data-driven medical decision-making. Due to advancements in DL and convolutional neural networks (CNNs), more advanced medical applications are now possible. For example, the application of AI to medical imaging has shown promise in improving diagnosis accuracy and speed.

In summary, the growth of AI in the field of medicine has been a slow process of growing acceptance and use, marked by significant technological advancements that have the potential to revolutionize the provision of healthcare. The integration of AI systems into healthcare has the potential to improve patient care by increasing disease diagnosing accuracy and streamlining clinical operations. Despite issues with data privacy, algorithmic bias, and the need for human expertise, AI has the potential to revolutionize healthcare practices and results if used wisely and effectively (Figure 14.1).

14.4 APPLICATION OF ARTIFICIAL INTELLIGENCE IN HEALTHCARE DIAGNOSIS AND TREATMENT

The integration of ML algorithms into medical practice has generated promising outcomes in enhancing diagnostic accuracy, reducing costs, and improving patient care quality. Notably, the use of AI-driven diagnostic instruments for diseases such as cancer has resulted in a 5.7% diminution in false-positive rates and a 9.4% decline in false-negative rates, thereby displaying its ability to surpass human capabilities in specific healthcare realms [8]. Further studies have reinforced the superior performance of AI in detecting breast cancer, with AI systems showing a sensitivity rate of 90% compared to 78% achieved by radiologists and successfully identifying early-stage breast cancer at a rate of 91% versus 74% achieved by radiologists.

Additionally, the incorporation of AI in dermatological diagnosis utilizing CNNs has demonstrated a degree of accuracy comparable to that of dermatologists, underscoring its capacity to identify and propose therapeutic strategies for melanoma cases [9, 10]. Furthermore, the utilization of AI in the diagnosis of diabetic retinopathy and cardiovascular diseases constitutes a paradigmatic illustration of its extensive applicability and effectiveness in healthcare settings [11].

Within the realm of clinical laboratory testing, AI has demonstrated a pivotal function in augmenting the accuracy, swiftness, and efficiency of diagnostic protocols.

Studies have consistently shown the importance of AI in identifying and enumerating microorganisms, diagnosing diseases, and predicting clinical outcomes with a high degree of precision and dependability, resulting in enhanced laboratory productivity and improved patient care [12, 13]. The integration of AI within emergency department (ED) settings has been explored, wherein AI-driven algorithms have shown significant improvements in patient outcomes and operational efficiency [14–16].

The integration of AI with genomic medicine presents auspicious prospects for monitoring, forecasting, and tailored healthcare interventions. The ability of AI to monitor nascent disease threats and pinpoint genetic indicators linked to disease susceptibility underscores its potential to propel healthcare toward more personalized and prophetic paradigms.

Within the world of gastroenterology, AI has been harnessed to augment the identification and characterization of colonic polyps, facilitate the distinction between chronic pancreatitis and pancreatic cancer, and forecast disease progression and therapeutic response. The integration of AI in endoscopic procedures has demonstrated significant potential, as evidenced by advancements such as ENDOANGEL and GI Genius, which have been shown to enhance the detection of adenomas during colonoscopic examinations.

Combining surgical instruments with preoperative planning optimized by AI can improve the accuracy of implant placement in total hip arthroplasty (THA). This customized method allows surgeons to place prosthetic implants with enhanced precision, thereby allowing patients to achieve optimal limb length and providing valuable guidance for managing intricate anatomical variations or complex cases [17].

Unlike the Bing model, which exhibits a complete inability to recognize scoliosis, ChatGPT showcases impeccable precision in diagnosing scoliosis from X-ray images. Notwithstanding, the accuracy of this method drastically declines to 43.5% when determining Cobb angles, thereby exposing a significant discrepancy relative to human assessments. Additionally, ChatGPT encounters difficulties in identifying axial vertebral rotation, categorizing the specific classification of scoliosis, and ascertaining the orientation of spinal curvature. In conclusion, although ChatGPT demonstrates promise in identifying scoliosis, its accuracy in quantifying Cobb angles and other metrics is limited and inconsistent with evaluations performed by experts [18] (Figure 14.2).

> Artificial intelligence possesses considerable capacity for enhancing the management of sepsis in intensive care units (ICUs). Notwithstanding, the persistent moral quandaries and obstacles stemming from the untrustworthiness and lack of transparency of AI algorithms impede the present state of AI research in this realm, thereby rendering it inadequate for routine clinical application. The integration of artificial intelligence in sepsis management may facilitate the mitigation of current knowledge deficiencies, specifically in the context of corticosteroid therapy. The results of our study suggest that integrating artificial intelligence-derived insights with corticosteroid therapy may lead to more personalized and efficacious sepsis treatments [19].
>
> The integration of artificial intelligence-driven predictive modeling constitutes a vital component of electronic health records (EHR) systems.

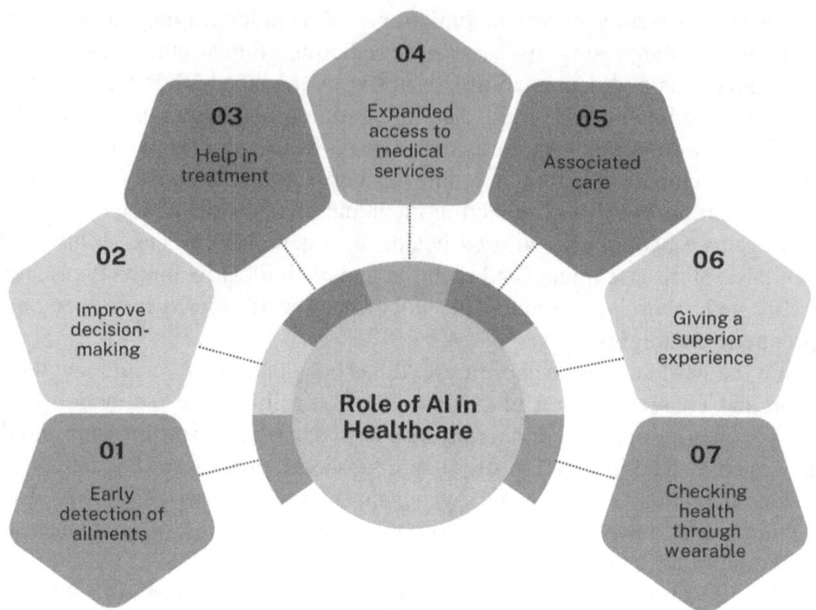

FIGURE 14.2 AI in Health Care.

Through the examination of archival patient data, artificial intelligence is capable of predicting forthcoming health patterns and enabling prompt identification of illnesses For instance, prophetic models can identify individuals susceptible to contracting persistent conditions such as diabetes or cardiovascular diseases, thereby facilitating timely interventions and precautionary steps [2–4].

14.5 ARTIFICIAL INTELLIGENCE IN MEDICAL IMAGING AND RADIOLOGY

AI has played a pivotal role in radiology and pathoradiology by augmenting image interpretation, with DL models proving exceptionally adept at recognizing anomalies, pinpointing fractures, tumors, and other conditions from medical images such as X-rays, computed tomography (CT) scans, and magnetic resonance imaging (MRIs) [1]. This capacity not only enhances diagnostic precision but also facilitates the early identification of diseases, which is vital for achieving successful treatment outcomes [20]. We can readily categorize fracture patterns and develop treatment plans tailored to specific fracture patterns using AI-driven tools. The application of AI in skeletal metastasis and radio-diagnosis further demonstrates its potential to transform healthcare. AI algorithms can scrutinize imaging data to identify metastatic involvement, thereby enabling early intervention and personalized treatment plans [21].

In radiology, DL and ML are being leveraged to create innovative solutions that will improve the detection of colon polyps and cancer diagnosis and classification via CT colonography. Additionally, DL algorithms have the capability to rapidly and efficiently automate the extraction and categorization of images, which can aid in the diagnosis of stroke when combined with neuroimaging techniques utilizing MRI and CT scans. The quality of scan images, often compromised due to time constraints in managing stroke patients, can also be enhanced using AI-driven super-resolution algorithms. AI can facilitate the diagnosis of tuberculosis by automatically detecting tumors when paired with MRI and X-ray imaging. Furthermore, Alzheimer's disease can be diagnosed at an early stage with the assistance of positron emission tomography (PET).

The incorporation of AI in radiology has become a game changer, poised to tackle the global radiologist shortage and boost diagnostic precision and speed. Neves et al. conducted a systematic review to clarify the role of eye-tracking data in enhancing DL models for radiology, uncovering a landscape marked by both opportunities and obstacles. This literature review consolidates findings from key studies, focusing on the integration of AI in radiology, with a particular emphasis on utilizing eye gaze data to improve transparency and performance in DL models. The shortage of radiologists, exacerbated by an aging population and the COVID-19 pandemic, has highlighted the need for innovative solutions in diagnostic medicine. AI, particularly DL, has been identified as a crucial technology capable of transforming radiology by enhancing workflow efficiency, reducing reading times, and improving diagnostic accuracy [22, 23]. However, the opaque nature of DL models, the Blackbox Problem, has hindered their widespread acceptance among healthcare professionals. Their systematic review, conforming to the PRISMA guidelines, analyzed 60 studies to assess the impact of incorporating eye-glancing data into DL models across various radiological tasks. The review revealed a taxonomy that categorizes the literature by application goals, such as error detection, classification, and fatigue estimation, offering a nuanced understanding of how eye gaze data can enhance AI models' performance and explainability. Their findings suggest that integrating eye gaze data can lead to more human-centric AI models, mirroring the diagnostic process of radiology and thus can be helpful in enhancing the radiologic diagnostic process through AI-driven insights and fostering transparency in AI decision-making. Although incorporating eye gaze data into radiology AI holds great potential, obstacles remain. Further studies are necessary to determine the most effective way to leverage eye gaze data in improving the transparency and precision of DL models in radiology.

14.6 ARTIFICIAL INTELLIGENCE IN ONCOLOGY

Noteworthy advancements have been made in the realm of AI, specifically in the realm of early lymphoma detection and diagnosis, facilitated by cutting-edge medical imaging modalities. To assess the accuracy of AI in detecting lymphoma, Bai et al. undertook an exhaustive examination and meta-analysis, underscoring the technology's capability to transform the landscape of medical diagnostics. The utilization of AI in medical imaging for the identification of lymphoma, a multifaceted neoplasm comprising lymphocytes, presents substantial diagnostic hurdles attributable to its intricate categorization and diverse spectrum of physiological immune functions. The disparity in opinions among specialists results in substantial discrepancies in the identification of characteristic symptoms. Within this framework, the integration of AI, specifically ML and DL, presents an innovative methodology for augmenting diagnostic capabilities [24–26].

The integration of ML algorithms, specifically AI, has led to a significant advancement in the detection and management of skeletal metastases, thereby revolutionizing the fields of medical imaging and oncology. The imperative requirement for precise identification of bone metastasis, typically a hallmark of advanced cancer, underscores the importance of leveraging cutting-edge technologies to enable prompt diagnosis and therapeutic strategy development for patients afflicted with this condition. Research has extensively explored the application of AI in this field, highlighting its ability to improve diagnostic accuracy, expedite the process, and mitigate the subjective nature of image interpretation. ML algorithms have been evaluated across various radiological modalities, including whole-body bone scintigraphy (WBS), CT, MRI, and PET, with each modality presenting distinct hurdles and prospects for AI integration. The creation and utilization of AI in skeletal metastasis imaging have produced encouraging outcomes, notably in enhancing the identification of metastatic lesions, which is vital for prompt and suitable cancer management (1). A seminal investigation was conducted by Dong et al. [22] Within this domain, researchers have employed a DL paradigm to facilitate the analysis of WBS images, with a specific focus on identifying bone metastases. This investigation incorporated a comprehensive dataset comprising 12,222 cases, which revealed the AI model's exceptional diagnostic capabilities surpassing those of seasoned nuclear medicine physicians, achieving an accuracy of 93.5% compared to 89.00% and a sensitivity of 93.5% versus 85.00%. This substantial enhancement in diagnostic efficacy not only underscores the capability of AI in alleviating the workload of healthcare practitioners but also emphasizes its capacity to enhance the quality of patient care by expediting the identification of metastatic lesions. Additionally, the utilization of AI in whole-slide biopsy has been broadened to encompass distinct cancer types, including prostate and breast cancer, with investigations employing CNNs to attain high classification accuracy. For instance, a CNN architecture specifically designed for prostate cancer patients on whole-body MRI (WBS) yielded an accuracy of 91.42% ± 1.64%, demonstrating the proficiency of AI in differentiating between cancerous and non-cancerous bone lesions. Likewise, for breast cancer patients, the classification precision was found to be higher in RGB images at 92.50% compared to other prominent CNN architectures. Progress in AI technologies has also enabled the creation of models with reduced computational demands, allowing their deployment on mobile and embedded devices. The lightweight model LB-FCN, designed for categorizing WBS images from prostate cancer patients, achieved a classification precision of 97.41%, substantially surpassing state-of-the-art networks such as InceptionV3, ResNet50, and Xception when tested on the same dataset. This underscores the potential of AI in making high-quality diagnostic tools more accessible and viable for widespread adoption [22].

14.6.1 Radiology-Based Applications

Thoracic Imaging: One of the deadliest and most prevalent types of tumors is cancer of the lungs. The identification of pulmonary nodules is possible through lung cancer screening, and early detection often proves to be a lifesaver. AI can lend a hand by automatically categorizing these nodules as either harmless or malignant.

Abdomino-Pelvic Imaging: The swift progress of medical imaging technology, particularly in CT and MRI, has resulted in a rise in unintended consequences, including liver lesions. AI can enable the distinction between benign and malignant classifications for certain lesions.

Colonoscopy: The likelihood of developing colorectal cancer is substantially heightened by unnoticed or misclassified colonic growths. Although the majority of these growths are initially harmless, they possess the capacity to become malignant with the passage of time. Consequently, it is crucial to employ trustworthy AI-driven methods for ongoing surveillance and prompt detection.

Mammography: It can be challenging to technically analyze screening mammograms. AI can assist in the interpretation process by identifying and characterizing minute calcium accumulations in the breast tissue.

Radiation Oncology: Through dividing tumors into targeted areas for optimal radiation dosage, AI can automate radiation treatment planning. Additionally, AI can track treatment response over time, thereby enhancing the accuracy and efficiency of evaluating radiation therapy outcomes.

Brain Imaging: Brain tumors can be classified as primary, secondary, non-cancerous, or cancerous. They are characterized by unusual cell proliferation. AI can be utilized to predict the diagnosis of these tumors.

14.6.2 Non-Radiology-Based Application

Dermatology: Expert dermatologists must conduct thorough visual examinations to identify skin cancer in suspicious areas. The diverse array of dimensions, hues, and surface irregularities makes it challenging to analyze skin abnormalities. With their immense ability to learn, DL algorithms can process this variability and detect characteristics that even evade human experts.

Pathology: Accurate identification of various cancer types relies on measuring digital whole-slide images of biopsy samples. Because of the broad spectrum of variations in imaging equipment, staining methods, slide preparation, and magnification, traditional AI methods often require substantial modifications to address this challenge. Advanced AI can detect cell division, segment histologic building blocks (such as tubules, epithelium, and nuclei), tally events, and provide more detailed descriptions and classifications of tissue.

Genomic Analysis: The increasing availability of sequencing data is providing more opportunities to utilize genomic endpoints in cancer diagnosis and treatment. AI-driven approaches can predict the effects of mutations on the binding specificities of RNA and DNA-associated proteins, as well as identify and extract high-level features linking somatic point mutations and cancer types.

14.7 ARTIFICIAL INTELLIGENCE IN DRUG DISCOVERY AND DEVELOPMENT

The incorporation of AI into the healthcare sector, particularly in the realm of drug discovery and development, has garnered growing attention and investments. This fusion has emerged as a game-changing force, seeking to tackle the challenges of escalating costs and dwindling efficiency plaguing the pharmaceutical industry. AI, encompassing its subfields of ML and DL, has been recognized as a crucial technology in augmenting various stages of the drug development pipeline. ML, through its trifecta of supervised, unsupervised, and RL, provides tools for diagnosing diseases, predicting drug efficacy, and uncovering disease subtypes and targets. DL, leveraging artificial neural networks, has shown promise in processing vast amounts of experimental data to potentially unearth new drugs or repurpose existing ones for more effective treatments. The drug development process, characterized by a feedback-driven cycle of induction and deduction, benefits from AI through the automation of certain stages, leading to reduced randomness and errors. The role of AI extends from the identification of novel compounds to the optimization of hit and lead compounds, demonstrating its ability to streamline the drug discovery process and improve the selection of promising drug candidates [27].

The COVID-19 pandemic has highlighted the urgent requirement to accelerate the drug discovery process, which is typically a time-consuming, costly, and intricate endeavor with a low success rate. AI has emerged as a vital contributor in this field by introducing novel computational approaches for de novo drug design, property prediction, and drug response analysis. These approaches have enhanced the efficacy and success rates of drug development pipelines. The application of AI in drug development has proven instrumental in overcoming the challenges associated with data collection, labeling complexity, and molecular representation. Graph neural networks (GNNs), generative models, and RL have shown promise in repurposing medications, predicting disease associations, and optimizing molecular properties for improved treatment outcomes. Open-source databases and AI-based software tools have facilitated drug design, despite challenges related to data disparity and labeling inconsistencies [28].

In the domain of pharmaceutical research, AI enabled the shift from traditional quantitative structural activity/property relationship (QSAR/QSPR) modeling to more advanced methods that harness DL for enhanced predictive precision. For example, GNNs have been utilized to produce latent representations of molecular structures, thereby enhancing the modeling of intricate molecules like peptides and macrocycles [29].

14.8 ARTIFICIAL INTELLIGENCE IN ELECTRONIC HEALTH RECORD AND CLINICAL DECISION SUPPORT SYSTEM

The incorporation of ML into digital medical files (DMF) and medical guidance systems (MGS) signifies a substantial breakthrough in medical innovation. ML has the capability to transform healthcare by augmenting the speed, precision, and excellence of patient treatment.

14.8.1 Artificial Intelligence in Electronic Health Record

Digital patient charts, also known as electronic health records (EHRs), store a vast array of patient information, including diagnoses, medication regimens, immunization dates, allergies, radiological images, and test results. The wealth of data in EHRs presents an opportunity for AI to improve healthcare delivery. Specifically, AI technologies such as ML and DL are designed to process and analyze large volumes of EHR data. By leveraging these technologies, hidden patterns and trends that may not be apparent through manual review can be uncovered. For example, AI can facilitate patient identification, personalized treatment planning, and disease outbreak prediction. A key subset of AI, NLP, plays a vital role in extracting meaningful insights from unorganized EHR data. NLP tools can decipher and condense medical records, thereby improving the precision and speed of clinical record-keeping. Consequently, healthcare professionals are relieved of administrative burdens, allowing them to focus more on delivering quality patient care.

14.8.2 Artificial Intelligence in Clinical Decision Support System

Computerized decision support systems (CDSS) are innovative tools created to aid healthcare experts in their diagnostic deliberations. By integrating data from diverse sources, these systems offer guidance grounded in empirical evidence to inform patient treatment. The integration of AI into CDSS amplifies their ability to deliver precise and prompt assistance.

Diagnostic Support: AI-driven clinical decision support systems can markedly enhance diagnostic precision by scrutinizing patient information and cross-referencing it with extensive medical knowledge repositories. For instance, AI-powered algorithms can facilitate the diagnosis of intricate conditions by detecting faint patterns in imaging data or laboratory results that might elude human clinicians. This minimizes diagnostic mistakes and guarantees prompt treatment.

Treatment Recommendations: AI can facilitate the development of personalized treatment plans. By analyzing a patient's genetic profile, medical background, and relevant data, AI can provide targeted therapeutic suggestions. This customized approach reduces the need for experimentation and enhances patient results, outperforming traditional treatment methods.

Workflow Optimization: AI-powered CDSS can simplify clinical workflows by automating mundane tasks such as prescription management, scheduling appointments, and notifications for preventive measures. This not only boosts productivity but also minimizes the risk of human mistakes, guaranteeing that patients receive prompt and suitable care.

14.8.3 Advantages of Artificial Intelligence in Electronic Health Records and Clinical Decision Support Systems

The fusion of AI with EHR and CDSS provides a multitude of benefits:

Enhanced Healthcare Results: AI facilitates prompt identification and timely intervention, tailored therapy approaches, and precise diagnostic assessments, resulting in superior patient results.

Improved Productivity: By automating repetitive tasks and streamlining data analysis, healthcare professionals can devote more time and attention to delivering quality patient care.

Lower Expenses: By streamlining processes and enhancing diagnostic precision, AI can decrease healthcare expenditures related to avoidable tests, treatments, and hospital re-admissions.

Data-Driven Insight: AI delivers healthcare professionals evidence-informed guidance, amplifying their critical-thinking abilities.

14.9 CHALLENGES AND ETHICAL CONSIDERATIONS

The utilization of AI in the healthcare sector gives rise to numerous concerns and moral dilemmas, notwithstanding its several benefits [30–32].

Protecting Patient Information: The utilization of AI in healthcare necessitates handling large quantities of sensitive medical data, thereby introducing concerns about privacy and security. Implementing robust safeguards is essential to prevent unauthorized access and protect patient data from potential breaches.

Prejudice and Impartiality: If AI systems are trained on imbalanced data, they may inadvertently perpetuate existing prejudices in the healthcare sector. It requires meticulous consideration and the use of comprehensive and varied datasets to guarantee the impartiality and fairness of AI systems. An imbalanced dataset may lead models to prefer certain eye movement patterns, which may put specific radiologists or patients at a disadvantage.

Responsibility and Openness: As many DL models are opaque, issues of accountability may emerge. It is essential to ensure that the deployment of these models in radiography does not undermine the responsibility of healthcare professionals in making medical judgments. Clarity regarding the implementation and timing of these models is also vital to empower patients and healthcare providers to make informed decisions about patient care.

Human Autonomy: The automation of radiology jobs can boost efficiency and help address the lack of skilled radiologists; however, care must be taken to avoid undermining the independence of healthcare professionals. Striking a balance that enables these technologies to augment radiologists' judgment rather than replace them is essential.

Security and Regulatory Compliance: Ensuring the well-being of patients and the efficacy of AI-driven healthcare solutions hinges on adherence to established regulatory guidelines and standards. Robust security safeguards are essential to mitigate the substantial risk of data compromise and unauthorized use. These safeguards entail limited access, secure data encryption, and protected transmission protocols.

Healthcare Integration: Integrating AI into existing healthcare systems can be a daunting task. Ensuring seamless implementation requires that healthcare professionals undergo comprehensive training, and intuitive interfaces must be developed.

14.10 FUTURE DIRECTIONS AND EMERGING TRENDS IN ARTIFICIAL INTELLIGENCE HEALTHCARE APPLICATIONS

Notwithstanding these breakthroughs, the incorporation of AI in healthcare encounters obstacles, notably the scarcity of AI-driven, Food and Drug Administration (FDA)-sanctioned medications available on the market. This highlights the imperative of supplementing AI-based analytics with conventional experimental methods, such as clinical trials and regulatory approvals, to unlock the full potential of AI in drug discovery and development. Further research is still required to enhance the reliability of AI models and to achieve a robust level of empirical evidence. The opaque nature of DL networks, which often lacks transparency in decision-making processes, remains a crucial area for future investigation. There is still a need for pioneering approaches, such as AI, to enhance the drug development process and mitigate the high attrition rates in clinical trials. The attrition rate, particularly in late-stage clinical trials, remains a pressing concern, with a significant proportion of new chemical entities failing to reach the clinic due to various factors, including lack of efficacy and safety concerns. All these areas remain the domains for future research in the realm of AI.

14.11 CONCLUSION

In the healthcare sector, AI holds immense potential to substantially improve patient outcomes and treatment plans. The integration of AI-powered predictive analytics can refine the accuracy, efficacy, and cost-effectiveness of clinical testing and disease diagnosis. Furthermore, AI can facilitate the development of guidelines and population health management by providing timely and accurate information to optimize pharmaceutical choices. Its application in mental health and virtual health support services has yielded positive outcomes in patient treatment. However, to ensure the equitable and effective utilization of AI, it is essential to address issues like bias and customization flaws. To guarantee the ethical and successful integration of AI in healthcare, several measures must be taken. Firstly, to safeguard patient data and vital healthcare operations, comprehensive cybersecurity plans and robust security measures must be developed and implemented. To facilitate the use of AI algorithms in clinical decision-making, rules and standards must be established in collaboration with healthcare organizations, regulatory agencies, and AI specialists. Moreover, investing in research and development is crucial for the advancement of AI solutions designed to overcome challenges in healthcare. By continuously monitoring variables like disease prevalence, population demographics, and geographic distribution, AI algorithms can identify individuals who are more likely to develop a particular condition, thereby informing treatment or preventative efforts. Additionally, edge analytics can predict future healthcare events, ensuring that resources like vaccines are distributed fairly. The general public holds diverse opinions about AI in healthcare; some individuals are willing to utilize AI for health-related tasks, but they still prefer to collaborate with human experts on complex issues. For AI to be successfully integrated into healthcare procedures, patient education and trust-building are essential. The ethical and successful integration of AI requires overcoming obstacles such as privacy concerns, data quality, bias, and the need for human skills. Effective collaboration among stakeholders is crucial for establishing ethical guidelines, developing trust between patients and caregivers, and developing viable AI systems. Unleashing AI's full potential in the healthcare industry demands persistent research, innovative thinking, and interdisciplinary collaboration. AI has the potential to revolutionize healthcare through improved patient outcomes, increased efficiency, and increased accessibility to individualized care and high-quality therapy upon effective integration [33].

REFERENCES

1. Alowais SA, Alghamdi SS, Alsuhebany N, Alqahtani T, Alshaya AI, Almohareb SN, Aldairem A, Alrashed M, Bin Saleh K, Badreldin HA, Al Yami MS. Revolutionizing healthcare: the role of artificial intelligence in clinical practice. *BMC Medical Education*. 2023 Sep 22;23(1):689.
2. Mak KK, Pichika MR. Artificial intelligence in drug development: present status and future prospects. *Drug Discovery Today*. 2019 Mar 1;24(3):773–80.
3. Suleimenov IE, Vitulyova YS, Bakirov AS, Gabrielyan OA. Artificial intelligence: what is it? *Proceedings of the 2020 6th International Conference on Computer and Technology Applications*. 2020;22–5. https://doi.org/10.1145/3397125.3397141.
4. Davenport T, Kalakota R. The potential for artificial intelligence in healthcare. *Future Healthcare Journal*. 2019;6(2):94–8. https://doi.org/10.7861/futurehosp.6-2-94.
5. Russell SJ. *Artificial intelligence a modern approach*. Pearson Education, Inc.; 2010.
6. Badnjević A, Avdihodžić H, Gurbeta Pokvić L. Artificial intelligence in medical devices: past, present and future. *Psychiatria Danubina*. 2021 May 19;33(suppl 3):101–6.
7. McCorduck P, Cfe C. *Machines who think: a personal inquiry into the history and prospects of Artificial Intelligence*. AK Peters; 2004.
8. McKinney SM, Sieniek M, Godbole V, Godwin J, Antropova N, Ashrafian H, Back T, Chesus M, Corrado GS, Darzi A, Etemadi M, Garcia-Vicente F, Gilbert FJ, Halling-Brown M, Hassabis D, Jansen S, Karthikesalingam A, Kelly CJ, King D, Ledsam JR, Melnick D, Mostofi H, Peng L, Reicher JJ, Romera-Paredes B, Sidebottom R, Suleyman M, Tse D, Young KC, De Fauw J, Shetty S. International evaluation of an AI system for breast cancer screening. *Nature*. 2020 Jan;577(7788):89–94. doi: 10.1038/s41586-019-1799-6. Epub 2020 Jan 1. Erratum in: *Nature*. 2020 Oct;586(7829):E19. doi: 10.1038/s41586-020-2679-9. PMID: 31894144.
9. Han SS, Park I, Chang SE, Lim W, Kim MS, Park GH, Chae JB, Huh CH, Na JI. Augmented intelligence dermatology: deep neural networks empower medical professionals in diagnosing skin cancer and predicting treatment options for 134 skin disorders. *Journal of Investigative Dermatology*. 2020 Sep 1;140(9):1753–61.
10. Haenssle HA, Fink C, Schneiderbauer R, Toberer F, Buhl T, Blum A, Kalloo A, Hassen AB, Thomas L, Enk A, Uhlmann L. Man against machine: diagnostic performance of a

deep learning convolutional neural network for dermoscopic melanoma recognition in comparison to 58 dermatologists. *Annals of Oncology*. 2018 Aug 1;29(8):1836–42.

11. Li S, Zhao R, Zou H. Artificial intelligence for diabetic retinopathy. *Chinese Medical Journal* (English). 2021;135(3):253–60. https://doi.org/10.1097/CM9.0000000000001816.
12. Peiffer-Smadja N, Dellière S, Rodriguez C, Birgand G, Lescure FX, Fourati S, et al. Machine learning in the clinical microbiology laboratory: has the time come for routine practice? *Clinical Microbiology and Infection*. 2020;26(10):1300–9. https:// doi.org/ 10.1016/j.cmi.2020.02.006.
13. Smith KP, Kang AD, Kirby JE. Automated interpretation of blood culture gram stains by use of a deep convolutional neural network. *Journal of Clinical Microbiology*. 2018;56(3):e01521–17. https://doi.org/10.1128/JCM.01521-17.
14. Panch T, Szolovits P, Atun R. Artificial intelligence, machine learning and health systems. Journal of Global Health. 2018;8(2). https://doi.org/10.7189/ jogh.08.020303.
15. Berlyand Y, Raja AS, Dorner SC, Prabhakar AM, Sonis JD, Gottumukkala RV, et al. How artificial intelligence could transform emergency department operations. *The American Journal of Emergency Medicine*. 2018;36(8):1515–7. https://doi.org/10.1016/j.ajem.2018.01.017.
16. Matheny ME, Whicher D, Thadaney Israni S. Artificial intelligence in health care: a report from the National Academy of Medicine. *JAMA*. 2020;323(6):509–10. https://doi.org/10.1001/jama.2019.21579.
17. Zheng H, Feng E, Xiao Y, Liu X, Lai T, Xu Z, Chen J, Xie S, Lin F, Zhang Y. Is AI 3D-printed PSI an accurate option for patients with developmental dysplasia of the hip undergoing THA? *BMC Musculoskeletal Disorders*. 2024 Apr 22;25(1):308.
18. Fabijan A, Zawadzka-Fabijan A, Fabijan R, Zakrzewski K, Nowosławska E, Polis B. Artificial intelligence in medical imaging: analyzing the performance of ChatGPT and Microsoft Bing in Scoliosis Detection and Cobb Angle Assessment. *Diagnostics*. 2024 Apr 5;14(7):773.
19. Liang C, Pan S, Wu W, Chen F, Zhang C, Zhou C, Gao Y, Ruan X, Quan S, Zhao Q, Pan J. Glucocorticoid therapy for sepsis in the AI era: a survey on current and future approaches. *Computational and Structural Biotechnology Journal*. 2024 Apr 12.
20. Hosny A, Parmar C, Quackenbush J, Schwartz LH, Aerts HJ. Artificial intelligence in radiology. *Nature Reviews Cancer*. 2018 Aug;18(8):500–10.
21. Dong X, Chen G, Zhu Y, Ma B, Ban X, Wu N, Ming Y. Artificial intelligence in skeletal metastasis imaging. *Computational and Structural Biotechnology Journal*. 2023 Nov 4.
22 Shih G, Wu CC, Halabi SS, Kohli MD, Prevedello LM, Cook TS, Sharma A, Amorosa JK, Arteaga V, Galperin-Aizenberg M, Gill RR. Augmenting the national institutes of health chest radiograph dataset with expert annotations of possible pneumonia. *Radiology: Artificial Intelligence*. 2019 Jan 30;1(1):e180041.
23. Neves J, Hsieh C, Nobre IB, Sousa SC, Ouyang C, Maciel A, Duchowski A, Jorge J, Moreira C. Shedding light on AI in radiology: a systematic review and taxonomy of eye gaze-driven interpretability in deep learning. *European Journal of Radiology*. 2024 Feb;1:111341.
24. Bai A, Si M, Xue P, Qu Y, Jiang Y. Artificial intelligence performance in detecting lymphoma from medical imaging: a systematic review and meta-analysis. *BMC Medical Informatics and Decision Making*. 2024 Jan 8;24(1):13.
25. Peng Y, Deng H. Medical image fusion based on machine learning for health diagnosis and monitoring of colorectal cancer. *BMC Medical Imaging*. 2024 Jan 24;24(1):24.

26. Obaid AM, Turki A, Bellaaj H, Ksantini M. Diagnosis of gallbladder disease using artificial intelligence: a comparative study. *International Journal of Computational Intelligence Systems*. 2024 Mar 14;17(1):46.
27. Qureshi R, Irfan M, Gondal TM, Khan S, Wu J, Hadi MU, Heymach J, Le X, Yan H, Alam T. *AI in drug discovery and its clinical relevance*. Heliyon; 2023 Jul.
28. Agrawal PJ. Artificial intelligence in drug discovery and development. *Journal of Pharmacovigilance*. 2018;6(2):1000e173.
29. Jiménez-Luna J, Grisoni F, Weskamp N, Schneider G. Artificial intelligence in drug discovery: recent advances and future perspectives. *Expert Opinion on Drug Discovery*. 2021 Sep 2;16(9):949–59.
30. Karimian G, Petelos E, Evers SM. The ethical issues of the application of artificial intelligence in healthcare: a systematic scoping review. *AI and Ethics*. 2022 Nov;2(4):539–51.
31. Naik N, Hameed BM, Shetty DK, Swain D, Shah M, Paul R, Aggarwal K, Ibrahim S, Patil V, Smriti K, Shetty S. Legal and ethical consideration in artificial intelligence in healthcare: who takes responsibility? *Frontiers in Surgery*. 2022 Mar 14;9:266.
32. Farhud DD, Zokaei S. Ethical issues of artificial intelligence in medicine and healthcare. *Iranian Journal of Public Health*. 2021 Nov;50(11):i.
33. Johnson KB, Wei WQ, Weeraratne D, Frisse ME, Misulis K, Rhee K, Zhao J, Snowdon JL. Precision medicine, AI, and the future of personalized health care. *Clinical and Translational Science*. 2021 Jan;14(1):86–93.

15 The Road Ahead

Forecasting the Future Impact of HealthTech Innovations

Shaik Khaja Mohiddin and Shaik Sharmila

15.1 INTRODUCTION

The landscape of the healthcare sector is changing with lightning speed as a technology-enabled revolution takes place, which was made possible through rapid advancement in digital technology and an innate tendency towards more personalized, convenient, and efficient patient care (i.e., personalized digital health). This transition is being driven by technologies such as artificial intelligence (AI), blockchain, genomics, the Internet of Things (IoT), and telemedicine. They note how each solution has unique functions that complement the accuracy, speed, and availability of healthcare services, thereby enriching patient care as well as operational efficiencies across the healthcare ecosystem [1]. There is now an opportunity to address these issues head-on with the integration of HealthTech solutions globally for a world that faces challenges related to aging demographics and rapidly increasing costs in healthcare systems.

HealthTech has helped transform the healthcare domain altogether, given that digital technology is advancing quickly today and people are seeking more personalized and on-demand care. This change is also led by technologies such as AI, blockchain, genomics, IoT, and telemedicine. Each of the three innovations and developments provides distinct aspects that enable accuracy, speed, and reach in issuing medical services to patients, which cascade down further supporting healthcare systems processes and adding impetus across the healthcare landscape. The aging and costs of the expanding population thereof are causing stress on global healthcare systems; HealthTech solutions have the potential to tackle that burden, mitigating it more effectively [2].

The diagnostic ability and treatment planning have gone through a paradigm shift because of AI. Machine learning algorithms could mine large datasets for patterns and predict patient outcomes more accurately than conventional methods. The use of genomics in personalized medicine enables the tailoring of treatment to an individual's genetic code, with a potential for better therapeutic efficacy and fewer adverse events. However, the use of blockchain technology also exposes a secure and transparent way to manage patient data that protects their privacy from risks of breaches arising in an increasingly digital healthcare system [3].

DOI: 10.1201/9781003516163-15

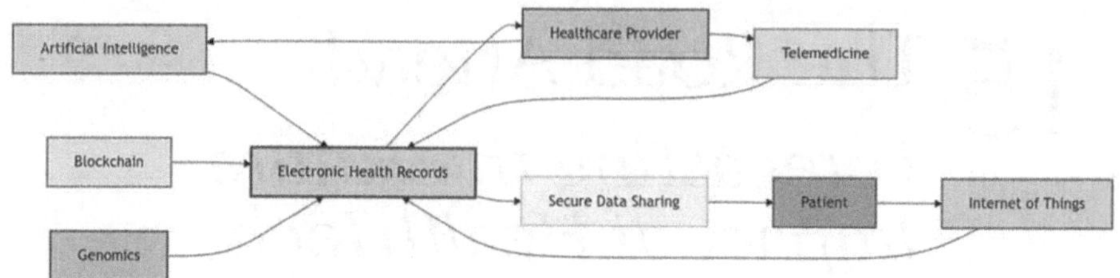

FIGURE 15.1 The Role of HealthTech in Modern Healthcare: A Holistic View of EHR, AI, and IoT.

IoT devices in healthcare allow the provision of health monitoring services in real time and remote patient management, creating new opportunities for early intervention treatments as well as easier treatment of a chronic illness that offers to be more proactive adjust the course work. Telemedicine, facilitated by the COVID-19 pandemic, has expanded access to medical care among underserved and remote populations, suggesting its ability as a tool for reducing healthcare inequities. Given the rapid progress within these technologies, it is important to explore their potential synergies and address some of the ethical and regulatory challenges they present to ensure a sustainable future for HealthTech [4]. Figure 15.1 shows a holistic view of electronic health record (EHR), AI, and IoT.

15.2 CURRENT TRENDS IN HEALTHTECH

Healthcare has seen rapid technological adoption of AI, blockchain technology, genomics, IoT, and telemedicine in recent advancements. There are a ton of healthcare applications that will be optimized with AI diagnostic instruments, predictive analytics, and therapeutic recommendations. Machine learning algorithms can already identify abnormalities in medical imaging, helping improve diagnosis accuracy for diseases like cancer and cardiovascular disease. In addition, genomics is revolutionizing the field of personalized medicine, which allows physicians to tailor treatments based on an individual's genome. Clustered Regularly Interspaced Short Palindromic Repeats (CRISPR) technology is changing the game of gene editing and holds promise for treating a range of genetic diseases. The IoT, through wearable devices and sensors, supports the management of chronic diseases by enabling continuous real-time patient monitoring [5].

The use of AT has grown substantially in the last few years, being propelled not only by COVID-19 (accelerated demand for telemedicine and remote care) but also due to a steady increase over time. Telemedicine systems have played a crucial role in ensuring the availability of healthcare services during lockdowns, and their usage is growing even more in the post-pandemic era, especially with regard to rural and underserved regions. Latest data shows short-term growth in telemedicine use soared 35.3% of office visits to be handled via telehealth in the US last year, a trend physicians and consumers are likely to continue as they see its convenience but also realize it is working well for many needs. IoT technologies, such as wearable health monitors and smart medical devices, have been rapidly adopted for remote monitoring to considerably improve the management of chronic diseases like diabetes and hypertension [6]. Despite the clear benefits, many challenges remain in these technologies becoming more widespread. The integration of AI, blockchain, and IoT into traditional healthcare is impeded by continued concerns over data security, data privacy, and legal compliance. Further, the costs to deploy these new technologies can be prohibitive for small healthcare providers and low-income countries. Addressing these issues is vital in ensuring the continued growth and successful implementation of HealthTech solutions globally.

15.3 ARTIFICIAL INTELLIGENCE IN HEALTHCARE

Table 15.1 shows an overview of current trends in HealthTech. The healthcare industry is being reshaped by AI on a large scale when it comes to diagnosis and treatment. AI-enabled diagnostic tools can process large datasets to expedite and enhance disease diagnosis. In the medical imaging field, these models are extremely efficient in detecting disorders like cancer and cardiovascular diseases as well as diabetic retinopathy. Broadly speaking, AI models are used in radiological imaging to identify tumours with remarkable accuracy, often surpassing human performance. In addition, AI tools are used with predictive analytics to predict which patients will develop specific diseases so that they can receive earlier interventions and more targeted treatment methodologies. AI is also powerful in personalized medicine, where it uses genetic and health history to provide patient-tailored drugs [7].

While there are many successful applications of AI use cases in healthcare. In another area, such as image analysis for diabetic retinopathy, using AI tools to help diagnose the disease early through deep learning algorithms that analyse retina images and significantly reduce blindness. IBM Watson Health helps oncologists select a best-fit cancer therapy option by analysing patient data and medical literature extensively. In practice, robotic surgical equipment such as the acai Surgical System uses AI to help achieve better outcomes in complex surgeries by making surgeons more precise and controlled [8].

Figure 15.2 shows the integration of AI, IoT, blockchain, and genomics with EHR. The opportunities for AI in healthcare are mammoth. AI-driven drug discovery deploys machine learning algorithms to screen potential drug candidates, thereby accelerating the development of new therapeutic agents and reducing costs. Predictive healthcare and AI are among the most promising areas for the use of artificial intelligence in health, as they enable models to predict patient outcomes, alerting doctors to intervene early before a person gets sick. . Inarguably, the growth in natural language processing (NLP) will undoubtedly empower AI to expose nuggets of wisdom from both clinical notes and research publications containing unstructured data about patient treatment. Due to the current problems, AI technologies are expected to become instrumental in addressing modern issues such as increasing healthcare access and availability and reducing costs while improving health outcomes [9].

TABLE 15.1
Overview of Current Trends in HealthTech: Technologies, Applications, Benefits, Challenges, Adoption Rates, and Future Potential

Technology	Application	Key Benefits	Challenges	Adoption Rate	Future Potential
AI	Diagnostic tools, predictive analytics	Increased diagnostic accuracy, personalized treatment	Data privacy, regulatory concerns	High in diagnostics (e.g., radiology)	AI-driven personalized medicine
Blockchain	Secure patient data, healthcare transactions	Enhanced data security, transparency	Complex implementation, regulatory barriers	Moderate in pilot programs	Secure global health data management
Genomics	Personalized medicine, gene editing	Targeted treatments, fewer side effects	Ethical concerns, high cost	Growing in personalized medicine	Gene-based treatments for chronic diseases
IoT	Remote monitoring, wearable health devices	Real-time health tracking, chronic disease management	Data security, device interoperability	Rapid growth in chronic disease management	Comprehensive remote care
Telemedicine	Remote consultations, telehealth services	Expanded access to healthcare, convenience	Limited in rural areas, regulatory challenges	High due to COVID-19 pandemic	Long-term integration in global healthcare
CRISPR	Gene editing, treatment of genetic disorders	A potential cure for genetic diseases	Ethical issues, regulatory delays	Emerging in research and pilot programs	Revolutionize the treatment of genetic conditions

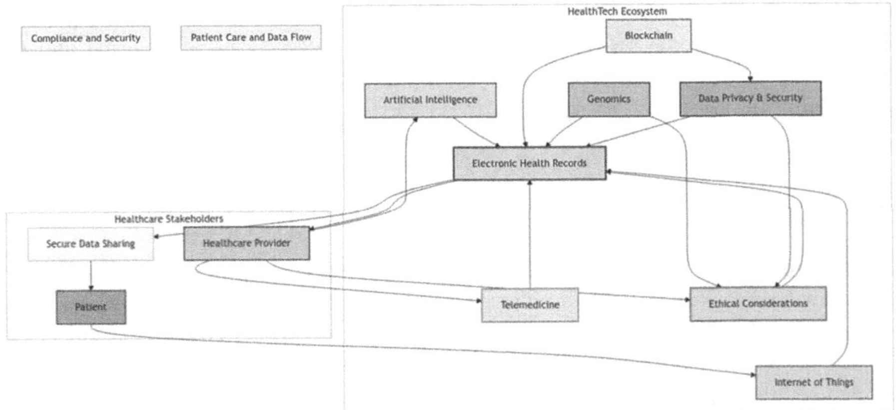

FIGURE 15.2 Integration of AI, IoT, Blockchain, and Genomics with EHR for Secure and Ethical Healthcare Delivery.

15.4 BLOCKCHAIN TECHNOLOGY

Blockchain technology has been rapidly emerging as a potent tool for securing patient data and ensuring the privacy and durability of medical records in healthcare. The World Health Organization Consulting report mentions that blockchain serves as a decentralized and unchanging ledger that boosts trust and lessens the exchange of data between healthcare providers and patients, without relying on central authorities vulnerable to breaches. All processing of the transaction will be done with a cryptographic behaviour; it is almost impossible to apply machines to alter data without a guarantee. Blockchain technology offers immense scope in securing patient data, preventing fraud, and delivering transparency to healthcare transactions, vital components of the increasingly digital health [10].

Blockchain in healthcare has provided many use cases and pilot projects that underscore the benefits of blockchain for better health outcomes. The Estonia e-Health Foundation has already successfully used blockchain to secure more than a million health records for its patients, in the process restoring data control to individuals. The United Arab Emirates has taken a step further in the Ministry of Health and Prevention using blockchain technology to prevent them from distributing counterfeit medicines among their patients. The US Food and Drug Administration (FDA) launched a major blockchain-based trial to secure the healthcare data exchange among providers, patients, and researchers in collaboration with IBM, aiming toward more effective clinical trial management as well as patient outcomes [11].

Despite the promise, blockchain lacks standards in healthcare. The major concern is the scalability of blockchain systems that are quite resource-consumptive and can take a long time to process huge data volumes. Also, the implementation of blockchain in existing healthcare IT structures faces several technical and regulatory challenges on its way, especially in jurisdictions with strict data protection laws. In addition, the cost of deploying blockchain systems may be prohibitive for many smaller healthcare organizations. Still, the future is bright for this project, especially as technology improves. Research of more efficient consensus algorithms and the definition of blockchain interoperability standards is expected to allow new ways in which data can be exchanged safely, with potential alternative applications across the healthcare sector that could revolutionize patient empowerment [12].

15.5 GENOMICS AND PERSONALIZED MEDICINE

By revealing what underpins the diseases that we study, genomics is revolutionizing healthcare and making it both more targeted and personalized. Genomics plays a role in healthcare that goes beyond just diagnosis – it also involves helping us predict risk, prevent problems, and personalize our approach to treatment. Genetic information can be used to predict the risk of certain diseases, such as cancer or heart disease, and healthcare providers may use this data for targeted interventions. This genomic data can be used to facilitate the development of pharmacogenomics, which looks at how genes influence a patient's response towards drugs. As a result, it can lead to more specific prescriptions and less of medication errors that minimize the side effects of drugs while increasing the treatment efficacy [13].

It is one of the most dramatic advances resulting from introducing genomics into healthcare personalized medicine. Individualized therapy: As the therapies are designed based on individual genetic profiles, patients get the most appropriate therapies with the least side effects. Genomic sequencing can be used to sequence the DNA of tumours and take their mutations into account when choosing targeted therapies, for instance, in oncology. The strategy has proven useful in cases such as melanoma and lung cancer that have not responded to traditional treatments. Finally, personalized medicine has also emerged in chronic disease treatment as the ability to tailor therapies from a genetic standpoint, which ultimately leads to improved long-term patient outcomes [14].

Advances in genomics, along with precision and personalized medicine, are already transforming how we treat illness today. Emerging technologies such as CRISPR gene editing and other advanced sequencing techniques will take our understanding of the genome to new heights. For one, CRISPR shows some potential for tinkering with the genes that go awry in genetic diseases to correct them. A breakthrough of unrivalled significance would be an actual cure for genetic stuff like sickle cell anaemia or cystic fibrosis. In addition, the rapid pace of innovation in next-generation sequencing (NGS) is dramatically reducing costs and improving turnaround time for genome sequencing, making personalized medicine more affordable. The future implications of these technologies would drive a radical change in the way diseases are diagnosed, treated, and prevented, leading to the healthcare system being predictive, preventive, as well as precise [15].

15.6 ETHICAL CONSIDERATIONS AND CHALLENGES

HealthTech has been expanding rapidly, yet there is a need for ethical considerations to avoid unethical implementations. A key concern is maintaining patient privacy and securing sensitive health data. As healthcare systems depend on AI, IoT, and other digital tools for better support from automated data feeds (HealthTech), a massive volume of health-related personal information is amplified across all fronts, seeming to open wide doors to persecuted privacy leaks or malicious data-used practices. Yet another question is the inherent bias possibility in AI, due to some of its algorithms being machine learning models that can take on their training data biases. Unless the models are trained with diverse datasets, this might result in disparate healthcare outcomes within marginalized populations. Developers and healthcare organizations are being asked to ensure that these AI systems remain bias-free, transparent, and secure as various ethical standards around the use of technology within the medical practice [16].

Regulatory and compliance challenges further complicate the landscape of HealthTech. The pace of innovation in AI, telemedicine, and genomics often exceeds the capacity of existing regulatory frameworks. As a result, healthcare regulators must rapidly adapt to new technologies while ensuring safety and efficacy. Compliance with regulations, such as the General Data Protection Regulation (GDPR) in Europe and the Health Insurance Portability and Accountability Act (HIPAA) in the United States, remains a significant hurdle. Ensuring that HealthTech companies adhere to data protection laws, especially when handling cross-border data transfers, is essential to maintaining patient trust and safeguarding their rights in the digital healthcare environment [17].

Ensuring equitable access to HealthTech solutions is a pressing ethical challenge. Advanced healthcare technologies, such as AI diagnostics and wearable health devices, have the potential to improve healthcare outcomes globally, but they are not always accessible to disadvantaged populations. Economic, geographic, and infrastructural barriers often prevent people in low-income or rural areas from benefiting from these innovations. Addressing this disparity requires collaborative efforts between governments, healthcare providers, and technology developers to create scalable, affordable solutions. Actions such as expanding into telemedicine in rural locations or reducing the costs of wearable HealthTech can help to address this issue and ensure that we all benefit from HealthTech. Table 15.2 shows key applications of genomics in personalized medicine and their future impact.

15.7 INTERNET OF THINGS IN HEALTHCARE

The Healthcare of Things: How IoT is transforming the connected patient experience and the IoT and leveraging interconnected devices to collect, stream, and analyse patient health data immediately. Such devices that range from wearable health monitors to sophisticated medical equipment are transforming how patient care is redefined, monitored on a 24/7 basis, diagnosed quicker, and diseases treated more optimally. For example, wearable devices like smartwatches and fitness trackers can track vital signs such as heart rate, blood pressure, and oxygen saturation, which helps patients better manage chronic diseases such as diabetes or hypertension. Other than this, IoT-based devices are also being used in institutions to monitor patients remotely and keep them out of frequent hospital visits [18].

Improved patient monitoring is probably the biggest gift of IoT to healthcare. Remote patient monitoring (RPM) systems leverage IoT devices to remotely monitor

TABLE 15.2
Key Applications of Genomics in Personalized Medicine and Their Future Impact

Genomic Application	Disease Area	Personalized Treatment Approach	Key Benefits	Emerging Technologies	Future Impact
Pharmacogenomics	Cancer, cardiovascular diseases	Tailoring drug prescriptions based on genetic profile	Reduced adverse drug reactions, higher treatment efficacy	CRISPR, gene therapy	Personalized drug development
Genetic risk assessment	Cancer, Alzheimer's, diabetes	Genetic screening for predisposition to diseases	Early intervention, prevention strategies	NGS	Prevention of hereditary conditions
Tumour genomics	Oncology (breast, lung, etc.)	Targeted therapies based on tumour mutations	More effective treatment, fewer side effects	Liquid biopsy, NGS	Customized cancer therapies
Inherited genetic disorders	Cystic fibrosis, sickle cell anaemia	Gene editing to correct mutations	Potential cure, elimination of genetic disorders	CRISPR, gene editing	Eradication of inherited genetic diseases
Prenatal genomics	Congenital disorders	Genetic testing for foetal health and abnormalities	Early diagnosis, informed pregnancy decisions	Non-invasive prenatal testing (NIPT)	Early prevention and intervention
Preventative genomics	Cardiovascular, diabetes	Personalized lifestyle and dietary recommendations	Improved chronic disease management	AI-powered genomic analysis	Predictive and preventative healthcare

TABLE 15.3
Key IoT Devices and Their Applications in Healthcare

IoT Device	Application	Key Benefits	Challenges	Future Trends	Impact on Healthcare
Wearables	Monitoring vital signs (e.g., heart rate, blood pressure)	Continuous monitoring, improved chronic disease management	Data security, battery life	Integration with AI for predictive health	Reduced hospital visits, early diagnosis
Smart glucose monitors	Diabetes management	Real-time glucose monitoring and reporting	Device interoperability, cost	Advanced sensors, real-time adjustments	Better control of diabetes, fewer complications
Smart implants	Post-surgery monitoring	Continuous internal health data collection	Invasiveness, regulatory hurdles	Miniaturization, improved accuracy	Proactive post-surgery care reduces risks
Ingestible sensors	Digestive health tracking	Real-time data on gastrointestinal conditions	Cost, patient compliance	Expanded use for various internal conditions	Enhanced precision in internal diagnostics
Hospital asset tracking	Monitoring medical equipment	Increased efficiency, reduced loss of assets	Cost of implementation	AI-driven equipment management	Improved hospital resource allocation

the health status of patients outside traditional hospital settings, which is particularly beneficial for chronic disease management. Monitor blood sugar levels and wirelessly transmit results to a clinician so that treatment plans can easily be adjusted. IoT-enabled gadgets facilitate the continuous monitoring of post-operative patients, alerting healthcare providers to any detected irregularities, hence enabling prompt interventions. Furthermore, IoT systems can enhance the efficiency of care delivery in hospitals by monitoring the location and status of medical equipment and assisting in the management of hospital bed occupancy [19].

Anticipated advancements in IoT healthcare technology are predicted to significantly improve patient care. An emerging trend is the advancement of smart implants and ingestible sensors, which will yield more accurate health data from within the body. The integration of IoT devices with AI enables the prediction of prospective health difficulties and the recommendation of preventive measures before the escalation of problems. The progression of 5G technology will significantly facilitate expedited and more dependable data transmission between IoT devices and healthcare systems, hence enhancing the overall quality of remote treatment. As these technologies advance, IoT in healthcare is poised to transition from reactive care to proactive and predictive healthcare, enhancing patient outcomes and decreasing healthcare expenditures. Table 15.3 shows key IoT devices and their applications in healthcare.

15.8 TELEMEDICINE AND REMOTE CARE

The proliferation of telehealth services has markedly accelerated in recent years, especially because of the global COVID-19 pandemic. Telemedicine allows healthcare professionals to conduct remote consultations, diagnoses, and treatments via digital communication systems. However, this shift to telemedicine has also improved the ability of those in underutilized or remote areas without nearby medical facilities. It is not only primary care, but patients are also taking advantage of the telehealth opportunity for dermatology appointments or psychiatric counselling and their post-surgical follow-ups. Effective systems of telemonitoring to assess the health condition at a distance have been implemented by hospitals and clinics, reducing person-to-person exposure in diagnostic steps and ensuring follow-up for chronic patients from afar [20].

From the patient's perspective, telemedicine has several clear benefits. This offers a distinct advantage of convenience for patients who would otherwise have to travel quite far to see their consultant or even just for routine follow-ups. It also reduces the chances of exposure to disease in hospitals and clinics, an enormous ripe fruit for such seasons. Other benefits of telemedicine include reducing congestion in emergency rooms and outpatient departments, which can improve the efficiency and functioning of health systems. However, challenges exist – notably about data protection issues and also with the digital divide (unequal access to technological devices), as well as legislative barriers. A lack of access to telehealth technologies, for example, high-speed internet or cell phones in rural areas, may lead to patients being left behind simply because they cannot afford new systems, and the lightning-fast changes required by healthcare are beyond them with their desktop devices.

TABLE 15.4
Key Aspects of Telemedicine and Remote Care Applications

Aspect	Details	Benefits	Challenges	Future Trends	Potential Impact
Remote consultations	Doctor–patient interactions via video/audio	Increased access to healthcare	Digital divide, tech literacy	5G-powered high-quality video consultations	Improved access to specialists
Telemonitoring	Monitoring patients with chronic conditions	Continuous health tracking	Data security, integration with EHR	AI-enhanced monitoring devices	Reduced hospital admissions
Virtual diagnostics	Remote diagnosis of medical conditions	Quicker diagnosis, reduced travel time	Diagnostic accuracy in virtual settings	VR/AR for immersive consultations	Early intervention, improved outcomes
Post-surgical care	Remote follow-ups and health tracking	Reduced hospital visits, convenience	Compliance with telehealth regulations	Smart wearable integration	Better post-operative care
Mental health services	Virtual therapy and psychiatric consultations	Increased access to mental health support	Confidentiality, patient engagement	AI-driven mental health assessments	More widespread mental healthcare

Furthermore, challenges concerning data privacy and confidentiality while providing telehealth consultation need to be addressed [21].

Telemedicine has a promising future, driven significantly by advancements in technology and evolving patient needs. . 5G networks and AI are expected to markedly improve the speed and reliability of telemedicine services, thus boosting the quality of remote diagnoses, consultations, etc. Virtual reality (VR) and augmented reality (AR): Already well on the rise, VR and hopefully soon Extended Reality (XR) will play a bigger role in enhancing telehealth experiences with an already increased focus on remote surgical assistance to Physical Therapy (PT) sessions. Further, as telemedicine moves into the mainstream of healthcare delivery, it is expected to reduce healthcare disparities by increasing access to specialist services in underserved communities. Table 15.4 shows key aspects of telemedicine and remote care applications.

15.9 INTEGRATION OF HEALTHTECH SOLUTIONS

15.9.1 Combining Technologies for Holistic Care

This possibility exists when it comes to the integration of HealthTech solutions in an even more comprehensive and systematic healthcare campaigning. Note this enables healthcare providers to use technology such as AI, blockchain, genomics, and IoT systems so that they can work together delivering holistic, patient-centric care. Real-time patient data is captured by wearable IoT devices, and the AI systems analyse it to look for trends and emerging health concerns. It serves as storage of genomic data, which can be used to make more personalized treatment plans for patients and use network security functions at a slightly higher cost than the previous system. This comprehensive model has improved outcomes via supported ongoing monitoring and tailored management [22].

15.9.2 Interoperability and Data Sharing

HealthTech integration needs to be interoperable and enable data exchange between various platforms. Variations between systems for healthcare must interface, and the repeated disparate data formats have a detrimental effect when we are trying to build an ecosystem of shared situational awareness across a continuum of sites of care. Only then can HealthTech solutions truly fulfil their potential by ensuring smooth data streamlines between systems and devices. One way to accomplish this is through blockchain technology, which can be used as a secure chain for health records so that only the right people have access to important patient data. There is a shared standardization to establish common data formats and communication protocols. Other than the integration of individual technologies like A1 or IoT should be placed within an overarching framework.

15.9.3 Future Integration Strategies

Future integration techniques will likely emphasize the development of interconnected ecosystems that unify various HealthTech solutions. Cloud-based solutions can host

TABLE 15.5
Integration of HealthTech Solutions

Technology	Application	Benefits	Challenges	Interoperability Solutions	Future Integration Strategies
AI	Predictive analytics, diagnostics	Improved accuracy in diagnosis, early interventions	Algorithmic bias, data privacy	Standardized data formats, API integrations	Cloud-based platforms integrating AI, IoT, EHRs
Blockchain	Securing patient data, data sharing	Enhanced data security, transparency	High cost, scalability issues	Blockchain-based interoperability frameworks	Secure decentralized platforms for health records
IoT	Remote patient monitoring	Real-time health data, continuous monitoring	Device interoperability, data security	Unified communication protocols	Integration with 5G for faster data transmission
Genomics	Personalized treatment, gene therapies	Tailored therapies, precise medicine	Ethical concerns, data sensitivity	Genomic data integration with EHR systems	AI-powered genomic analysis for personalized care
Telemedicine	Remote consultations, virtual care	Increased access to care, convenience	Technology access, regulatory compliance	Improved cross-platform communication tools	AI and AR/VR-enhanced telehealth consultations
Wearable devices	Fitness tracking, chronic disease monitoring	Continuous data collection, proactive care	Battery life, data integration challenges	IoT standardization for wearables	Predictive analytics for personalized health insights

AI, IoT, and genetic data, allowing healthcare providers to access and analyse information from a unified interface. The integration of 5G networks will enhance the real-time interchange of health data, ensuring expedited reactions in urgent scenarios. Advancements in AI-driven predictive analytics may furnish clinicians with real-time information, enabling more informed decision-making. Ethical frameworks need to be developed that should encourage transparency, protect data, and ensure the fairness of AI applications in healthcare. Table 15.5 shows integration of HealthTech solutions.

15.10 ETHICAL CONSIDERATIONS AND CHALLENGES

15.10.1 Addressing Ethical Concerns

The incorporation of sophisticated HealthTech solutions raises ethical issues, especially with data protection and the application of AI in decision-making processes. Data from patients gathered by IoT devices and analysed by AI systems must be safeguarded against breaches and unauthorized access. Concerns regarding algorithmic bias in AI may result in disparate healthcare results. If AI models are trained on homogeneous datasets, they may produce erroneous diagnoses for specific demographic groups. To mitigate these issues, ethical frameworks must be established that emphasize openness, data protection, and the assurance of fairness in AI applications [23].

15.10.2 Regulatory and Compliance Issues

HealthTech has rapidly developed in many places, faster than legal frameworks, bringing data protection, patient consent, and compliance challenges. To securely and legally process patient data, healthcare organizations need to comply with complex legislation such as HIPAA in the United States or GDPR in Europe. As new digital technologies such as AI, blockchain, and the IoT become commonplace in our society, regulators also need to adapt by amending existing laws or creating norms where they were not before. Confronting these regulatory obstacles will be essential for the secure and extensive implementation of HealthTech solutions, especially in cross-border healthcare contexts.

15.10.3 Ensuring Equitable Access to HealthTech

Equitable access to HealthTech is a significant issue, given the advantages of sophisticated technologies such as AI, IoT, and personalized medicine are frequently concentrated in metropolitan or affluent areas. Facilitating access to these breakthroughs for underprivileged communities is essential for mitigating healthcare inequities. Telemedicine and mobile health (mHealth) platforms can address this disparity by delivering remote healthcare services to rural or economically disadvantaged populations. Governments and healthcare organizations must cooperate to guarantee the availability of essential infrastructure, including internet connectivity and access to inexpensive HealthTech equipment, hence fostering inclusivity in healthcare. Table 15.6 shows ethical considerations and challenges in HealthTech.

TABLE 15.6
Ethical Considerations and Challenges in HealthTech

Ethical Concern	Description	Challenges	Proposed Solutions	Regulatory Frameworks	Future Strategies
Data privacy	Protecting sensitive patient information	Data breaches, unauthorized access	Strong encryption, blockchain technology	HIPAA (US), GDPR (Europe)	Strengthening patient consent and data encryption
Algorithmic bias	Bias in AI algorithms affecting treatment outcomes	Inaccurate diagnoses, unequal healthcare access	Training AI on diverse datasets, transparent algorithms	AI regulatory standards	Continuous AI model audits for bias prevention
Informed consent	Obtaining consent for data usage and AI decision-making	Complexity in AI-driven care, patient understanding	Clear consent forms, explainable AI (XAI)	National HealthTech regulations	Educating patients about AI decision-making
Accessibility	Ensuring equitable access to HealthTech	Socioeconomic and geographic barriers	Government subsidies, affordable tech solutions	Telemedicine expansion laws	Expanding infrastructure in underserved regions
Ownership of health data	Determining ownership of personal health data	Ambiguity over patient vs. provider ownership	Clear legal frameworks, blockchain for data control	Global health data sharing regulations	Patients controlling their health records via blockchain
Transparency in AI decisions	Explaining how AI arrives at healthcare decisions	Lack of transparency in AI-driven diagnosis and treatment	Development of XAI frameworks	Ethical AI guidelines for healthcare	Mandatory transparency reports for AI systems

15.11 FUTURE OUTLOOK AND PREDICTIONS

HealthTech is poised to significantly influence the future of healthcare, propelled by the growing incorporation of AI, genomics, and the IoT into routine medical practice. A significant forecast is the widespread implementation of AI-driven predictive healthcare, facilitating early diagnosis and tailored therapies. In the future, when wearable tech and IoT solutions continue to advance, these technologies will play a crucial role in managing chronic diseases and improving patient outcomes. Additionally, AI will solidify its position in healthcare systems around the world due to its ability to optimize clinical operations, reduce physician burnout, and improve diagnostic accuracy. Especially in underserved and rural areas, telemedicine is expected to progress with the help of 5G technology, allowing for more extensive virtual care and real-time patient monitoring [24].

Still, HealthTech has a long way to go before it can reach its full potential. Because of the large amounts of patient data collected by AI and IoT devices, there is a pressing need to protect this data from unauthorized access or disclosure. Comments: Today, blockchain looks like a promising high-tech way to keep all the data on one patient in need of that lockable and key-protected room for those excess records. 2021 will be another year where we just have promises as the complexities are not something you can tackle with a simple web portal on your smartphone either; back-end logic is complex. Regulatory frameworks must also evolve to keep pace with advances in technology, and innovations such as genomics and AI should be integrated into healthcare practices ethically and safely. Regulatory policies are often slower to change than technology development; thus lawmakers and regulators need to balance the promotion of innovation with ensuring patient safety.

Education, partnerships, and research and development should be the pillars of any long-term strategy for HealthTech progress. For global adoption, governments and businesses must work together to create solutions that are both scalable and cost-efficient. In addition, medical professionals need education on how to use these emerging technologies so they can be seamlessly integrated into patient treatment. Everyone, especially in areas with little resources, should be able to take advantage of HealthTech advancements, making equity a key consideration. HealthTech has the potential to revolutionize healthcare, but to overcome present challenges and ensure the industry's future success, careful planning and collaboration are required [25].

15.12 CONCLUSION

HealthTech is unequivocally transforming the healthcare sector, with innovations such as AI, blockchain, genomics, IoT, and telemedicine facilitating substantial progress in diagnoses, treatment, patient management, and data protection. AI technologies are improving diagnostic precision and facilitating individualized therapies, whereas IoT devices provide real-time patient health monitoring, resulting in more proactive care. Blockchain technology guarantees secure and transparent handling of sensitive health data, while telemedicine has expanded access to healthcare services, particularly during the global epidemic. Despite significant advancements in these technologies, problems persist, including data security issues, legal obstacles, and the necessity for equal access across diverse groups.

The next era of HealthTech development will be defined by a plethora of important areas for improvement. The use of AI and machine learning with sophisticated predictive analytics might benefit individualized treatment, hence offering, in addition, accurate preventive medicine. Additionally, advancements in blockchain technology could potentially improve data security and interoperability within healthcare systems to enable the safe and smooth transition of patient records among various platforms. Moreover, we can expect the IoT and wearable technology to evolve further and provide higher levels of reportable data for better chronic disease management or post-surgical follow-up. The system can provide a far more immersive version of telemedicine, an area where VR or AR remains barely explored. We need to discuss how these technologies should channel ethical and regulatory challenges into a sustainable, equitable resolution using HealthTech solutions. This will entail setting up the right frameworks and protocols to drive innovation and ensure patient outcomes are responsibly guarded and afforded by many.

REFERENCES

1. J. Smith, J. Brown, and M. Taylor, "The role of digital technologies in modern healthcare: Trends and future directions," *J. Healthcare Technol.*, vol. 15, no. 3, pp. 112–125, 2022.
2. R. Jones and K. Lee, "Emerging technologies in HealthTech: From AI to blockchain," *Int. J. Health Informatics*, vol. 28, no. 4, pp. 215–229, 2021.
3. S. Patel, "Digital transformation in healthcare: The impact of AI, IoT, and genomics," *Health Informatics J.*, vol. 12, no. 2, pp. 89–102, 2020.
4. E. Clark, G. Roberts, and D. Fisher, "Telemedicine in the age of COVID-19: Lessons learned and future directions," *J. Telehealth Med.*, vol. 11, no. 4, pp. 145–158, 2020.
5. L. Brown, P. Williams, and T. Zhang, "HealthTech innovations: Meeting the challenges of an ageing population," *Global J. Med. Res.*, vol. 19, no. 1, pp. 45–60, 2023.
6. P. Williams and Z. Zhang, "Healthcare challenges and solutions: The rise of digital health," *J. Health Technol.*, vol. 17, no. 2, pp. 88–97, 2022.
7. H. Kim, R. Davis, and J. Lee, "Machine learning in medicine: Advancing diagnostics and treatment," *J. Med. Artif. Intell.*, vol. 9, no. 1, pp. 34–47, 2021.
8. T. Nguyen, A. Kumar, and S. Davis, "AI in healthcare: Enhancing diagnostic accuracy and efficiency," *AI Med. J.*, vol. 10, no. 3, pp. 76–91, 2021.
9. A. Kumar and R. Davis, "Machine learning applications in healthcare: Predicting outcomes," *J. Med. Computer Sci.*, vol. 11, no. 1, pp. 22–35, 2022.
10. J. Lee, "Personalized medicine: The role of genomics in treatment optimization," *Personalized Med. J.*, vol. 7, no. 2, pp. 53–68, 2020.
11. D. Green, M. Hernandez, and N. Cole, "Genomics and health: A new era of personalized medicine," *J. Genetic Res.*, vol. 14, no. 2, pp. 101–118, 2023.
12. M. Hernandez and N. Cole, "Pharmacogenomics and its role in personalized medicine," *J. Precision Med.*, vol. 11, no. 1, pp. 45–59, 2021.
13. R. Evans, "Blockchain for healthcare data security: Current trends and prospects," *J. Blockchain Res.*, vol. 5, no. 4, pp. 256–270, 2020.
14. W. Fang, P. Johnson, and L. Reed, "Securing health data: The role of blockchain technology," *J. Health Data Security*, vol. 8, no. 1, pp. 12–25, 2022.
15. P. Johnson and L. Reed, "Blockchain in healthcare: Security and transparency," *J. Digital Health*, vol. 13, no. 2, pp. 78–89, 2021.

16. K. Martin, “Blockchain and its impact on healthcare data management,” *J. Digital Health*, vol. 6, no. 2, pp. 45–59, 2020.
17. P. White, H. Anderson, and Y. Kim, “IoT in healthcare: Enhancing patient monitoring and management,” *J. Healthcare IoT*, vol. 4, no. 3, pp. 78–92, 2021.
18. H. Anderson and Y. Kim, “IoT applications in healthcare: Revolutionizing patient care and monitoring,” *J. Health Informatics*, vol. 6, no. 2, pp. 102–118, 2022.
19. J. Park, “Internet of Things (IoT) and its applications in healthcare,” *IoT J. Med. Sci.*, vol. 2, no. 1, pp. 22–36, 2023.
20. G. Roberts and D. Fisher, “Expanding telemedicine access in underserved areas: Opportunities and challenges,” *J. Remote Healthcare*, vol. 8, no. 2, pp. 65–74, 2021.
21. S. Moore, “Reducing healthcare disparities through telemedicine: Evidence from recent studies,” *J. Telemedicine e-Health*, vol. 9, no. 2, pp. 50–64, 2022.
22. W. Johnson, R. Thompson, and F. Garcia, “Ethical considerations in HealthTech: Balancing innovation with regulation,” *J. Med. Ethics*, vol. 18, no. 1, pp. 88–102, 2023.
23. R. Thompson and F. Garcia, “HealthTech ethics: Addressing privacy and equity in digital healthcare,” *J. Healthcare Ethics*, vol. 12, no. 3, pp. 190–202, 2021.
24. J. Baker, “HealthTech ethics: Addressing privacy and equity in a digital world,” *J. Healthcare Ethics*, vol. 13, no. 3, pp. 203–217, 2020.
25. J. Lee, “Blockchain and its role in healthcare data security,” *J. Healthcare IT*, vol. 8, no. 1, pp. 34–45, 2021.

16 Embracing HealthTech for a Healthier Tomorrow

Anurag Kumar, Parth Gharat, Ashwini Dattatraya Gopwad, Rahul Maurya, and Anuradha More

16.1 INTRODUCTION

The advancement of health technology is evolving from early innovations to the current digital health landscape. This journey highlights how biotechnology, digital solutions, and regulatory frameworks have shaped modern healthcare delivery. Innovation in health technology spans a wide range of domains, including but not limited to medical equipment, diagnostics, medicines, digital health solutions, telemedicine, health informatics, and many more [1] Artificial intelligence-driven decision support systems (AI-DSS) demonstrate how AI enhances decision-making and patient outcomes. AI-DSS technologies encompass machine learning (ML), natural language processing (NLP), and deep learning. They exhibit healthcare applications such as diagnostics, personalised treatments, and risk prediction, addressing challenges like interpretability and bias. Emphasising user-centred design, workflow integration, and ethical considerations are vital for successful adoption. AI-DSS enhances healthcare delivery by advocating for continued research, interdisciplinary collaboration, and innovation [2]. AI technologies, like deep learning, considerably enhance disease detection, especially in challenging conditions such as cancer and cardiovascular diseases [3]. By analysing large-scale patient data, AI systems can identify trends and abnormalities, leading to earlier interventions and improved patient outcomes [4]. AI combines various data sources to tailor treatment strategies, forecast patient responses, and enhance therapeutic approaches. Modern technologies have transformed healthcare delivery, providing new applications and benefits. Some commonly used technologies in various fields are the Internet of Things, artificial intelligence (AI), wearable devices, telemedicine, virtual reality, and robotics. These services support personalised health and well-being. The pharmaceutical industry is experiencing significant challenges and financial burdens in clinical trial retention and adherence. With modern technologies, individuals can conveniently participate in clinical studies. In today's digital age, patients can receive more comprehensive health information through these technologies. Additionally, these methods decrease the likelihood of mistakes and accurately assess the quantity of data for improved analysis. Healthcare service providers are increasingly adopting wearable technology to proactively monitor high-risk patients in real time and predict potential health crises

DOI: 10.1201/9781003516163-16

TABLE 16.1
A Brief Overview of the Types, Uses, and Challenges of AI in Healthcare [7–9]

Type	Description	Applications	Challenges
Predictive analytics [8, 9]	The use of statistics to anticipate the outcomes of patients and potential risks of illness	Utilisation of individualised treatment strategies and early disease detection	Data privacy concerns, algorithm bias
Medical imaging analysis	Examines medical images to arrive at a correct diagnosis	Cancer detection, neurological disorder diagnosis	High costs, need for extensive training data
Virtual health assistants [9]	AI chatbots provide instant medical information and support	Patient engagement, symptom checking	Limited understanding of complex queries, potential misinformation
Clinical decision support CDS further has below types • Rule-based systems • Probabilistic systems • Cognitive models • Data-based systems • Laboratory medicine [8, 9]	Analyses patient data to assist in diagnosis and treatment decisions	• Evidence-based decision-making, workflow optimisation • Alerts for vaccinations and medication reminders • Diagnostic support for complex cases • Personalised treatment plans • Glycaemic control in ICUs • Diagnostic support and clinical management	Integration with existing systems, regulatory compliance • Usability and user experience issues • Data access and integration with existing systems • Reliability and effectiveness concerns • Synchronisation with healthcare professionals • Lack of consensus on definitions and scope

[5]. Artificial intelligence and analytics (AIA) technology improves basic healthcare in the Azzi et al. design. This paradigm meets patient needs across health conditions, including complex chronic care with comorbidities. The system links AIA technology to health outcomes to improve patient representation and management [6]. AI-DSS are revolutionising healthcare by improving diagnostics, treatment planning, and patient management. These systems use AI technologies like ML and NLP to enhance patient outcomes and simplify healthcare processes. The types of AI, their applications, and the challenges they present in the healthcare industry are detailed in Table 16.1.

16.1.1 Brief History and Evolution of HealthTech

Artificial respiratory technology emerged in the late 1950s, while the 1970s and 1980s saw the proliferation of advanced medical technology. It generated economic and ethical concerns about stopping its usage when it no longer provided advantages. The 1960s saw the respirator's expensive therapy extended to include the artificial kidney, computed tomography (CT), and magnetic resonance imaging (MRI), which led to the present use of AI and ML. AI research in the 1960s focused on imitating human intelligence. Notably, DSS have advanced tremendously due to AI-DSS initially increased cognition via cognitive theories and unstructured decision-making in 1972 and 1977. Affordable technology changed technical health care's nature and cost. Furthermore, 20–40 lab tests may run on automated analysers. Pharmaceuticals for functional and pathological sickness rose. Various developments led to AI/ML integration in health technologies [10]. The emergence of data mining and ML has revolutionised DSS, facilitating dynamic decision-making using sophisticated algorithms and neural networks [11].

16.2 THE ADOPTION OF NEW TECHNOLOGY IS CRUCIAL FOR ADVANCING FUTURE HEALTH

The chapter explores the intersection of AI and ML with healthcare technologies, highlighting their significant influence on diagnostics, treatment, and patient care. The chapter provides a comprehensive overview of the integration of AI and medical devices, showcasing their applications in various fields such as radiology, pathology, prosthetics, drug delivery, and more. The chapter covers AI-driven image interpretation, diagnostics, wearable health monitoring, and telehealth systems. Big data and computational approaches have transformed all knowledge-based professions. These developments transformed modern medicine. The COVID-19 epidemic changed diagnosis, treatment, and care. Several AI-based medical applications are evaluated for transformational potential. Clinical data patterns are used by ML algorithms to predict patient outcomes. By detecting anomalies quicker, AI aids in X-ray, CT, and MRI evaluation. AI's NLP simplifies electronic health record (EHR) data extraction for clinicians and reduces administrative work. This assists students, researchers, record-keepers, and billers [12].

16.2.1 The Current Landscape of Health Technology

The healthcare sector benefits significantly from innovations that can improve health, increase access to services, lower costs, and contribute to medical advancements. The advancements in medical technology, such as implantable devices, robotic surgery systems, prosthetics, and wearable detectors, have significantly improved patient care and medical interventions. Furthermore, various tools and methods, such as inheritable testing, point-of-care diagnostics, imaging technologies, and lab-on-a-chip bias, have significantly transformed the early detection and precise assessment of conditions, resulting in improved treatment outcomes [13]. Thinking about a product from concept to commercialisation is difficult. The majority of innovators fail to finish this complicated procedure. The innovation process might fail at any point. Early-stage startups are at high risk of failure. Product life cycles might be shorter due to fast-changing market needs and tastes, necessitating ongoing innovation and adaptation for survival [14].

16.2.2 Electronic Health Records

The combination of AI-DSS and EHRs is revolutionising healthcare. This integration is significantly enhancing clinical decision-making, leading to better patient outcomes, and making processes more efficient. This collaboration enables the efficient use of extensive health data, resulting in predictive analytics and tailored treatment approaches. EHRs are digital representations of patients' paper charts intended to enhance the collection, storage, and dissemination of health information among healthcare professionals. EHRs improve clinical decision-making, enhance patient care, and support research by providing comprehensive patient interactions and outcomes data. EHRs function as a clinical data storage tool, facilitating medical recordkeeping and decision-making procedures [15]. EHRs function as a repository for clinical data, facilitating medical documentation and decision-making procedures. They play a crucial role in maintaining structured data input and standardising medical terminology, both of which reduce errors and increase efficiency [16]. Bennett et al. conducted a case study with 423 patients treated by Centerstone in Indiana. The study showed that predictive algorithms based on EHR data could effectively predict patient treatment responses, reaching an accuracy of 72% [17]. Innovative healthcare solutions influence health outcomes, access to services, costs, and medical research. Electronic medical records (EMRs) reflect clinicians' work styles, specialties, and expertise and are used to improve diagnosis and treatment precision. EMRs integrate patient data, enabling medical professionals to make informed decisions based on comprehensive medical histories. Random forests and support vector machines enhance disease detection using EHR data [18]. EHRs make it possible to gather organised data, which is very useful for treating rare diseases [19]. This systematic method facilitates early diagnosis and focused therapy via multidisciplinary case management. EU-PEARL represents European Patient-Centric Clinical Trial Platforms.EU-PEARL simplifies protocol feasibility, site selection, patient pre-screening, and data-driven platform trial recruitment. Automated technologies and algorithms may influence healthcare providers' suggestions and actions. Personalised education, alerts, reminders, and constraints in EHRs may influence doctors' behaviours. However, these chances have not been fully utilised. EHR implementation for interventions, research, and clinical treatment is hindered by many difficulties. These include increased upfront expenses, cost–benefit symmetry uncertainty, and technical infrastructure shortages. Scientific publications have published COVID-19 research utilising real-world data, including EHR databases. As statistics and clinical epidemiology are insufficient for understanding EHR-based research's advantages and drawbacks, interpreting and using this data are difficult [20].

Fu et al. discuss the longitudinal study of disease progression, particularly Alzheimer's disease (AD), to develop personalised treatment strategies. The study examined disease trajectories, including chronological aspects and connections between events, to improve understanding of AD types, risk measurement, and development. The findings enhance patient care and medical research by enabling earlier, more accurate diagnoses and specialised care, such as managing risk factors and lifestyle changes. The study used International Classification of Diseases, 10th Revision (ICD-10) to analyse patient data from UC Health's EHRs, applying the Fine and Gray model to identify critical time-related risk factors and map diagnostic paths [21]. EHRs should allow authorised healthcare personnel to share patient data. In the best-case scenario, patients may choose any hospital, provide authorisation, and talk to a very experienced doctor. EHRs must be securely linked to the Internet and integrated with medical data to educate doctors and patients [22]. Chelladurai et al. describe the architecture of a blockchain-based EHR management system. The system provides a high-level view of how the health blockchain manages data for individuals in the healthcare system, facilitating data exchange between patients and providers. All participants must first complete a registration process to transmit data. The healthcare provider entity is divided into doctors, EHR managers, and a blockchain repository. Once registered, patients can visit any healthcare provider within the peer-to-peer (P2P) blockchain network for further care [23].

16.2.3 Telemedicine and Remote Patient Monitoring

AI-DSS and telemedicine considerably improve patient outcomes in managing chronic diseases by enhancing monitoring, adherence, and clinical decision-making. This collaboration enables quick actions and tailored support, resulting in improved health outcomes. Friedman et al. [24] developed telemedicine systems like the Telephone Linked Care (TLC system), which allow for ongoing monitoring of patient's health metrics, facilitating prompt physician interventions. This improves medication adherence and blood pressure control in hypertensive patients [25]. In today's academic landscape, advanced stand-alone systems can detect tones and analyse data to alert the user promptly. Telemedicine improves patient health and saves money. Telehealth treats diabetes and HbA1c. Telehealth for diabetic foot illness improves global access and patient satisfaction. Telehealth improves diabetes results, access, and satisfaction. Globally inclusive, patient-centred diabetic care may ensue.

16.2.4 Wearable Health Devices

Live data analysis and simple interfaces in AI-DSS linked to smartwatches are transforming several sectors. AI improves situational awareness and operational efficiency by analysing complex data. Wearable health devices enhance patient treatment by monitoring several health factors. Fitness trackers, smartwatches, and dermal wearables are their categories. They are used therapeutically in Figure 16.1. Smartwatches track heart rate (HR), activity levels, and sleep patterns. Fitness trackers emphasise physical activity and caloric expenditure. Skin-based wearables encompass tattoo-based and textile-based devices that continuously monitor physiological data [23]. Recent developments in battery technology, power recycling, and storage capacity have markedly improved the accessibility of wearable health procedures.

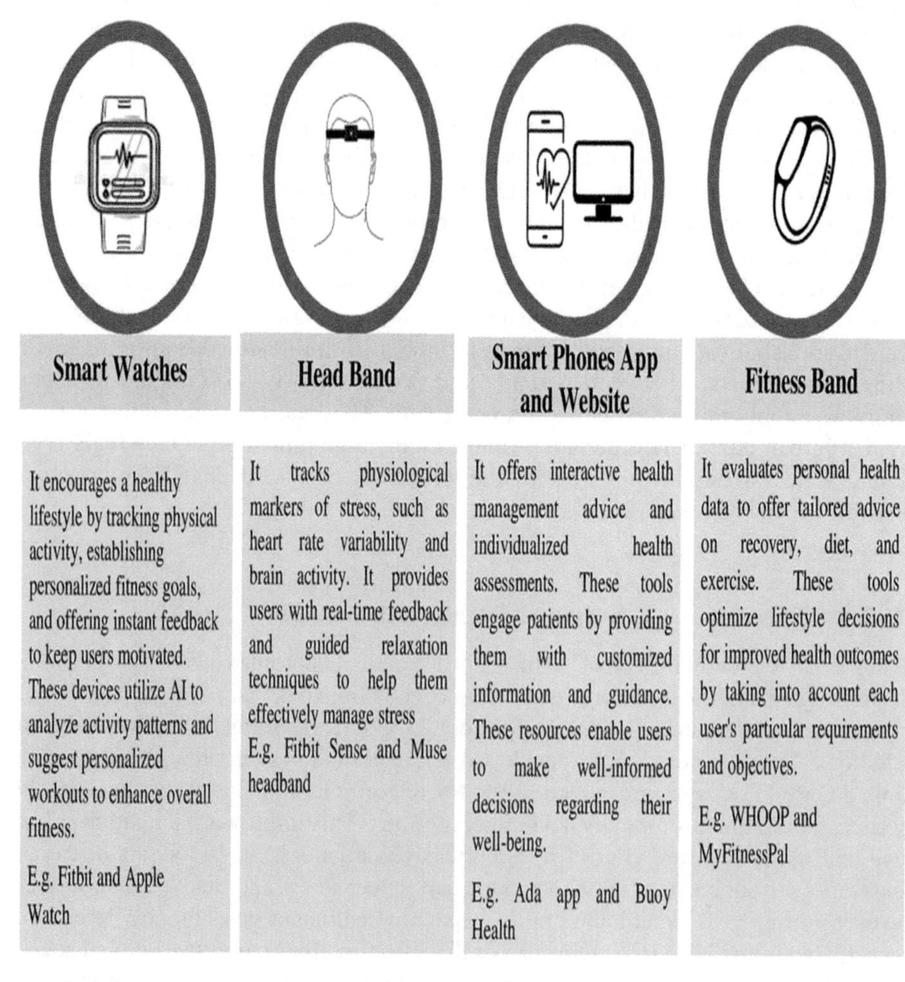

FIGURE 16.1 Examples of Healthcare Wearables with AI.

Nevertheless, there are a few drawbacks associated with these advancements. Wearable sensors have been utilised in oncology to monitor patients throughout their treatment. Although technological issues hampered patient participation, wearable technology has proven effective in managing non-coronary vascular diseases by allowing for pre-operative mobility monitoring and enhancing medication compliance. This method enables the use of patient-generated data in real time, which can improve clinical decision-making [26]. These devices use Newton's second law, wherein mass deflection in the opposite direction of motion, accompanied by a certain degree of acceleration, may be quantified electrically [27]. The smart wearable devices and their applications based on AI are shown in Figure 16.1. HR measurements during rest and activity may indicate cardiovascular disease risk. High resting HRs have been linked to an elevated risk of coronary artery disease and all-cause mortality in healthy populations. Additionally, they are widely acknowledged as a predictor of adverse outcomes in patients with heart failure (HF). Increased adverse cardiovascular events are associated with impaired HR recovery following exercise.

16.2.5 Impact on Healthcare: Cost Reduction

Reducing healthcare costs is a multifaceted challenge that can be addressed through various innovative strategies. Research indicates that implementing advanced technologies, multidisciplinary approaches, and targeted interventions can significantly lower expenses while maintaining or improving care quality. Advanced business intelligence (BI) enhances data integration and analytics, allowing healthcare firms to detect inefficiencies and improve operations. This may result in significant cost reductions and enhanced financial outcomes. Analytics helps healthcare providers make informed decisions that save money and improve operations. Data integration streamlines healthcare operations analysis by integrating processes and data sources. EHR, financial, and other data integration may give healthcare organisations a complete picture of their operations and reveal cost-cutting opportunities [28]. The GEstIC study, which stands for Grupo de Estudo da Insuficiência Cardíaca (Heart Failure Study Group), evaluated the impact of a multidisciplinary heart failure (HF) clinic on healthcare-related events and costs. GEstIC study showed that implementing a multidisciplinary clinic for HF management led to a significant decrease in all-cause hospitalisations by 53.7% and a substantial cost reduction of €1,561,213 within a year [29]. Predictive models targeting hospital readmissions have shown potential for substantial cost savings, with estimates exceeding $1 million by preventing readmissions through targeted intervention.

16.2.6 Genomics in Modern Healthcare

AI is becoming increasingly integrated into different areas of medicine, including genetics. AI algorithms can analyse large volumes of genetic data, identify patterns, and make fast and accurate predictions. The increasing involvement of AI in healthcare has the potential to revolutionise disease prevention, diagnosis, and treatment. It can provide valuable insights and enhance patient outcomes, particularly in genetic engineering and gene therapy research. AI is a valuable tool in generating hypotheses and aiding in experimental techniques. Prior genetic data can aid in identifying hereditary conditions and gene-related disorders. Drug development and discovery advancement heavily rely on using AI and ML technology. ML and AI are anticipated to have a significant influence on various aspects of the human experience, including genetics [30]. Advancements in AI have greatly enhanced the efficiency of genome sequencing, enabling scientists to accurately determine the sequence of nucleotides in an individual's DNA. AI plays a crucial role in genome sequencing. Accessing healthcare data has become more convenient by integrating medical electronic records into patient care operations. Most hospitals now offer computer-based access, making it the primary source for retrieving information. Past studies have shown that raw medical imaging data can be utilised to develop advanced and precise prognostic models. Sizeable integrated health systems can already use basic ML algorithms to automatically identify hospitalised patients at risk of being transferred to the intensive care unit (ICU) [31]. Computational tools have played a crucial role in revolutionising the drug design process, making it more efficient and effective. Traditional computational methodologies still have several issues, such as reliability, computational costs, and time costs. AI can potentially eliminate these obstacles to computational drug design, thus increasing the utilisation of computational techniques in drug development. It is also rapidly employed in the medical industry to enhance the success rates of in vitro fertilisation (IVF) procedures. AI has significantly transformed healthcare by making significant strides in genetics and disease diagnosis [32]. AI has been applied in several important domains:

- **Genomic Analysis and Sequencing:** Genomic analysis and sequencing benefit greatly from AI algorithms, which enable rapid and precise analysis of large volumes of genomic data. Researchers can now identify patterns, mutations, and genetic predispositions to diseases more efficiently than traditional methods.
- **Disease Diagnosis and Prediction:** AI algorithms can analyse complex medical data, such as genetic information, medical imaging, and patient records, to improve the early and precise detection of diseases. This may result in prompt treatments and improved patient outcomes.
- **Cancer Diagnosis and Monitoring:** ML algorithms may uncover cancer-related patterns in genomic data. Early diagnosis, subtype classification, and cancer recurrence risk prediction may all benefit from these models. Utilising AI technology for early diagnosis and monitoring improves treatment plans, resulting in better patient outcomes.
- **Patient Ancestry Prediction:** By analysing genetic markers, AI systems can predict an individual's ancestral ancestry. This is accomplished by comparing the genetic profile to reference databases of diverse demographic groupings. Ancestral prediction could have significant implications in personalised medicine considering the potential associations between different populations and genetic variants. In addition, it aids in personalised healthcare planning.
- **Genetic Engineering:** AI is vital for gene editing technologies like Clustered Regularly Interspaced Short Palindromic Repeats (CRISPR). ML techniques help to optimise the design of genetic alterations and forecast the results of gene edits.

- **AI-Integrated Personalised Medicine:** It allows healthcare practitioners to customise therapies based on individual genetic profiles. Genetic differences impact medication metabolism, and it is considered to optimise therapy effectiveness.
- **Precision Medicine:** AI assists in identifying subgroups within populations that may exhibit variable disease susceptibilities or respond differently to treatments, as determined by genetic markers. This enables more accurate and focused healthcare interventions.
- **Genetic Counselling:** AI technologies aid genetic counsellors in analysing complicated genetic data, leading to more accurate risk assessments and patient explanations.

16.2.6.1 Ethical Issues

AI in genetics has the potential to change healthcare by improving genetics and disease detection, but ethical issues such as patient privacy, genetic testing permission, and responsible data use must be addressed. Further research, cooperation among AI experts, healthcare practitioners, and ethical considerations are needed to advance AI in these fields. AI has influenced several scientific fields, including functional genomics, which manages massive data volumes. Sequencing advances have created massive functional genomics data. AI has made gene expression, epigenetic modifications, binding site locations, regulatory processes, and variation–disease connections easier to understand [33]. In recent decades, AI has gained popularity as a valuable tool in various life science disciplines, especially in fields with intricate mechanisms and extensive data production. Some critical applications include predicting DNA regulatory regions, discovering cell morphology and spatial organisation, identifying associations between phenotypes and genotypes, classifying DNA methylation and histone modifications, discovering biomarkers, detecting transcriptional enhancers, diagnosing cancer, and analysing evolutionary mechanisms [34]. Understanding the impact of genetic mutations on healthcare is crucial as they can influence an individual's vulnerability to diseases and how they respond to treatment. It is crucial to understand these mutations to make precise diagnoses and administer effective treatments. Although coding area mutations in the genome often get much attention, non-coding region mutations should also be acknowledged for their significance. Changes in these areas can impact how transcription factors bind and regulate genes. These mutations may play a role in the onset of disease. Having a clear understanding of the genetic basis of the disease is crucial for developing targeted therapies, identifying high-risk individuals, and advancing personalised treatment approaches. AI is the latest and most advanced approach to address these issues. AI models may analyse various types of biological data to identify genetic mutations and predict their potential effects [35]. There are numerous benefits to using this approach instead of traditional methods. These include enhanced accuracy, streamlined analysis, the ability to identify new mutations, integration with clinical data for personalised medicine, and the discovery of disease-related biomarkers. Despite being in its early stages, the application of AI/ML tools in genomics has already proven advantageous for researchers. They have been able to develop programmes that provide targeted assistance. Facial analysis can be used to examine people's faces. AI programmes can accurately identify genetic disorders. They are applying ML methods to determine the primary type of cancer from a liquid biopsy and to forecast the progression of a specific type of cancer in a patient. Using ML to differentiate disease-causing genomic variants from benign ones. Applying deep learning techniques to enhance the performance of gene editing tools like CRISPR. The combination of AI, genomics, and precision medicine has the potential to revolutionise healthcare by providing personalised treatment options and improved disease management. Through the utilisation of AI-driven drug discovery, integration of genomic data, advancement of precision medicine, the discovery of biomarkers, and adherence to ethical AI practices, the full potential of these technologies will be realised in the near future, resulting in improved patient outcomes and increased innovation in healthcare. This research is essential for the development of therapies that can effectively benefit diverse demographic groups.

Functional genomic data has contributed to the advancement of cancer precision medicine. Functional genomics has made significant progress in informing precision medicine for common non-cancer disorders, like kidney disease. Examples demonstrate the use of ML and statistical techniques to evaluate functional genomics data from disease-relevant tissues. This helps advance the field of precision medicine for common non-cancer disorders [36, 37].

16.3 THE USE OF ARTIFICIAL INTELLIGENCE AND MACHINE LEARNING IN THE PHARMACEUTICAL INDUSTRY, WITH A FOCUS ON DRUG DELIVERY SYSTEMS

Drug delivery technology has advanced to meet demand. The first-generation technology improved medication solubility, stability, and bioavailability. However, cell membranes and the blood–brain barrier were issues. Biological obstacles were overcome by second-generation drug delivery. Improved penetration, targeted tissue or cell dispersion, and bodily defence protection. Second-generation drugs worked better and had fewer negative effects. Second-generation drug delivery systems have improved yet have physicochemical and biological constraints. Innovative approaches in third-generation pharmaceutical delivery address complex biological and physicochemical obstacles.

Addressing biological obstacles and improving target site drug transport improve solubility, stability, and release kinetics [38]. AI is revolutionising drug discovery and delivery in the pharmaceutical industry, completely changing traditional approaches. AI algorithms in drug discovery rapidly analyse extensive biological and chemical datasets to identify potential drug candidates with exceptional accuracy. Software like stats Ease-DOE Pro®, Discovery Studio®, Chem draw, PubChem [39], etc. have proven useful. The database helps analyse drug molecules and their physiochemical properties. AI algorithms in drug discovery rapidly analyse extensive biological and chemical datasets to identify potential drug candidates with exceptional accuracy. ML techniques, such as Quantitative Structure–Activity Relationship (QSAR) models, predict physicochemical properties and biological interactions, streamlining the development process [40]. Three packages exist: MULTIVAR, PLANEX, and INTERLAB. These software programs serve distinct functions in statistical analysis, tailored for chemists and facilitating drug discovery [41]. AI can also help drug repurpose by discovering new therapeutic applications for existing medications. In drug delivery,

AI optimises formulations and systems, allowing for more precise and individualised approaches. Intelligent algorithms improve the comprehension of pharmacokinetics and pharmacodynamics, thus guiding the creation of precise medicine strategies [42]. Integrating AI and ML in the pharmaceutical industry is revolutionising drug delivery systems, enhancing efficiency and precision in drug development. AI algorithms analyse extensive biological data to identify drug candidates and optimise formulations, leading to targeted therapies and improved patient outcomes.

16.3.1 Integration of Artificial Intelligence and Machine Learning in Healthcare

Two subgroups of AI are ML and deep learning. They utilise multilayer neural networks and high-performance algorithms to address various problems effectively. Structured data, including genetic, electrophysical, and imaging data, undergoes a thorough examination in medical diagnosis using ML techniques. In healthcare, AI provides advanced tools and techniques for medication design, telemedicine, doctor–patient communication through chatbots, and intelligent machines for analysing disease causes and likelihood of occurrence. Large language models (LLMs) allow conversational bots to engage patients in meaningful discussions and provide individualised health advice and assistance [43]. Chatbots that use AI can look at a user's symptoms and medical history to make personalised suggestions that make patients happier. AI's predictive abilities enable healthcare providers to customise care plans using individual patient data, boosting patient autonomy and engagement [44]. ML algorithms can analyse patient feedback in real time, identifying themes and sentiments to drive improvements in care delivery. AI streamlines administrative tasks like scheduling appointments and allocating resources, resulting in more efficient healthcare systems and better patient experiences. While the integration of AI and ML in healthcare presents significant opportunities, it also raises concerns regarding data privacy and algorithmic bias, necessitating careful consideration and ethical oversight. AI field is dedicated to developing intelligent computer systems capable of recognising, processing, and responding to inputs [45]. Researchers believe that the sky is not the limit for new inventions. AI draws from various disciplines, such as mathematics, biology, philosophy, psychology, neuroscience, statistics, and computer science. AI aims to create transparent, interpretable, and explainable systems to improve intelligent agents' capabilities. The idea of trusting machines as human replicas began with the invention of the Turing test, which evaluates a machine's intelligence based on its ability to respond to instructions like a human. If the machine passes the test, it is deemed intelligent. AI has significantly impacted various aspects of society, ushering in a new era in this digital revolution.

16.3.2 Artificial Intelligence-Powered Genetic Mutation and Pattern Detection Tools

While AI algorithms take their cues from human intellect, their application in clinical genomics tends to focus on tasks that are both difficult for humans to complete and prone to mistakes when dealing with conventional statistical methods. Several methods discussed earlier have been adapted to address various aspects of clinical genomic analysis, including variant calling, genome annotation, variant classification, and phenotype-to-genotype correspondence. In the future, they could also be utilised to predict genotypes based on phenotypes. Therapeutic interpretation of genomes requires extreme accuracy in detecting individual genetic variants. Standard variant-calling techniques often face systemic errors due to sample preparation, sequencing technology, sequence context, and biological influences. AI algorithms, such as Convolutional Neural Network (CNN), can address these issues by understanding population-level dependencies and strand bias, leading to biased mistakes but high accuracy. Deep variant, a CNN-based variant caller, was trained on read alignments and has performed better than traditional techniques for specific variant-calling tasks. CNN's ability to recognise intricate relationships in sequencing data is believed to be the reason for increased accuracy. Deep learning has the potential to transform base calling and variant identification for nanopore-based sequencing technologies, which have traditionally struggled to compete with established sequencing technologies due to inaccuracies [46, 47]. In human genomics, it is still challenging to computationally identify and predict non-coding pathogenic variation [48]. Recent research suggests that AI systems will significantly enhance our understanding of non-coding genetic diversity. Splicing defects in genes are responsible for a significant portion, approximately 10%, of rare pathogenic genetic variation [49]. Identifying defects related to gene splicing can be challenging due to the complexity of various DNA interactions that influence the process, such as intronic and exonic splicing enhancers, silencers, and insulators. Splice-AI, a 32-layer deep neural network, can accurately predict canonical and non-canonical splicing using exon–intron junction sequence data [50]. Identifying these abnormalities may be problematic owing to the intricate nature of intronic and exonic splicing enhancers, silencers, insulators, and other DNA interactions that affect gene splicing, which include long-range and combinatorial mechanisms. A neural network, SpliceAI, can accurately predict canonical and non-canonical splicing using exon–intron junction sequence data, providing an excellent example of the corroboration of AI in healthcare. Molecular illness diagnosis requires identifying pathogenic variations and understanding how they influence the patient's phenotype [48]. AI algorithms may improve phenotype-to-genotype mapping, notably in extracting higher-level diagnostic ideas from medical images and EHRs. Various types of AI are shown in Figure 16.2. According to their functions, capabilities, and typical uses, Weak AI follows commands. For example. Siri, Alexa, Alpha Go, Watson, and Sophia robots do not think or behave like humans. Future events may alter this. Strong AI should compete with human intelligence. Outperforming others is difficult yet possible. Machines may replace humans. Stephen Hawking and others consider it a significant social danger.

16.3.3 Healthcare Machine Learning: A Necessary but Daunting Task

ML involves the creation of algorithms that allow computers to learn from their data and previous experiences [51]. Independently using this approach, the machine evaluates the training data, or accessible dataset, and uses algorithms to forecast the

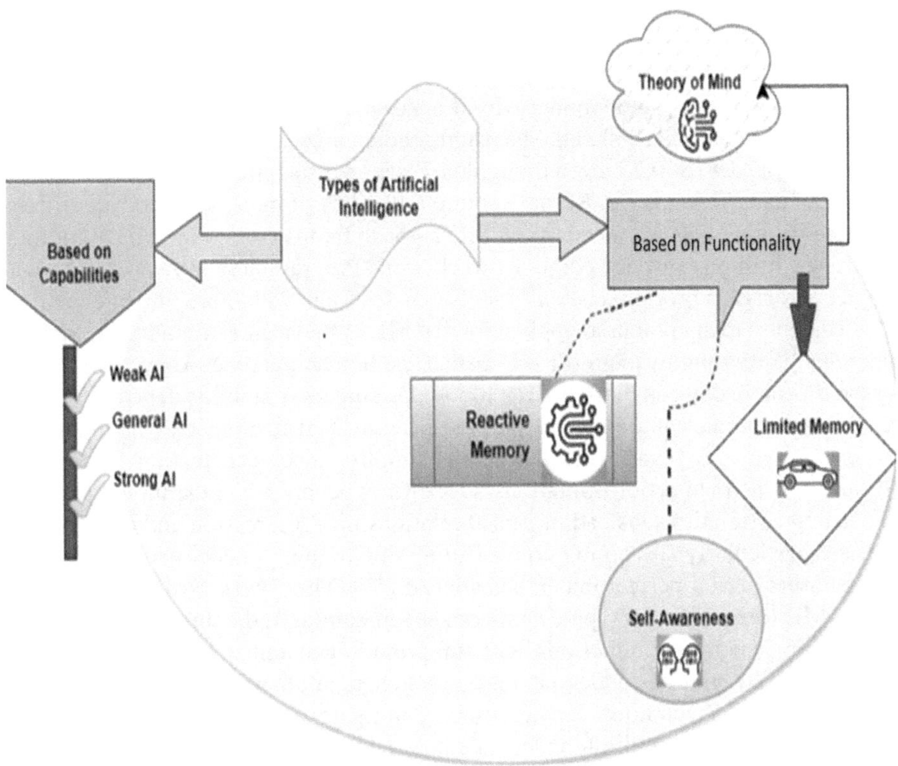

FIGURE 16.2 Types of AI Based on Function and Capabilities.

potential output based on the input. The more data provided, the better the performance or prediction becomes. Simply put, the more data the machine acquires, the more it can enhance its efficiency. It can learn from data and make automatic improvements. This resource is handy for managing large amounts of complex data and solving complicated problems that would otherwise be time-consuming for humans. The machine receives input data and produces results using a suitable algorithm. ML is a sophisticated procedure that uses data to acquire knowledge and enhance performance. There are three main types of categorisations: supervised learning, unsupervised learning, and reinforcement learning. Supervised learning is a process in which the machine is provided with labelled data to grasp various concepts [52, 53]. Unsupervised learning, in contrast, entails the machine training itself without any external guidance, utilising unlabelled or unclassified data. This method is effective in refining data to align with the desired outputs. Reinforcement learning is a feedback-based approach where the machine is rewarded for correct actions and penalised for wrong ones. Reinforcement learning encompasses various fascinating applications, such as robotic dogs learning from their mistakes and computers mastering video games [54]. ML is extensively utilised in many domains, including medical diagnosis, image processing, photo tagging applications, etc. The primary benefit of ML lies in its iterative nature and ability to learn autonomously [55]. If AI performed well in medical tests, one could wonder why it is not performing better. In one study that predicted cardiovascular risk, all AI systems had an areas under the receiver operator curve (AUC). AUC of 0.75, even though the researchers supplied the AI with practically all the data. To improve, AI may require more data or more advanced algorithms. Big data training sets are needed for ML algorithms to work well. ML algorithms often need millions of data points to work well. Programmers say more data with simpler algorithms produces better models than less data with more intricate methods [56]. There are many potential applications of ML in the healthcare industry. Medical data must be thoroughly examined. Consider the human genome. About 100 MB per person. Portable devices monitor HR, blood pressure, and mobility. The data reveals that ML can predict ailments and provide personalised treatments. ML algorithms can categorise X-ray and MRI images to simplify disease detection for doctors. ML also has its own set of limitations. Overfitting occurs when the model produces misleading correlations instead of causal relationships. Regression and classification trees are particularly susceptible to overfitting due to their tendency to continuously split datasets until a perfect match is achieved [57]. The "black box" is a constraint in ML. ML often involves inputting model specifications and data into the software, which then generates predictions without providing detailed explanations for its conclusions. Without this understanding, researchers might miss vital signs of flawed models. Validation techniques are necessary to mitigate the risks of black box analysis and overfitting. Using multiple independent patient cohorts to analyse the predictive capabilities of models can help determine the generalisability of study findings. The Clinical Bidirectional Encoder Representations from Transformers (Clinical BERT) model, utilising the first 3–5 days of clinical notes, omitting discharge notes, may predict hospital readmission risk using NLP [58]. Figure 16.3 demonstrates how during an outbreak like COVID-19, ML-based decision support systems may aid clinical practice. Accurate diagnosis and prediction of patient outcomes may improve medical resource management. In contrast to conventional methods, ML algorithms

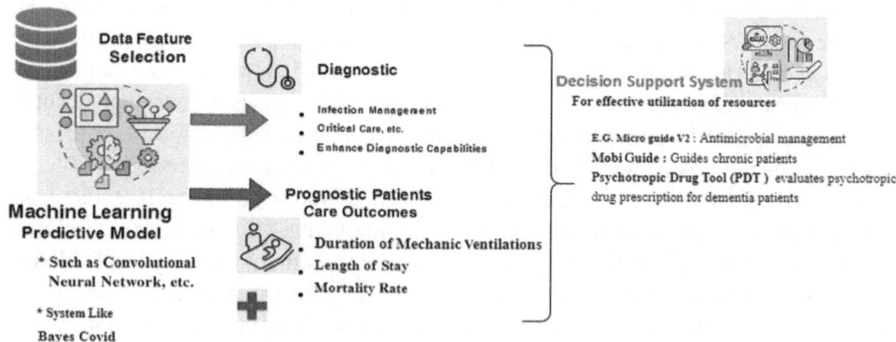

FIGURE 16.3 Effect of ML Model and Decision Support System Impact on Health Care.

enable non-linear model selection and prediction of clinical outcomes, while online training techniques upgrade DSS as epidemic data grows [59].

While AI holds promise for various health applications, researchers must also consider AI's broader social, ethical, and economic implications. Concerns about AI safety are growing as AI gains more autonomy. AI presents two additional challenges: defining personhood legally and understanding the psychological experience of human identity as AI becomes more human-like. The issue is exacerbated by the inevitable rise of more advanced human–machine hybrids.

16.4 OBSTACLES TO INTEGRATING ARTIFICIAL INTELLIGENCE AND MACHINE LEARNING

The integration of AI and ML in healthcare presents significant opportunities but also faces notable resistance and interoperability challenges. Understanding these dynamics is crucial for successful implementation.

16.4.1 Resistance from Healthcare Professionals

Healthcare professionals frequently resist due to worries about job security, trust in AI systems, and the risk of algorithmic bias [60]. AI acceptance delays and scepticism are everyday forms of pushback that reveal greater problems with trust and how these problems are seen to affect patient care [61].

16.4.2 Interoperability Challenges

Interoperability constitutes a significant obstacle, as heterogeneous systems fail to interact efficiently, impeding data exchange and integration [62].

- Limited standardisation hinders healthcare AI/ML technology use. According to Krones et al., applying AI models in low-income settings like rural Brazil might be challenging due to generalisation and practical application challenges. Fragmented data collection and storage hamper AI healthcare in high- and low-income countries [63].
- The integration of AI and ML across various sectors faces significant challenges due to the lack of comprehensive regulatory frameworks. This absence complicates compliance and accountability, particularly in critical areas such as law, drug development, and financial reporting. Lack of unified frameworks makes AI and ML integration across industries difficult. The absence of standardisation makes compliance and accountability difficult, especially in legislation, medication research, and financial reporting.
- The rigorous clinical validation of AI and ML technologies is crucial for their successful incorporation into healthcare. Nonetheless, existing approaches and criteria for testing these systems in practical clinical environments are still inadequately examined. A systematic review of 32 studies indicated that the majority of AI-enabled clinical decision support systems (CDSS) predominantly emphasise image recognition and risk assessment; however, only 12

studies documented real-world performance metrics, highlighting a substantial deficiency in validation practices [64].

16.5 FUTURE PROSPECTS AND INNOVATIONS

The future of healthcare innovations involving AI, EHR, and wearables is poised for significant transformation. These technologies promise to enhance patient care, streamline operations, and improve health outcomes. AI applications are expanding in diagnostics, treatment planning, and patient monitoring, demonstrating accuracy comparable to human specialist [65]. Algorithms based on ML within EHR systems have the capability to forecast comorbidities, thereby facilitating timely healthcare interventions [66]. Wearables equipped with AI can continuously monitor vital signs, alerting healthcare providers to potential health issues before they escalate Technological advances have revolutionised fields that seek to solve human issues. Non-invasive liquid biopsies may deliver precise diagnosis and disease stages using molecular biomarkers. ML, high-throughput sequencing techniques, and microRNA (miRNA) profiling help identify DNA alterations or discover new biomarkers. Biphotonic and Raman spectroscopy tissue examination using nanoparticles improves sickness diagnosis. Drug synthesis may be exact, stage-specific, structure-based, and targeted using in vitro and in vivo models. Bioinformatic tools for omics have simplified high-throughput data analysis and provide precise results in less time. ML algorithms understand drug binding kinetics and mechanics [67]. Collaborative research has developed an approach to enhance clinical research and trial procedures in cardiology. With short- and long-term suggestions, the collaborative promotes cardiovascular medication and device innovation. Strengthen trial patient-centeredness and involvement, real-world evidence, stakeholder needs, and the cardiovascular clinical research network of healthcare organisations [68]. Despite the challenges of Cardiovascular Disease (CVD), which is the most common cause of mortality and disability, the US has a low enrolment rate in drug and device studies and a lag in drug innovation. Innovative technologies can enhance patient engagement, produce high-quality evidence in practical contexts, and ensure that evidence meets the needs of all parties involved. Industry and authorities must commit to collaboration in early talks about trial innovation [69].

16.6 CONCLUSION

Health technology, genomics, novel drug delivery, and AI/ML are transforming the healthcare sector, leading to a healthier future with precision medicine and innovative treatment strategies. This collaboration improves the accuracy of diagnoses, tailors treatment plans, and expedites the process of discovering new drugs, all leading to better patient outcomes. Health technology, especially high-throughput sequencing, produces extensive genomic data to discover diseases, their associations, and biomarkers. AI applications in healthcare optimise data analysis, converting raw data into practical clinical insights. AI and ML enhance the analysis of intricate genomic data, leading to better risk prediction and clinical decision-making. These technologies enable the advancement of personalised medicine, with treatments customised to the genetic variations of individuals. Although these innovations hold great potential, addressing challenges like data privacy, algorithmic transparency, and robust clinical validation is crucial for their successful implementation in healthcare.

REFERENCES

[1] S. Sharma, R. Rawal, and D. Shah, "Addressing the challenges of AI-based telemedicine: Best practices and lessons learned," *Journal of Education Education Health Promotion*, vol. 1, pp. 338, Sept. 2023.

[2] M. Elhaddad and S. Hamam, "AI-driven clinical decision support systems: An ongoing pursuit of etpotential," *Cureus*, Apr. 2024, https://doi.org/10.7759/cureus.57728.

[3] P. Mathur, S. Srivastava, X. Xu, and J. L. Mehta, "Artificial intelligence, machine learning, and cardiovascular disease," *Clinical Medicine Insights: Cardiology*, vol. 14, p. 118954682092740, Jan. 2020, https://doi.org/10.1177/1179546820927404.

[4] I. Mishra, V. Kashyap, R. Pahwa, and R. Dheivanai, "Revolutionizing healthcare: The impact and growth of artificial intelligence (AI)," *International Research Journal on Advanced Engineering Hub (IRJAEH)*, vol. 2, no. 07, pp. 1875–1881, Jul. 2024, https://doi.org/10.47392/irjaeh.2024.0257.

[5] A. Haleem, M. Javaid, R. Suman, and R. Vaishya, "Exploring the capabilities of modern technologies for health care," *DOAJ: Directory of Open Access Journals*, Jan. 2022, https://doi.org/10.4103/am.am_128_21.

[6] S. Azzi, S. Gagnon, A. Ramirez, and G. Richards, Healthcare applications of artificial intelligence and analytics: A review and proposed framework. *Applied Sciences*, vol. 10, p. 6553, 2020.

[7] F. E. Ekpar, "A comprehensive artificial intelligence-driven healthcare system," *European Journal of Electrical Engineering and Computer Science*, vol. 8, no. 3, pp. 1–6, 2024.

[8] D. S. Gour, P. M. Joshi, and D. A. R. Qureshi, "Artificial intelligence and intelligent computing techniques for healthcare decision support," in *Artificial Intelligence and Their Applications*, Iterative International Publishers, Selfypage Developers Pvt Ltd, 2024, pp. 97–116.

[9] J. G. Carrasco Ramírez, "AI in healthcare: Revolutionizing patient care with predictive analytics and decision support systems," *Journal of Artificial Intelligence General science (JAIGS)*, ISSN:3006-4023, vol. 1, no. 1, pp. 31–37, 2024.

[10] E. Jonsson and S. J. Reiser, "The history of the International Journal of Technology Assessment in Health Care," *International Journal of Technology Assessment in Health Care*, vol. 25, no. S1, pp. 11–18, Jul. 2009, https://doi.org/10.1017/s0266462309090357.

[11] G. Phillips-Wren, M. Daly, and F. Burstein, "Support for cognition in decision support systems: An exploratory historical review," *Journal of Decision Systems*, vol. 31, no. suppl. 1, pp. 18–30, 2022.

[12] B. Asgarova, E. Jafarov, N. Babayev, A. Ahmadzada, V. Abdullayev, and T. Triwiyanto, "Development process of decision support systems using data mining technology," *Indonesian Journal of Electrical Engineering and Computer Science*, vol. 36, no. 1, p. 703, 2024.

[13] R. Kulshrestha, V. G. Shanmuga Priya, S. Awasthi, R. C. Prasad, and M. S. Sheeja, "AI & ML in medicine," in *Futuristic Trends in Biotechnology, Volume 3, Book 22* (pp. 233–245), IIP Series, Mar. 2024, https://doi.org/10.58532/v3bkbt22p5ch1.

[14] D. J. Devi, D. N. Jain, Z. N. Rodoshi, and A. Kumar G, *Advancements in Healthcare Technology*. Amkcorp Research Technologies Private Limited, 18 Apr. 2024.

[15] L. Burton, F. Milad, R. Janke, and K. L. Rush, "The landscape of health technology for equity deserving groups in rural communities: A systematic review," *Community Health Equity Research & Policy*, 2024.

[16] A. Bednorz, J. Mak, J. Jylhävä, and D. Religa, "Use of electronic medical records (EMR) in gerontology: Benefits, considerations and a promising future," *Clinical Interventions in Aging*, vol. 18, pp. 2171–2183, 2023.

[17] C. C. Bennett, T. W. Doub, and R. Selove, "EHRs connect research and practice: Where predictive modelling, artificial intelligence, and clinical decision support intersect," *Health Policy and Technology*, vol. 1, no. 2, pp. 105–114, 2012.

[18] I. Keshta and A. Odeh, "Security and privacy of electronic health records: Concerns and challenges," *Egyptian Informatics Journal*, vol. 22, no. 2, pp. 177–183, 2021, https://doi.org/10.1016/j.eij.2020.07.003.

[19] P. Kumar, V. Subathra, Y. Swasthika, and V. Vishal, 1. Disease diagnosis using machine earning on electronic health records. 2024, doi: 10.1109/ic3iot60841.2024.10550235

[20] R. Asarnusch, C. Daniela, B. Christoph, U. Melanie, and M. Tim, Practical use of electronic patient records: findings from two care projects in centres for rare diseases. *Bundesgesundheitsblatt-gesundheitsforschung-gesundheitsschutz*, 2022, doi: 10.1007/s00103-022-03599-8.

[21] C. Péter, and K. Matti, 4. Electronic health record databases provide a platform for intervention studies. *Acta Paediatrica*, 2022, doi: 10.1111/apa.16329.

[22] M. Fu and T. S. Chang, 5. Identifying common disease trajectories of Alzheimer's disease with electronic health records. *medRxiv*, 2024, doi: 10.1101/2024.07.26.24311084.

[23] U. Chelladurai and S. Pandian, "A novel blockchain based electronic health record automation system for healthcare," *Journal of Ambient Intelligence and Humanized Computing*, vol. 13, no. 1, pp. 693–703, 2022.

[24] R. H. Friedman, et al., "A telecommunications system to manage patients with chronic disease," *Studies in Health Technology and Informatics*, vol. 52, Pt 2, pp. 1330–1334, 1998.

[25] L. Li, J. Zhou, Z. Gao, W. Hua, L. Fan, H. Yu, L. Hagen et al. "A scoping review of using large language models (LLMs) to investigate electronic health records (EHRs)" ArXiv, (2024). Accessed December 25, 2024. https://arxiv.org/abs/2405.03066.

[26] H. Motahari-Nezhad, F. Zare, H. Akbari, and A. Sadeghdaghighi, "Health outcomes of Fitbit, Garmin or Apple watch-based interventions: A systematic review of systematic reviews," *Baltic Journal of Health and Physical Activity*, 2022.

[27] S. K. Shah, M. T. Mardini, and T. M. Manini, "Narrative review of advances in smart wearables for noncoronary vascular disease," *JVS-Vascular Insights*, vol. 2, p. 100103, 2024.

[28] K. Bayoumy, et al., "Smart wearable devices in cardiovascular care: where we are and how to move forward," *Nature Reviews Cardiology*, vol. 18, no. 8, pp. 581–599, 2021.

[29] N. T. Nwosu, "Reducing operational costs in healthcare through advanced BI tools and data integration," *World Journal of Advanced Research and Reviews*, vol. 22, no. 3, pp. 1144–1156, 2024.

[30] R. Rego, N. Pereira, A. Pinto, S. Pereira, and I. Marques, "Impact of a heart failure multidisciplinary clinic on the reduction of healthcare-related events and costs: the GEstIC study," *Frontiers in Cardiovascular Medicine*, vol. 10, 2023.

[31] A. Rajkomar, J. Dean, and I. Kohane, Machine learning in medicine. *New England Journal of Medicine*, vol. 380, 1347–1358, 2019. doi: 10.1056/NEJMra1814259.

[32] C. Caudai, A. Galizia, F. Geraci, L. L. Pera, V. Morea, and E. Salerno, "Allegra via, Teresa Colombo, AI applications in functional genomics," *Computational and Structural Biotechnology Journal*, vol. 19, pp. 5762–5790, 2021.

[33] R. Li, L. Li, Y. Xu, and J. Yang, "Machine learning meets omics: Applications and perspectives," *Briefings in Bioinformatics*, vol. 23, no. 1, 2022.

[34] M. Mann, C. Kumar, W.-F. Zeng, and M. T. Strauss, "Artificial intelligence for proteomics and biomarker discovery," *Cell Systems*, vol. 12, no. 8, pp. 759–770, 2021.

[35] G. Novakovsky, N. Dexter, M. W. Libbrecht, W. W. Wasserman, and S. Mostafavi. Obtaining genetics insights from deep learning via explainable artificial intelligence. *Nature Review Genetics*, 24(2), pp. 125–137, Feb 2023. doi: 10.1038/s41576-022-00532-2. Epub 2022 Oct 3. PMID: 36192604.

[36] C. Huang, R. Mezencev, J. F. Mcdonald, and F. Vannberg, "Open source machine-learning algorithms for predicting optimal cancer drug therapies," *PLOS ONE*, vol. 12, 2017.

[37] S. Huang, N. Cai, P. P. Pacheco, S. Narrandes, Y. Wang, and W. Xu, "Applications of support vector machine (SVM) learning in cancer genomics," *Cancer Genomics Proteomics*, vol. 15, pp. 41–51, 2018.

[38] A. D. Gholap, M. J. Uddin, M. Faiyazuddin, A. Omri, S. Gowri, and M. Khalid, "Advances in artificial intelligence in drug delivery and development: A comprehensive review." *Computers in Biology and Medicine*, 108702, 2024.

[39] E. E. Bolton, S. Kim, and S. H. Bryant. 3. PubChem3D: Similar conformers. *Journal of Cheminformatics*, 2011. doi: 10.1186/1758-2946-3-13.

[40] Haval Abhijeet Madhukar, Kumar Shwetabh, and Sushree Sasmita Dash. "Machine learning-based enhanced drug delivery system and its applications–a systematic review." *J Angiother,* vol. 642, 2023: 123098.

[41] D. Wienke, U. Wank, M. Wagner, and K. Danzer, "MULTIVAR, PLANEX, INTERLAB – from a collection of algorithms to an expert system: Statistics software written from chemists for chemists," in *Software Development in Chemistry 5*, Berlin, Heidelberg: Springer Berlin Heidelberg, 1991, pp. 113–127.

[42] K. Chinnaiyan, S. L. Mugundhan, D. Narayanasamy, and M. Mohan, "Revolutionizing healthcare and drug discovery: The impact of artificial intelligence on pharmaceutical development," *Current Drug Therapy*, vol. 19, 2024.

[43] B. Wen, R. Norel, J. Liu, T. Stappenbeck, F. Zulkernine, and H. Chen, "Leveraging large language models for patient engagement: The power of conversational AI in digital health," *arXiv [cs.AI]*, 2024.

[44] O. Johnson, The role of AI and mobile apps in patient-centric healthcare delivery. *World Journal of Advanced Research and Reviews*, 2024. doi: 10.30574/wjarr.2024.22.1.1331.

[45] M. Yakubova and Tashkent State University of Law. (2024). "The legal challenges of regulating AI in cybersecurity: A comparative analysis of Uzbekistan and global approaches. *International Journal of Law and Policy*, vol. 2, no. 7, 2024, pp. 7–9. https://app.paperpile.com/view/?id=0113999c-8deb-4bc1-b339-3333cd0e1f00

[46] H. Li, "Towards better understanding of artifacts in variant calling from high-coverage samples," *arXiv [q-bio.GN]*, 2014.

[47] E. Garrison and G. Marth, "Haplotype-based variant detection from short-read sequencing," *arXiv [q-bio.GN]*, 2012.

[48] O. Simeone, "A brief introduction to machine learning for engineers," *Foundations and Trends® in Signal Processing*, vol. 12, no. 3–4, pp. 200–431, 2018.

[49] R. Soemedi, et al., "Pathogenic variants that alter protein code often disrupt splicing," *Nature Genetics*, vol. 49, no. 6, pp. 848–855, 2017.

[50] A. Telenti, "Deep sequencing of 10,000 human genomes," *Proceedings of the National Academy of Sciences of the United States of America*, vol. 113, no. 42, pp. 11901–11906, 2016.

[51] X. Wang, X. Lin, and X. Dang, "Supervised learning in spiking neural networks: A review of algorithms and evaluations," *Neural Network*, vol. 125, pp. 258–280, 2020.

[52] F. Jiang, "Artificial intelligence in healthcare: Past, present and future," *Stroke and Vascular Neurology*, vol. 2, no. 4, pp. 230–243, 2017.

[53] O. Simeone, "A very brief introduction to machine learning with applications to communication systems," *IEEE Transactions on Cognitive Communications and Networking*, vol. 4, no. 4, pp. 648–664, 2018.

[54] A. Halevy, P. Norvig, and F. Pereira, "The unreasonable effectiveness of data," *IEEE Intelligent Systems*, vol. 24, no. 2, pp. 8–12, 2009.

[55] K. R. Foster, R. Koprowski, and J. D. Skufca, "Machine learning, medical diagnosis, and biomedical engineering research – commentary," *BioMedical Engineering OnLine*, vol. 13, no. 1, p. 94, 2014.

[56] O. M. Doyle, M. A. Mehta, and M. J. Brammer, "The role of machine learning in neuroimaging for drug discovery and development," *Psychopharmacology (Berl.)*, vol. 232, no. 21–22, pp. 4179–4189, 2015.

[57] B. D. Mittelstadt, P. Allo, M. Taddeo, S. Wachter, and L. Floridi, "The ethics of algorithms: Mapping the debate," *Big Data & Society*, vol. 3, no. 2, p. 205395171667967, 2016.

[58] L. Matondora, M. Mutandavari, and B. Mupini, "NLP based prediction of hospital readmission using ClinicalBERT and clinician notes," *International Journal of Innovative Science and Research Technology*, pp. 2549–2557, 2024.

[59] U. Demirbaga, N. Kaur, and G. S. Aujla, "Uncovering hidden and complex relations of pandemic dynamics using an AI driven system," *Scientific Reports*, vol. 14, no. 1, p. 15433, 2024.

[60] Y. Yang, E. W. T. Ngai, and L. Wang, "Resistance to artificial intelligence in health care: Literature review, conceptual framework, and research agenda," *Information & Management*, vol. 61, no. 4, p. 103961, 2024.

[61] R. Essex, "Resistance in health and healthcare," *Bioethics*, vol. 35, no. 5, pp. 480–486, 2021.

[62] B. Gopi, M. L. Sworna Kokila, C. V. Bibin, D. Sasikala, E. Howard, and S. Boopathi, "Distributed technologies using AI/ML techniques for healthcare applications," in *Social Innovations in Education, Environment, and Healthcare*, IGI Global, 2024, pp. 375–396.

[63] F. Krones and B. Walker, "From theoretical models to practical deployment: A perspective and case study of opportunities and challenges in AI-driven cardiac auscultation research for low-income settings," *medRxiv*, 2023.

[64] A. P. Susanto, D. Lyell, B. Widyantoro, S. Berkovsky, and F. Magrabi, "How well do AI-enabled decision support systems perform in clinical settings?, " *Studies in Health Technology and Informatics*, vol. 310, pp. 279–283, 2024.

[65] T. Annamalai, K. Rajeswari, E. Sowmiya, and A. Saranya, "Future perspective of artificial intelligence in healthcare and medical treatments," in *Advances in Systems Analysis, Software Engineering, and High Performance Computing*, IGI Global, 2024, pp. 206–214.

[66] K. P. Rahate and M. Karayat, "AI for public health and population health management," in *Advances in Healthcare Information Systems and Administration*, IGI Global, 2024, pp. 32–57.

[67] R. C. Sobti, J. Rai, and A. Prakash, "Introduction to emerging technologies in biomedical sciences," in *Biomedical Translational Research*, Singapore: Springer Nature Singapore, 2022, pp. 1–22.

[68] M. McClellan, N. Brown, R. M. Califf, and J. J. Warner, "Call to action: Urgent challenges in cardiovascular disease: A presidential advisory from the American Heart Association," *Circulation*, vol. 139, no. 9, pp. e44–e54, 2019.

[69] "Mobile fact sheet," *Pew Research Center*, 31 Jan. 2024. [Online]. Available: www.pewresearch.org/internet/fact-sheet/mobile.

Index

P

R

S

T

U

V

W

For Product Safety Concerns and Information please contact our EU representative GPSR@taylorandfrancis.com Taylor & Francis Verlag GmbH, Kaufingerstraße 24, 80331 München, Germany

Batch number: 10397790

Printed by Printforce, the Netherlands